Children with Vision Impairment
Assessment, Development, and Management

Children with Vision Impairment
Assessment, Development, and Management

Edited by

Naomi Dale
Consultant Clinical Psychologist and Paediatric Neuropsychologist, Great Ormond Street Hospital for Children; Professor of Paediatric Neurodisability, UCL Great Ormond Street Institute of Child Health, London, UK.

Alison Salt
Honorary Consultant Paediatrician, Neurodisability Service, Great Ormond Street Hospital for Children; Honorary Associate Professor, UCL Great Ormond Street Institute of Child Health, London, UK.

Jenefer Sargent
Consultant Paediatrician and Speciality Lead, Neurodisability Service, Great Ormond Street Hospital for Children, London, UK.

Rebecca Greenaway
Consultant Clinical Psychologist and Paediatric Neuropsychologist, Great Ormond Street Hospital for Children, London, UK.

2022
Mac Keith Press

© 2022 Mac Keith Press

Managing Director: Ann-Marie Halligan
Senior Publishing Manager: Sally Wilkinson
Publishing and Marketing Co-ordinator: Paul Grossman
Production Manager: Andy Booth

First published in this edition in 2022 by Mac Keith Press
2nd Floor, Rankin Building, 139–143 Bermondsey Street, London, SE1 3UW

British Library Cataloguing-in-Publication data
A catalogue record for this book is available from the British Library

Cover designer: Marten Sealby

ISBN: 978-1-911612-33-9

Typeset by Riverside Publishing Solutions Ltd
Printed by Hobbs the Printers Ltd, Totton, Hampshire, UK

Contents

Contents

Author Appointments

Kim Bates
Speech and Language Therapist, Neurodisability service, Great Ormond Street Hospital for Children, London, UK.

Richard Bowman
Consultant Ophthalmologist, Great Ormond Street Hospital for Children; Honorary Associate Professor, UCL Great Ormond Street Institute of Child Health, London School Hygiene Tropical Medicine, London, UK.

Giulia Cappagli
Post Doctoral Researcher, Unit for Visually Impaired People (UVIP), Istituto Italiano di Tecnologia (IIT), Genova, Italy.

Christopher Clark
Parent of a child with visual impairment, UK.

Kate Clark
Parent of a child with visual impairment, UK.

Michael Crossland
Specialist Optometrist, Moorfields Eye Hospital; Honorary Senior Research Associate, UCL Institute of Ophthalmology, London, UK.

Annegret Dahlmann-Noor
Consultant Ophthalmologist, Moorfields Eye Hospital; Honorary Associate Clinical Professor, UCL Institute of Ophthalmology, London, UK

Naomi Dale
Consultant Clinical Psychologist and Paediatric Neuropsychologist, Great Ormond Street Hospital for Children; Professor of Paediatric Neurodisability, UCL Great Ormond Street Institute of Child Health, London, UK.

Graeme Douglas
Professor of Disability and Special Educational Needs, University of Birmingham, Birmingham, UK.

Elisa Fazzi
Professor of Child Neurology and Psychiatry, Unit of Child Neurology and Psychiatry, ASST Spedali Civili of Brescia; Department of Clinical and Experimental Sciences, University of Brescia, Brescia, Italy.

Monica Gori
Principal Investigator, Unit for Visually Impaired People (UVIP), Istituto Italiano di Tecnologia (IIT), Genova, Italy.

Rebecca Greenaway
Consultant Clinical Psychologist and Paediatric Neuropsychologist, Great Ormond Street Hospital for Children, London, UK.

Andrea Guzzetta
Associate Professor of Child Neurology and Psychiatry, Department of Developmental Neuroscience, IRCCS Stella Maris Foundation; Department of Clinical and Experimental Medicine, University of Pisa, Pisa, Italy.

Jessica Hayton
Lecturer in Psychology; Programme Leader Graduate Diploma in Habilitation and Disabilities of Sight, UCL Institute of Education, London, UK.

Rachel Hewett
Research Fellow, Department of Disability and Special Educational Needs, University of Birmingham, Birmingham, UK.

M Cay Holbrook
Associate Professor, Educational and Counselling Psychology, and Special Education, University of British Columbia, Vancouver, British Columbia, Canada.

Clare Jackson
Clinical Psychologist, Addenbrookes Hospital, Cambridge, UK.

Sabina Kef
Assistant Professor, Faculty of Behavioural and Movement Sciences, Clinical Child and Family Studies, Vrije Universiteit, Amsterdam, the Netherlands.

Mike McLinden
Emeritus Professor of Education, University of Birmingham, Birmingham, UK.

Mariya Moosajee
Professor of Molecular Ophthalmology at UCL Institute of Ophthalmology and The Francis Crick Institute; Consultant Ophthalmologist in Genetic Eye Disease at Moorfields Eye Hospital and Great Ormond Street Hospital for Children, London, UK.

Susan Mort
Practical Skills Tutor, Graduate Diploma in Habilitation and Disabilities of Sight, UCL Institute of Education, London, UK.

Ngozi Oluonye
Consultant Paediatrician, Neurodisability service, Great Ormond Street Hospital for Children; Moorfields Eye Hospital, London, UK.

Els Ortibus
Professor of Child Neurology, Child Neurology Department, University Hospitals Leuven; Department of Development and Regeneration, KU Leuven, Leuven, Belgium.

Jackie Osborne
Qualified Teacher of Children and Young People with Vision Impairment (QTVI), Specialist Advisory Teacher and Vision Impairment Team Manager (Retired), UK.

Jugnoo Sangeeta Rahi
Professor of Ophthalmic Epidemiology, Population, Policy and Practice Research and Teaching Department, UCL Great Ormond Street Institute of Child Health; Honorary Paediatric Ophthalmologist, Great Ormond Street Hospital for Children, London, UK.

Steve Rose
Principal Speech and Language Therapist, Great Ormond Street Hospital for Children, London; Independent SLT and Deafblind Consultant, UK.

Elena Sakkalou
Senior Lecturer in Psychology, School of Psychology and Sports Science, Anglia Ruskin University, Cambridge, UK.

Alison Salt
Honorary Consultant Paediatrician Neurodisability Service, Great Ormond Street Hospital for Children; Honorary Associate Professor, UCL Great Ormond Institute of Child Health, London, UK.

Consultant Paediatrician, Paediatric Rehabilitation Service, Perth Children's Hospital; Clinical Associate Professor, University of Western Australia, Perth, Australia.

Jenefer Sargent
Consultant Paediatrician and Speciality Lead, Neurodisability Service, Great Ormond Street Hospital for Children, London, UK.

Julia Smyth
Occupational Therapist, Great Ormond Street Hospital for Children, London, UK.

Ameenat Lola Solebo
NIHR Clinician Scientist, Population, Policy and Practice Research and Teaching Department, UCL Great Ormond Street Institute of Child Health; Honorary Paediatric Ophthalmologist, Great Ormond Street Hospital for Children, London, UK.

Francesca Tinelli
Postdoctoral Neuropsychologist, Department of Developmental Neuroscience, IRCCS Fondazione Stella Maris, Pisa, Italy.

Holly Tuke
Person with visual impairment, UK.

Simon Ungar
Educational Psychologist, Schools and Community Psychology Service, Wandsworth Council; Academic and Professional Tutor, Department of Clinical, Educational and Health Psychology, University College London, London, UK.

Mathijs Vervloed
Associate Professor, Behavioural Science Institute, Radboud University, Nijmegen, the Netherlands.

Kim T Zebehazy
Associate Professor, Department of Educational and Counselling Psychology, and Special Education, University of British Columbia, Vancouver, British Columbia, Canada.

Foreword

Worldwide the causes of impaired vision are changing, with some ocular causes diminishing and cerebral aetiologies increasing in prevalence. Impairment of sight, or blindness, is rare in children but poses enormous challenges for the affected young people and their families, who very much depend upon skilled professional support from a range of agencies to optimise their chances in life. This book, with its up-to-date broad collection of salient information about the diverse characteristics and needs of children with vision impairment and how to cater for them, provides a welcome contribution to the knowledge and skills needed by the multidisciplinary health, education, and social care practitioners and all those working with children with visual impairment.

The book is divided into four sections which address in turn the range of causes of vision impairment, the impact of vision impairment on child development, approaches to habilitation, and the social consequences of low vision and ways to address them.

Part 1 addresses the wide range of causes and manifestations of low or no vision. An effective way to think about the visual system is from front to back. For children with vision impairment, the optics of the cornea, lens, and the ability to optically accommodate are the first thing to consider. The retina, pixelated as it is by cones for day vision and rods for night vision, digitally converts the focussed visual scene projected upon it into pre-processed electrical data. This information is conducted along the visual pathways to the occipital lobes for primary visual processing of visual clarity, contrast, brightness, colour, visual depth, and visual field perception. Further image processing takes place in the temporal lobes and the posterior parietal lobes. These processes are supported by additional processing in the pulvinar of the thalamus and superior colliculi (injury of which severely compounds cerebral visual impairment). Vision impairments can be due to disorder of any element of this overall process affecting any of the many complex networks involved in the processing of visual information. Part 1 highlights that lack of vision in infants and young children fundamentally impacts upon their learning, and it explains the strategies needed to deal with this risk. During early development the brain has an enormous capacity to adapt and develop, a phenomenon that can potentially be harnessed and encouraged by skilled care and parenting. This fascinating phenomenon is also well reviewed.

As vision is integral to multiple developmental processes, reduced vision may have a wide variety of consequences. For these reasons part 2 of the book highlights the potential impact that impaired vision can have upon social, motor, and language development as well as cognition, and addresses these issues in a clearly presented series of chapters. Identifying, greeting, and meeting up with friends is largely contingent upon vision in the typically sighted person. Much communication, whether in person or online, is enhanced by facial expression and gesture which the listener detects and understands visually. So it is not surprising that reduced vision can interfere with social engagement, with the potential risk of social isolation and consequent mental health issues. Recognition of such risks and ensuring that appropriate advance action is taken is clearly essential. For example, communicating using language and touch that describes the environment to the child or teaching the child's contemporaries about how vision impacts upon communication and what they can do to help prevent such problems arising in the first place. Consequently part 2 culminates in highlighting the fundamental role that parents and other caregivers and educators have in saliently rendering their child's experiences accessible and meaningful.

Children with vision impairments need to gain a range of special skills. Freedom to move around and find one's way gives autonomy and is of course an essential skill, while access to the printed word whether in print or in braille is another fundamental need. Ways to address these challenges are well addressed in part 3.

Part 4 focuses on social participation and quality of life. This section highlights how important it is for those with vision impairment to feel understood, included, and respected, culminating in gaining the sense of self-worth needed to successfully progress into adult life. Children with vision impairments, whether ocular or cerebral in origin, can only learn from what is accessible to them, often relying greatly upon the nature of their soundscape for example. Yet impairment of vision is a hidden disability, meaning that a person with typical sight can easily be unaware or forget that children with vision impairment have different experiences to their own. It is therefore essential that for every child with vision impairment their functional vision is known and understood by as many people as possible, including their school contemporaries. It is essential that their visual needs are understood at a fundamental level and taken into account as comprehensively as possible.

This book is a 'must read' for all developmental and neurodisability paediatricians, paediatric and educational psychologists, occupational therapists, physiotherapists, speech and language specialists, ophthalmologists and eye clinic staff, paediatric neurologists, specialist teachers of the visually impaired child and other educationalists, and family support and social care workers with responsibility for optimising the development and life opportunities of children with no or low vision in order to help bring about this aspiration.

Gordon N Dutton
Emeritus Professor of Visual Science
Glasgow Caledonian University, UK

Preface

Children with vision impairment are children first. They deserve equal rights and opportunities in the contemporary world, from birth to adulthood. This includes access to learning and development of skills for everyday living to enable full participation in social, educational, community, and occupational possibilities (United Nations Convention on the Rights of the Child, 1989). Children with vision impairment need additional support and management of care to achieve these aspirations and ambitions. The physical and social environment must be adapted and structured to support the child's growth, functioning, and participation in society.

This book is designed as a Practical Guide to support practitioners in their management of care of children who have long-term vision impairment and disability. Its main themes are *assessment of the child, the child's function and activity, and habilitation or remedial intervention.*

This Practical Guide aims to provide knowledge and guidance to support practitioners and researchers from all disciplines and backgrounds who need to come together to assist the child and their family from birth until early adulthood. This involves practitioners across health, education, and social care, and is designed to assist those who have specialist skills in vision impairment and those who have other specialist or more generalist skills but need to gain more insights. The book is also relevant to researchers in ophthalmological and vision science, neuroscience, and psychological and social science.

The development of this book was driven by the recognition of the need for a contemporary Practical Guide to support evidence-based practice that would reflect the many developments in theory, research, and practice in the field. Many of us were assisted in our formative years by the ground-breaking textbook of the time, *The Management of Visual Impairment in Childhood,* by Alistair Fielder, Anthony Best, and Martin Bax (Mac Keith Press, 1993). We thank Mac Keith Press, including Ann-Marie Halligan, Sally Wilkinson, Paul Grossman, and Andrew Booth, and Ting Baker and Duncan Potter at Riverside Publishing Solutions, for assisting us in the original vision of the book and their commitment to its development.

Many other people and organisations have also inspired the thinking and content of this book, including Patricia Sonksen, developmental paediatrician, who developed and was first director (1973–2000) of the multidisciplinary Developmental Vision Clinic service at Great Ormond Street Hospital for Children, London, UK. The Developmental Vision Clinic has been running for over 40 years and was one of the first multidisciplinary paediatric neurodisability service to focus on the functional vision and developmental needs of children with severe visual impairment and their families. We aim to bring the ongoing expertise and research insights from this team and that of other international experts to a broad multidisciplinary audience of professionals to assist them in their work with children with vision impairment. We are grateful to the collective faculty of authors of the chapters who have shared their expert knowledge and wisdom, and invested much time in helping advance the current ways of thinking in the book. The unique interdisciplinary academic contexts of the Mary Kitzinger Trust and the European Academy of Childhood Disability have enabled us to learn and grow together.

Our work has been inspired by thousands of children, parents, colleagues in the Developmental Vision Clinic service, and hospital and community practitioners who share their insights and have taught us so much over the years; we thank them all. Thank you to the parents and young people who have generously permitted their photographs and to Medical Illustrations of Great Ormond Street Hospital for photography. Last but not least, we wish to thank our families and friends who have provided loving care, support, practical help, patience, and understanding throughout the writing of the book.

Naomi Dale, Alison Salt, Jenefer Sargent,
and Rebecca Greenaway
November 2021

REFERENCES

Fielder AR, Best AB, Bax MCO (1993) *The Management of Visual Impairment in Childhood*. London: Mac Keith Press.

United Nations Convention on the Rights of the Child. Available at: https://www.ohchr.org/en/professionalinterest/pages/crc.aspx

CHAPTER 1

Introduction

Naomi Dale, Alison Salt, Jenefer Sargent, and Rebecca Greenaway

Vision impairment is a long-term condition, arising from multiple disorders of the eye, optic nerve, and brain. The child's vision may range from no functional vision (profound vision impairment) to severe, moderate, or mild levels of impairment. It is estimated that in 2015 there were 1.14 million children worldwide with profound visual impairment and blindness, though causes and prevalence vary between countries with avoidable causes being higher in those with lower incomes (Gilbert et al. 2017; see further Chapter 2). Although these children may face many potential barriers and limitations, with the support of parents, friends, and professionals, many of these children are able to fully participate in their society and achieve their aspirations.

There are many challenges for the child's learning and activity due to the significant impact of vision reduction on development and learning. Genetic and other biological factors may influence the child's eyes and brain, development, and learning. This very diverse population of children has varying intellectual abilities and may have co-occurring conditions including cerebral palsy, autism spectrum disorder, attention-deficit/hyperactivity disorder, epilepsy, and hearing impairment. They may have neuropsychiatric and behavioural disorders, as well as mental health issues. Some rare eye disorders are associated with neurometabolic and neurodegenerative conditions. Cerebral visual impairment may lead to disorders in basic and higher vision processing including visual perceptual problems.

The functional needs and habilitation of children with vision impairment are the main emphasis of this book. The focus is primarily on those with very early causation and onset of vision impairment as the majority of childhood vision impairment is congenital (Teoh et al. 2021). However, the needs of children with progressive vision impairment of later onset and children with acquired vision impairment are also considered in the relevant chapters.

GUIDING PRACTICE

This book is designed as a Practical Guide to support practitioners in their management of care of children who have long-term vision impairment and disability. Its main themes are *assessment of the child, the child's function and activity, and habilitation or remedial intervention.*

Assessment is key to understanding the child's current vision and developmental needs and establishing any co-occurring issues, such as intellectual or motor disability or autism spectrum disorder, and for guiding habilitation and intervention. A focus on the child's **function and activity** guides what needs to be assessed and possibly targeted for support, such as vision, motor function, cognition, language and social functions, and mental health. **Habilitation** covers the range of interventions and supports for everyday living and learning, from early years' intervention to mobility and navigation, everyday living skills, social relationships and participation, and augmentative and assistive technological supports. To cover the breadth of topics of relevance, we bring together an international group of leading multidisciplinary experts from health, education, habilitation, and social care.

A number of conceptual models are adopted to shape the content and consideration of the issues covered:

- First, the World Health Organization International Classification of Functioning, Disability and Health: Children and Youth Version (ICF-CY) informs practice and the short- and long-term goals for the child and their family. In contrast to a disability focus that is primarily biomedical, this model takes us to a *bio-functional-social (or biopsychosocial)* perspective that aims to enhance the child's and their family's function and participation in everyday life and society (see Fig. 1.1).

- Second, a multi-factorial model of risk and protective factors (Pennington 2006) considers multiple and interacting factors of risk and protection for the child and how they may influence the child's developmental progress and resilience. This model supports a *holistic multidisciplinary* approach and can inform timely preventative and interventionist strategies to meet the child's needs and to minimise longer-term risks and improve outcomes.

- Third, a family capacity-building model (Dunst et al. 2014) includes *family-centred partnerships* between children/young users, parents and practitioners and advocates for listening to the voices of the child or young person and parents. All practice is more effective if it is well communicated to the parents and child/young person, their viewpoint is heeded and a *negotiation approach* is undertaken to bring the perspectives of the parent and child/user when appropriate and professional together, and differences are resolved constructively (Dale 1996). This approach aims to empower the child or young person and their family and inclusion and participation in society. Chapters from a young person and from parents provide this important perspective.

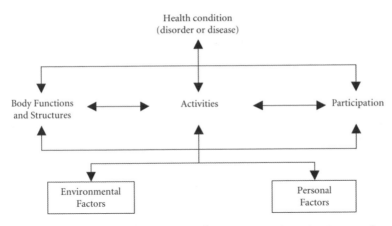

Figure 1.1 ICF-CY model for health or disability (World Health Organization 2007)

- Fourth, a *habilitation* model focussing on the child's developmental growth and optimising the child's strengths and outlook. This approach includes preventative and interventionist strategies to support the child thriving and learning, and overcoming challenges arising from the vision disability. Rehabilitation is also relevant to those children when vision has become impaired at a later age through late onset or acquired disorders and compensatory strategies are required.

- Finally, the book is *evidence-based* in that it draws on recent and contemporary scientific research to support practice and each chapter covers the relevant research available to support developments in practice. Areas that would be useful for future research are also highlighted, reflecting that practice methods are changing, dynamic, and ongoing.

SERVICE DELIVERY AND CONTEXT

Each country has different models of service delivery and degrees of resources, but all children with vision impairment are likely to need inputs from a range of health, education, and social care practitioners at primary, secondary, and tertiary levels to comprehensively meet their changing needs. This book endeavours to be of international relevance and has authors from different countries.

Whether in higher or low-moderate income countries, the most appropriate model of delivery is the World Health Organization pyramid of service delivery, which has been developed in the NHS tiered health care system (United Kingdom). Figure 1.2 highlights the delivery needed at each tier. Tiers 2 and 3 will need practitioners who have more training and experience and expertise in childhood vision impairment. Screening for vision and developmental disability is often likely to start in neonatal and maternity centres/hospital and in the community in Tier 1. Multidisciplinary specialist and diagnostic services at Tier 3 and targeted interventions from Tier 2 support the inclusion and

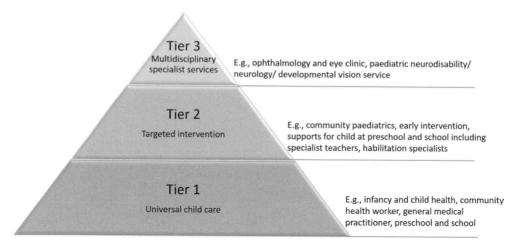

Figure 1.2 Tiered model of child care services for children with visual impairment

participation of the child and family in universal services at Tier 1. Tier 3 will include specialist paediatric and ophthalmological services for diagnostic and highly specialist care and management of the eye and vision disorder. Tier 2 ideally provides specialist community out-reach services such as specialist early intervention, habilitation, and education for children with vision impairment to support the child developing and learning and supporting the family in their daily lives. As countries further build their services in this field they can increase the expertise and specialisation of professionals in Tiers 2 and 3, along the lines of suggestions in this book.

In a lower-resourced country, a vision service to support children and families through the lifespan may be set up. This could run in conjunction with a specialist ophthalmology and paediatric service, with community outreach workers. Some key areas that may be relevant to start with are *early intervention* (Chapter 8), *habilitation* (Chapter 14), *psychological wellbeing and mental health* (Chapter 18), and *adolescence and transition* (Chapter 20). These chapters provide accessible practice tips and guidance that may be useful for the more generalist community or outreach practitioner from health or education who is starting off in the field.

ORGANISATION OF BOOK

The book is divided into four parts following the ICF-CY model (see Fig. 1.1): **Part 1 Eye Disorders, Vision, and Brain** focussing on body functions and structure; **Part 2 Child Development and Learning From Birth to Older Childhood** focussing on child function and development and learning across childhood; **Part 3 Further Approaches to Habilitation** focussing on functional activity and leisure and participatory activities; and **Part 4 Social Relationships and Participation** focussing on social relating and participation in everyday contexts.

Part 1 Eye Disorders, Vision, and Brain has chapters on causes, vision functions, and classification of childhood vision impairment; genetics and phenotype presentations of congenital eye disorders; cerebral visual impairment: identification, assessment, and management; brain plasticity and vision impairment; vision assessment of children with complex disorders; and assessment and habilitation of vision in infants and young children.

Part 2 Child Development and Learning From Birth to Older Development has chapters on early years, early intervention, and family support; motor development and hand skills; language and communication development; social communication and autism spectrum disorder; cognition; and the parental perspective.

Part 3 Further Approaches to Habilitation has chapters on orientation, mobility, and adaptive behaviour; low vision aids and assistive technologies; reading approaches for braille users and technological aids for spatial perception and mobility.

Part 4 Social Relationships and Participation has chapters on behaviour, psychological wellbeing, and mental health; quality of life, self-concept, and social relationships; towards autonomy and independence in adolescence; and the young person's experience and perspective.

Each chapter, after an introduction, is divided into four areas. The first sections cover relevant theory, contemporary research evidence, and practice insights. Scientific research provides the systematic evidence to inform, validate, and guide evidence-based practice that is effective. We have focussed on research published since 2000 but this does not deny the importance of earlier research and insights that these studies build on. Some earlier seminal studies are included where appropriate. The next sections provide practical guidance and strategies for assessment and management including for multidisciplinary management of care. As this is a continually changing field, each chapter concludes with signposts for ways forward for future research and practice. A reference list of the research cited and for further reading is available at the end of each chapter.

LANGUAGE USE AND DEFINITIONS

To clarify the language terms used in the book, the term *parent* refers to the mother, father, and/or significant caregiver as an inclusive term for all adults who regularly look after the child in the home environment. Where research has been carried out with the mother or father specifically, this is denoted. The term *child* refers to children of all ages up to late adolescence unless a particular age range is specified. Throughout this book, we refer to *habilitation*, a process aimed at helping people with a disability attain, consolidate, or improve skills and functioning for daily living, and which is particularly applicable to those children with very early onset of vision impairment. Rehabilitation may be considered more appropriate for those children who lose vision later in childhood and may be referred to specifically in some chapters. In this scenario, rehabilitation refers to regaining skills, abilities, or knowledge, and learning compensatory strategies for those that may have been lost or compromised.

Although there are different references and traditions in the field in relation to terminology regarding vision disability, we have chosen to mainly use the term *vision impairment*. A vision impairment is any visual condition that impacts on an individual's ability to successfully complete the activities of everyday life. At different points in the book, the term 'vision impairment' may be replaced by related terms such as 'blindness', 'vision disability', and 'severely visually impaired' or 'severe/profound visual impairment', according to terms used in a research study or the author's preference.

SUMMARY

This Practical Guide aims to support and equip practitioners to provide quality interventions and practice to achieve the most reliable assessments, effective interventions, and successful outcomes in life opportunities and quality of life for children with vision impairment and their families, in partnership with the child/young person and family. We and all the authors hope that this Practical Guide will be helpful in this endeavour.

REFERENCES

Dale N (1996) *Working with Families of Children with Special Needs: Partnership and Practice*. London: Routledge.

Dunst CJ, Bruder MB, Espe-Sherwindt M (2014) Family capacity-building in early childhood intervention: do context and setting matter? *School Community Journal* 24(1): 37–148.

Gilbert C, Bowman R, Malik ANJ (2017) The epidemiology of blindness in children: changing priorities. *Community Eye Health* 30(100): 74–77.

Pennington BF (2006) From single to multiple deficit models of developmental disorders. *Cognition* 101: 385–413. doi: 10.1016/j.cognition.2006.04.008.

Teoh LJ, Solebo AL, Rahi JS et al. (2021) Visual impairment, severe visual impairment, and blindness in children in Britain (BCVIS2): a national observational study. *The Lancet* 5(3): 190–200.

World Health Organization (2007) *ICY-CY: International Classification of Functioning, Disability and Health: Children and Youth Version*. Switzerland: World Health Organization Publications.

PART 1

Eye Disorders, Vision, and Brain

CHAPTER 2

Vision Functions, Classification, and Causes of Childhood Vision Impairment

Ameenat Lola Solebo and Jugnoo Sangeeta Rahi

INTRODUCTION

Vision comprises several different integrated vision functions (Braddick and Atkinson 2011), which together contribute to a child's health, developmental and social experiences, and learning (Rahi et al. 2009).

Visual acuity (the resolution of detail) is the primary function, with several important secondary functions including depth perception, visual field, and colour and contrast sensitivity. These permit higher-order visual processes, such as perception of faces, motion, or environment mapping. Abnormalities of visual function can range in type and severity, affecting one or both eyes, and can be due to eye or brain and visual pathway disease.

Severe bilateral impairment of acuity potentially confers significant everyday living demands or 'burden' for the child, family, and society (Rahi et al. 2003). Across the world the pattern of causes for vision impairment and blindness vary, reflecting the regional balance of the determinants of diseases and resources. The most significant global causes of severe vision impairment are retinal disorders, corneal scarring, congenital ocular structural anomalies, cataract, and brain disorders (Solebo et al. 2017). This chapter explores the different vision functions, the anatomy of the eye, causes of vision impairment, and the identification of vision disorders.

VISION AND VISION IMPAIRMENT

The eyes process light, turning it into neural signals that are transmitted to the brain via the visual pathways. The brain translates these signals into meaningful perceptions of the physical or social world, such as mapping one's environment and picking out objects within a crowded scene or interpreting the facial expressions of another person. Very poor vision is caused by impaired functioning of the eyes or by damage to the visual pathways of the brain (see Chapter 5).

Vision Functions

Acuity is the ability of the functioning visual system to 'resolve' edges in space, which is essential for analysis of detail. It is measured in terms of the degree of separation (or resolution) of the component parts of the images needed for them to be seen distinctly and separately. Secondary visual functions are largely dependent on acuity, with significantly impaired visual acuity leading to deficits of all other visual functions (Braddick and Atkinson 2011).

3D vision or depth is perceived using discrepancies between images generated by information from each of the eyes. It is also possible to detect depth with vision in only one eye, using cues such as shade and perspective (Harris and Wilcox 2009). Depth perception (stereopsis) also relies on higher-order processing of spatial information (see Chapter 5). Other visual functions such as perception of movement, visual guidance of movement, visual search, visual attention, and visual recognition, also require higher visual processing in vision association areas in the brain and are addressed in this chapter (see Chapter 5).

Eye movements enable tracking of moving objects and relocation of gaze (smooth pursuit and saccades respectively). There are six cardinal eye movements, in both directions horizontally (left and right) and vertically (up and down), and two additional rotatory movements (incyclotorsion and excyclotorsion), which stabilise an individual's eyes during head tilting. These movements are enacted by six muscles attached to each eye and choreographed by the central nervous system.

The visual field is the total area of space perceived when the eyes and head are still and typically extends furthest temporally (to the sides). The quality of acuity is distributed unequally with the central field being the most sensitive area (Patel et al. 2015). The peripheral visual field is also of importance as this is needed to perceive moving targets, and to guide and facilitate movement through 3D visual space.

Colour vision and contrast sensitivity are the ability to discriminate between different hues and areas of different luminance respectively. Perception of large differences in luminance, such as a black font on a white background, require less contrast sensitivity than perception of grey images on lighter grey background. Poor environmental lighting

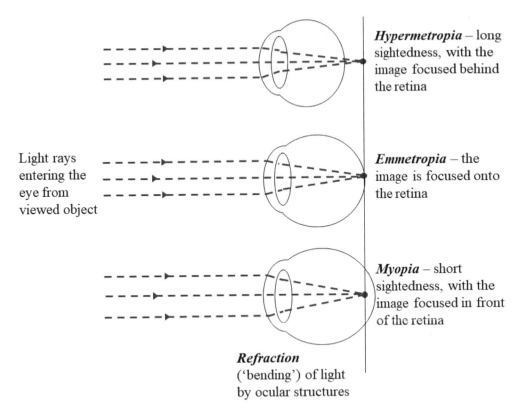

Hypermetropia – long sightedness, with the image focused behind the retina

Light rays entering the eye from viewed object

Emmetropia – the image is focused onto the retina

Myopia – short sightedness, with the image focused in front of the retina

Refraction ('bending') of light by ocular structures

Figure 2.1 Refractive errors and emmetropia

has significant negative impact on contrast sensitivity (Braddick and Atkinson 2011). The retina can also automatically adjust to accommodate to light intensity, known as light and dark adaptation.

In order to perceive clarity of 'form', the curved surfaces on and within the eyeball bend (refract) light as it enters the eye so that a focussed image is formed upon the retina (Fig. 2.1). Refraction can also be an active process, called accommodation, when a person changes their focus from a more distant to a nearer object. The optical or refractive power of the eye alters with lens shape, while the eyes converge, and this dual process of accommodation and convergence ensures that the image remains in focus and singular irrespective of its distance from the eyes.

The common refractive errors (Fig. 2.1) are:

- *Hypermetropia.* Due to the higher curvature and shorter length of a smaller child's eye, a degree of hypermetropia is the natural state in many children until age 4 or 5 years of age.

> **Box 2.1** Amblyopia
>
> *There are three forms of amblyopia.*
>
> *Deprivational:* where there is obscuration of the image coming into the brain, due to for instance cataract or retinal abnormality, and preventing formation of the pathways necessary for processing of detailed images.
>
> *Refractive:* where an out-of-focus image is presented to the brain, preventing the normal development of vision.
>
> *Strabismic:* where one eye is directed away from central gaze ('squint') preventing that eye from presenting a detailed image to the brain.
>
> *Amblyopia can be unilateral or bilateral. Unilateral amblyopia is more common and results in more severe impairment of the affected eye, due to competition for neural pathways serving the better seeing eye.*

- *Myopia* occurs when the eyeball is too long or when the cornea is less curved and may be associated with a family history of myopia (being 'short-sighted').
- *Astigmatism*, in which there are different degrees of refraction within an individual eye as measured at separate axes.

Amblyopia

In typically developing children, visual functions, particularly acuity, rapidly improve during the first years of life as a result of the maturation of ocular anatomy and neural pathway circuitry (Lewis and Maurer 2005). Sensory and motor functions have a sensitive window, which is a finite early developmental period during which high quality stimuli must be experienced in order for the function to fully develop. Consequently, any disorder that impedes the presentation of a clear focussed image to the brain in early childhood can lead to delayed or abnormal development of the visual system (see Box 2.1). This abnormal development (amblyopia) can be reversed in children with sufficient vision potential and the developmental trajectory reset if treatment is undertaken during the sensitive window (Holmes and Clark 2006). Prevention of permanent amblyopia where feasible lies at the heart of the management of childhood eye and vision disease and disorder (see Chapter 4).

Measuring Vision in Childhood

Visual acuity is recorded numerically using fractions (e.g. 20/20 or 6/6 vision) or decimal scores, or is estimated in gross terms (e.g. able to fix gaze on external stimuli or able to perceive light). The preferred scale for quantifying visual acuity is the logarithm of the Minimum Angle of Resolution or logMAR because of its standardised charts and its linear arithmetic progression, which enables robust quantification of acuity (vs the historical Snellen geometric scale and non-standardised charts) (Rosser et al. 2001). Vision of 0.0 logMAR is the normal adult level, with vision of 1.0 logMAR (a logarithm unit of change) being 10 times worse.

A full-term infant will be able to perceive and show attention preference for human facial features and high contrast (black on white) patterns within a few hours of birth. However, neonates typically have an acuity of only 1.5 logMAR. This rapidly improves to 1.0 logMAR at 1 month of age and 0.5 logMAR by 12 months of age. 'Adult' levels of acuity (0.0–0.1 logMAR) are reached by 5 to 6 years of age (Sonksen et al. 2008). Accompanying this rapid improvement in acuity are developing cognitive and motor skills and therefore choice of the appropriate tests to assess a child's vision requires understanding of their current developmental status (Chapter 4).

In infants and pre-verbal children, it is not possible to measure recognition acuity using optotypes (letters, shapes, or pictures). Resolution acuity can be measured through observation of preferential looking responses to boards with high contrast gratings on one half and grey background on the other (Teller et al. 1986). A recent innovation reports on the presentation of stimuli on a touchscreen device (Livingstone et al. 2018). Once children can match or name optotypes, recognition acuity can be measured using standardised charts. Systematic assessment of detection vision is useful when acuity is below the range of resolution or recognition testing materials (Sonksen and Dale 2002; see Chapter 4).

Other visual functions can be assessed using validated tools such as formal perimetry (to map the visual field) or Ishihara plates (colour vision) or stereoscopic testing plates.

Definition and Classification of Childhood Vision Impairment

Acuity is the primary visual parameter used in formal national and international definitions of visual impairment (Table 2.1). It is difficult to apply these taxonomies to children when recognition acuity at distance cannot be measured (see Chapter 4).

Practical methods of quantifying detection vision such as the Near Detection Scale (Sonksen and Dale 2002) have been developed for clinical and research purposes with infants and children with no or very low levels of vision (Sonksen and Dale 2002). This includes measurement and categorisation of profound vision impairment (no vision or light perception at best) and severe vision impairment (basic non-light reflecting 'form' vision; see Chapter 4).

New empirically driven methods of classification of cerebral vision impairment that do not rely on acuity alone are now also being developed (Sakki et al. 2021; see Chapter 5).

Prevalence and Incidence of Childhood Vision Impairment

In the UK, as in other high-income countries, childhood vision impairment is uncommon. The annual incidence of childhood vision impairment, severe visual impairment,

Table 2.1 Classification of vision impairment (World Health Organization 2006)

WHO level of visual impairment	Category of impairment (ICD–10 code)	Best achievable distance acuity with both eyes open		Visual field (around central fixation)
		Worse than:	Better than or equal to:	
No visual impairment	–	–	0.5 LogMAR	–
Moderate visual impairment	1 (Low vision)	0.5 LogMAR	1.0 LogMAR	–
Severe visual impairment	2 (Low vision)	1.0 LogMAR	1.3 LogMAR	–
Blindness	3 (Blindness)	1.3 LogMAR	1.8 LogMAR	10 degrees or less, but better than 5 degrees
	4 (Blindness)	1.8 LogMAR	Light perception	5 degrees or less
	5 (Blindness)	No light perception		–

or blindness (VI/SVI/BL, using ICD-10 definitions) is estimated at 5 to 6 per 10 000 in the first year of life, with a cumulative incidence of 10 per 10 000 by the child's 16th birthday (Rahi et al. 2003; Teoh et al. 2021). Half of these children will have severe visual disability (SVI/BL). The majority of the children with SVI/BL have additional non-ophthalmic disorders or impairments and/or present before their first birthday, and almost 10% of those with SVI/BL will die in the first year following diagnosis. In the UK, certain ethnic minority groups, or lower socioeconomic strata, are over-represented amongst children with SVI/BL (Rahi et al. 2003; Teoh et al. 2021).

Childhood blindness is more common in lower and middle-income countries due to dietary and infection-related disorders but with universal prevention programmes the rates of preventable disorders are reducing. The prevalence of global childhood blindness is between 0.3 and 1.2 per 1000 individuals aged 0 to 16 years, with an estimated 1.4 million children who are blind and 14 million children with vision impairment (Solebo et al. 2017).

Causes of Childhood Vision Impairment

Vision impairment is classified according to the anatomical site of the impaired eye or visual system, recognising that most children have more than one site affected (Rahi et al. 2003). The eye is divided into three coats (see Fig. 2.2):

1. The external coat, comprising the transparent cornea anteriorly and the thick white outer supportive layer of the sclera.
2. The middle coat, comprising the uvea, which holds much of the blood supply in the eye and which is visible anteriorly as the pigmented iris.

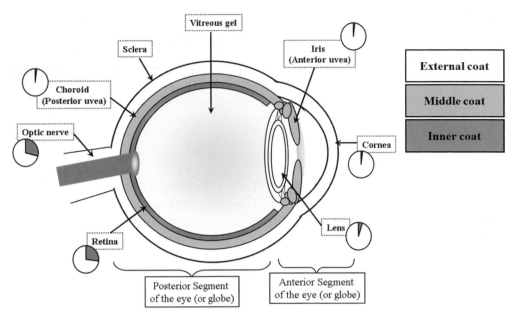

Figure 2.2 The anatomy of the eye, with indicative pie chart showing relative contribution of each site to childhood severe visual impairment or blindness (Rahi et al. 2003)

3. The inner coat, the retina, which holds the neurosensory cells which detect light. The centre of the retina is called the macula, which contains the highest concentration of cone cells and therefore provides fine visual discrimination. Temporal (towards the temples, away from the nose) to this is the opening in the coats through which passes the ganglion fibres from cells in the retina that make up the optic nerve.

The conjunctiva is a thin fibrovascular sheet coating the inside of the eyelids and the front surface of the sclera. The eye has anterior and posterior segments divided by the natural intraocular crystalline lens. Understanding the anatomy of the eyes and optic nerves enables the understanding of the impact of congenital and early ocular disease (or congenital disorders of the peripheral visual system) on childhood visual functions (see Fig. 2.2).

This chapter highlights the most impactful disorders at population level, but is not intended to be a comprehensive list of all visually disabling conditions of childhood, nor intended to describe the treatment or management of individual disorders.

Refractive Error

Globally, refractive error is one of the most important preventable and readily treatable causes of mild and moderate childhood visual impairment (Malik et al. 2018). Sensory stimulus plays a potentially important role in the growth of the eye but the mechanism is not yet understood (Mutti et al. 2009). All children with eye or vision disorders are at greater risk of refractive errors, which can, if not corrected with glasses or contact lenses, be an additional avoidable cause of permanent reduced vision due to refractive amblyopia. However, for some of these children vision can be so poor that correction of refractive error does not result in benefit.

Corneal Disorders

In high-income countries such as the UK, corneal diseases accounts for 2% of childhood 'blindness' (WHO definition), and can be congenital, such as the anterior segment dysgenesis anomalies, secondary to trauma, a sequelae of inflammatory disorders such as atopic conjunctivitis, or due to idiopathic progressive disorders such as keratoconus. Congenital and acquired infections, and nutritional and genetic disease can also lead to corneal scarring. Once present, the scarring is permanent. Corneal disorders are an important contributor to childhood blindness in low-income countries (Foster et al. 2008), with vitamin A deficiency being a key factor in the development of xerophthalmia (severely dry eye) and resultant corneal scarring (Solebo et al. 2017).

Globe Anomaly

Congenital anomalies of globe development, which occur in almost 10% of children with severe-profound vision impairment (Rahi et al. 2003) include poor overall formation of the eye (microphthalmia or anophthalmia) or poor formation of the anterior segment of the eye (anterior segment dysgenesis). These changes are not surgically reversible. Over half of these children will have an associated systemic disorder (Shah et al. 2012).

Cataract

Childhood cataract is the most common *avoidable* cause of childhood blindness worldwide (Solebo et al. 2017). It accounts for only 5% of children with severe-profound vision impairment in the UK, as public health interventions such as measles and rubella vaccination have reduced the incidence of disease. Diagnosis through newborn screening programmes affords infants the chance of early intervention to restore visual function. Where congenital cataract is diagnosed late, irreversible amblyopic visual loss occurs (Chak et al. 2006). At least one in four children with bilateral cataract will have a more general systemic disorder and will therefore need other medical care, increasing the importance of early detection (Rahi et al. 2000).

Uveal Disorders

Across lower, middle, and high-income countries, congenital uveal disorders such as coloboma and aniridia are the most common causes for childhood visual impairment (Rahi and Gilbert 2015; Teoh et al. 2021). Acquired childhood uveal disorders, such as uveitis (intraocular inflammation) are uncommon causes of bilaterally poor vision. Uveitis is, however, recognised as an important cause of avoidable childhood unilateral visual loss (Edelsten et al. 2003).

Retinal Disorders

About a third of children with severe-profound vision impairment have retinal disorders (Rahi et al. 2003), and these disorders are likely to account for an even higher proportion of children with moderate sight impairment (Mitry et al. 2013). Of these children, about half have inherited retinal dystrophy, with another prominent cause being retinopathy of prematurity (ROP). Potential treatments for a small number of inherited retinal dystrophies have emerged, but the remaining disorders remain untreatable (Solebo et al. 2017). ROP screening and treatment programmes with children born very preterm or very low birthweight have contributed to a global reduction of preventable ROP (Fierson et al. 2018).

Optic Nerve Disorders

About a third of children with severe-profound vision impairment in the UK surveillance study had optic nerve disorders due to either congenital disease (such as optic nerve hypoplasia), progressive disorders (inherited/primary congenital optic neuropathy), or disease acquired during childhood. The latter could comprise damage to the optic nerve or the optic chiasm due to disorders such as raised intracranial pressure) (Rahi et al. 2003), pituitary tumours, or optic pathway gliomas. Optic nerve and cerebral visual impairment often co-exist (Ryabets-Lienhard et al. 2016) and visual loss due to optic nerve disease is irreversible.

Cerebral Visual Pathway Disorders

A UK study of children with severe-profound vision impairment found almost half had cerebral visual pathway disorders, but population level prevalence rates are not reliable due to changing definitions and measurement of cerebral visual impairment (see Chapter 5). The rate may also be increasing globally with improved neonatal and paediatric care and increased survival of those born preterm or who suffer perinatal insult such as hypoxic-ischaemic encephalopathy (Rahi et al. 2003; Pehere et al. 2018). Children with acquired brain injury later in infancy or childhood (e.g. following head injury, cerebrovascular accident, or post-surgical hypoxia) may also have subsequent visual impairment. Many of these children also have complex additional health needs and impairments (see Chapter 5).

SCREENING, IDENTIFICATION, AND MANAGEMENT OF VISION IMPAIRMENT

Early detection and prompt identification of childhood vision impairment and its causes is essential for preventing or intervening with treatable conditions or for introducing early habilitation.

Primary prevention strategies aim to prevent the occurrence of disease causing avoidable vision impairment. In countries unable to provide these interventions, corneal scarring is still responsible for up to half of all childhood blindness (Malik et al. 2018).

Secondary medical prevention strategies aim to prevent or reduce the severity of the vision impairment occurring when eye disease cannot be prevented. They include prompt detection and adequate medical treatment. Two whole-population childhood eye and vision screening programmes are currently recommended by NHS England. The first is ocular examination as part of the Public Health England National Screening Committee's Newborn and Infant Physical Examination programme (NIPE). NIPE includes eye examination in the first 72 hours following birth, and a second 'safety net' examination between 6 and 8 weeks of age (Public Health England 2016). Most low- and middle-income countries, and some high-income countries, including the USA, do not have uniform implementation of neonatal ocular screening.

Apart from obvious signs of eye defects at birth, there are also other signs indicating a significant impairment of visual acuity (Blohme and Tornqvist 1997). These include absence of vision-directed behaviour (such as smiling in response to silent parental smiles, following the parent moving, and looking at the parent's face), nystagmus (constant or cyclical involuntary oscillatory movements of the eyes), and 'roving' eye movements (purposeless irregular intermittent movements in all directions). Parents and carers may be the first to notice these behaviours and their early concerns must be heeded quickly to ensure prompt referral to ophthalmological services for earliest investigation and potential diagnosis. Methods of improving this early identification at community health level are now being encouraged in low- and middle-income countries (Malik et al. 2018).

A significant high-risk group is children born preterm. In high-income countries infants born earlier than 32 weeks gestational age or with birthweights of less than 1500g are considered to be at risk of developing ROP (Solebo et al. 2017) and should be examined and monitored by ophthalmologists (Royal College of Ophthalmologists, Royal College of Paediatrics and Child Health 2018). In low- and middle-income countries, screening criteria and national programmes differ as larger and older infants are also considered to be at risk (Solebo et al. 2017). It is recommended that high-risk groups, such as children with a family history of ocular disorders, those with systemic disorders with known ophthalmic associations, or with neurological disorder, and those with sensorineural hearing loss undergo targeted ophthalmic assessment for early diagnosis and intervention (Solebo 2019).

Many countries undertake later childhood vision screening in order to detect treatable vision-related disorders (Solebo et al. 2015). The UK programme, which acts as a model internationally (United States Preventive Services Task Force et al. 2017), includes a check of vision at school entry (at 4–5 years of age) (Public Health England 2017). A range of resources are made available by Public Health England to support programme implementation.

The Role of the Multidisciplinary Team

The primary team for diagnosing eye disease and vision impairment is the multidisciplinary paediatric ophthalmology team comprising ophthalmologists, optometrists, orthoptists, and visual electrophysiologists. They work closely with other paediatric clinicians including neonatologists, neurodevelopmental/neurodisability paediatric teams, and neuroimaging and genetic teams for measuring vision functions, identifying vision impairment, and diagnosing child paediatric ophthalmic conditions and disorders. After birth, the primary care team in the community will be active in screening and detecting challenges in vision function and potential vision impairment. A well-integrated pathway to community health and educational services is essential (see Chapters 1 and 8). The specialist tertiary ophthalmological centre will continue to be involved and aim to minimise the impact of established visual impairment. This may include the prevention of further vision loss, the provision of low vision aids (see Chapter 16), guidance on educational support, and habilitation to assist activities of daily living and family support. The hospital family-liaison worker and local key worker can play an important role in facilitating communications between specialist and community care and jointly supporting the family through the difficult diagnosis-giving and early treatment period (Rahi et al. 2005).

IMPLICATIONS FOR RESEARCH AND PRACTICE

The rarity and variety of the conditions that cause childhood vision impairment are a challenge to research. Collaborative clinical research networks, including multi-centre or population-based disease cohorts, have successfully undertaken studies of rare eye disease, overcoming these obstacles by using detailed harmonised descriptions of each disease (Chak et al. 2006; Rahi et al. 2000; Rahi et al. 2010). However, many evidence gaps remain and many conditions remain untreatable medically. Emerging technologies such as ocular imaging (which allows improved phenotyping), genomics, and 'big data' may lead to improved outcomes through deeper understanding of the causes and mechanisms of each disorder, its natural history, and therapeutic targets (see Chapter 3).

At international level, robust screening and evidence-based surveillance, including consensus in, and harmonisation of assessment methods, classification, and data sets at population level, are needed. This has public health relevance that will lead to greater understanding of the health economic needs and resource planning for paediatric eye care services, children with vision impairment, and their families in each country. Future clinical practice needs improved screening and paediatric ophthalmological diagnostic services and specialist-community pathways globally, to ensure that all children receive the earliest identification of vision impairment and rapid access to preventative or treatable medical interventions or early intervention/habilitation to support optimal visual and developmental outcomes. This continues to be a priority of the World Health Organization and associated organisations like UNICEF.

SUMMARY

Vision requires the integration of a number of visual functions, with central visual acuity and detection vision in the peripheral visual field being particularly important. The frequency and causes of visual impairment vary significantly across the world, reflecting the global patterns of the overall health and survival of children as well as the socio-economic developmental status of the region. Children with visual and ocular disorders form a heterogeneous group, with differing ocular and systemic disorders, and other sensory, motor, and global developmental impairments. Tertiary health and community multidisciplinary care is necessary to enable them to function to their full capabilities to allow effective participation in society.

Key Points

- ✓ Vision depends on related vision functions, including acuity, which need systematic assessment that takes into account the child's developmental level.
- ✓ Children with vision impairment comprise a very heterogeneous group with regards to causes and available treatments.
- ✓ Amblyopia is a neurodevelopmental disorder in which a child does not 'learn to see', and its timely management is central to all other conditions.
- ✓ Many causes of childhood visual impairment are preventable and amenable to treatment, but in higher income countries, approximately 80% of childhood blindness is currently untreatable.
- ✓ Early detection and prompt identification of childhood vision impairment and its cause is essential for preventing or intervening with treatable conditions or for introducing early habilitation to minimise the impact of vision impairment.
- ✓ Prevention and intervention need to occur at primary, secondary, and tertiary levels of health care with defined methods and pathways of screening, treatment, and intervention.

REFERENCES

Blohme J, Tornqvist K (1997) Visual impairment in Swedish children. III. Diagnoses. *Acta Ophthalmol Scand* **75**: 681–687.

Braddick O, Atkinson J (2011) Development of human visual function. *Vision Res* **51**: 1588–1609. doi: 10.1016/j.visres.2011.02.018.

Chak M, Wade A, Rahi JS (2006) British Congenital Cataract Interest Group. Long-term visual acuity and its predictors after surgery for congenital cataract: findings of the British congenital cataract study. *Invest Ophthalmol Vis Sci* **47**: 4262–4269.

Edelsten C, Reddy MA, Stanford MR, Graham EM (2003) Visual loss associated with pediatric uveitis in English primary and referral centers. *Am J Ophthalmol* **135**(5): 676–680. doi: 10.1016/s0002-9394(02)02148-7.

Fierson WM, American Academy of Pediatrics Section on Ophthalmology, American Academy of Ophthalmology, American Association for Pediatric Ophthalmology and Strabismus, American Association of Certified Orthoptists (2018) Screening examination of premature infants for retinopathy of prematurity. *Pediatrics* **142**(6): e20183061. doi: https://doi.org/10.1542/peds.2018-3061.

Foster A, Gilbert C, Johnson G (2008) Changing patterns in global blindness: 1988–2008. *Community Eye Health* **21**: 37–39.

Harris JM, Wilcox LM (2009) The role of monocularly visible regions in depth and surface perception. *Vision Res* **49**: 2666–2685. doi: 10.1016/j.visres.2009.06.021.

Holmes JM, Clarke MP (2006). Amblyopia. *The Lancet* **367**: 1343–1351.

Lewis TL, Maurer D (2005) Multiple sensitive periods in human visual development: evidence from visually deprived children. *Dev Psychobiol* **46**: 163–183.

Livingstone I, Butler L, Misanjo E et al. (2018) Testing pediatric acuity with an iPad: validation of 'Peekaboo Vision' in Malawi and the UK. *Transl Vis Sci Technol* **8**: 8. doi:10.1167/tvst.8.1.8.

Malik ANJ, Mafwiri M, Gilbert C (2018) Integrating primary eye care into global child health policies. *Arch Dis Child* **103**: 176–180.

Mitry D, Bunce C, Wormald R et al. (2013) Causes of certifications for severe sight impairment and sight impairment in children in England and Wales. *Br J Ophthalmol* **97**: 1431–1436.

Mutti DO, Mitchell GL, Jones LA et al. (2009) Accommodation, acuity, and their relationship to emmetropization in infants. *Optom Vis Sci* **86**: 666–676. doi:10.1097/OPX.0b013e3181a6174f.

Patel DE, Cumberland PM, Walters BC et al. (2015) Study of Optimal Perimetric Testing in Children (OPTIC): Normative Visual Field Values in Children. *Ophthalmology* **122**: 1711–1717. doi: 10.1016/j.ophtha.2015.04.038.

Public Health England (2016) *Newborn and Infant Physical Examination: Programme Handbook.* Available at: <https://www.gov.uk/government/publications/newborn-and-infant-physical-examination-programme-handbook> [Accessed 11 December 2019].

Public Health England (2017) *Child Vision Screening Resources.* Available at: <https://www.gov.uk/government/consultations/child-vision-screening-resources> [Accessed 11 December 2019].

Rahi JS, Dezateux C, the British Congenital Cataract Interest Group (2000) Congenital and infantile cataract in the United Kingdom: underlying or associated factors. *Invest Ophthalmol Vis Sci* **41**: 2108–2114.

Rahi JS, Cable N, British Childhood Visual Impairment Study Group (2003) Severe visual impairment and blindness in children in the UK. *Lancet* **362**: 1359–1365. doi:10.1016/S0140-6736(03)14631-4.

Rahi J, Cumberland P, Peckham C (2009) Visual function in working-age adults early life influences and associations with health and social outcomes. *Ophthalmology* **10**: 1866–1871. doi:10.1016/j.ophtha.2009.03.007.

Rahi JS, Cumberland PM, Peckham CS (2010) British Childhood Visual Impairment Interest Group. Improving detection of blindness in childhood: the British Childhood Vision Impairment study. *Pediatrics* **126**: e895–903. doi: 10.1542/peds.2010-0498.

Rahi JS, Manaras I, Tuomainen H et al. (2005) Health services experiences of parents of recently diagnosed visually impaired children. *Br J Ophthalmol* **89**: 213–218.

Rosser DA, Laidlaw DA, Murdoch IE (2001) The development of a 'reduced logMAR' visual acuity chart for use in routine clinical practice. *Br J Ophthalmol* **85**(4): 432–436.

Royal College of Ophthalmologists, Royal College of Paediatrics and Child Health (2008) *Guideline for the Screening and Treatment of Retinopathy of Prematurity*. Available at: <https://www.rcophth. ac.uk/wp-content/uploads/2014/12/2008-SCI-021-Guidelines-Retinopathy-of-Prematurity.pdf> [Accessed 6 October 2019].

Ryabets-Lienhard A, Stewart C, Borchert M et al. (2016) The optic nerve hypoplasia spectrum: review of the literature and clinical guidelines. *Adv Pediatr* **63**: 127–146. doi: 10.1016/j.yapd.2016.04.009.

Sakki H, Bowman R, Sargent J, Kukadia R, Dale N (2021) Visual function subtyping in children with early-onset cerebral visual impairment. *Dev Med Child Neurol* **63**: 303–321. doi.org/10.1111/dmcn.14710.

Shah SP, Taylor AE, Sowden JC et al. (2012) Anophthalmos, microphthalmos, and coloboma in the United Kingdom: clinical features, results of investigations, and early management. *Ophthalmology* **119**(2): 362–368.

Solebo AL (2019) Identification of visual impairments. In: Edmond A (ed.), *Health for all Children*, 5th Edition. Oxford: Oxford University Press, pp. 246–261.

Solebo AL, Cumberland PM, Rahi JS (2015) Whole-population vision screening in children aged 4–5 years to detect amblyopia. *Lancet* **385**: 2308–2319.

Solebo AL, Teoh L, Rahi J (2017) Epidemiology of blindness in children. *Arch Dis Child* **102**: 853–857. doi: 10.1136/archdischild-2016-310532.

Sonksen PM, Wade AW, Proffitt R, Heavens S, Salt AT (2008) The Sonksen logMAR test of visual acuity (II): age norms from 2 years 9 months to 8 years. *J AAPOS* **12**(1): 18–22.

Sonksen PM, Dale N (2002) Visual impairment in infancy: impact on neurodevelopmental and neurobiological processes. *Dev Med Child Neurol* **44**: 782–791.

Teller DY, McDonald MA, Preston K et al. (1986) Assessment of visual acuity in infants and children: the acuity card procedure. *Developmental Medicine & Child Neurology* **28**: 779–789. doi:10.1111/j.1469-8749.1986.tb03932.x.

Teoh LJ, Solebo AL, Rahi JS; British Childhood Visual Impairment and Blindness Study Interest Group (2021). Visual impairment, severe visual impairment, and blindness in children in Britain (BCVIS2): a national observational study. *Lancet Child Adolesc Health* **5**(3): 190–200. doi: 10.1016/S2352-4642(20)30366-7.

United States Preventive Services Task Force, Grossman DC, Curry SJ et al. (2017) Vision screening in children aged 6 months to 5 years: US Preventive Services Task Force recommendation statement. *JAMA* **318**: 836–844. doi: 10.1001/jama.2017.1126.

World Health Organization (2006) *International Statistical Classification of Diseases and Related Health Problems, Tenth Revision*. Geneva: World Health Organization Available from: <http://apps.who.int/classifications/apps/icd/icd10online/> [Accessed 11 December 2019].

CHAPTER 3

Congenital Eye Disorders

Genetics and Clinical Phenotypes

Mariya Moosajee and Ngozi Oluonye

INTRODUCTION

Congenital eye disorders are responsible for more than one-third of blindness and severe visual impairment in children worldwide, and encompass structural globe anomalies (including microphthalmia [small underdeveloped eye]), anophthalmia [complete absence of the eye], ocular coloboma [cleft in the inferior part of the eye], anterior segment dysgenesis (including corneal opacities, iridocorneal anomalies, and aniridia), primary congenital glaucoma, congenital cataracts, retinal dysplasia, vitreoretinopathies, retinoblastoma, and optic nerve anomalies. Recent advances in ocular genetics have advanced the understanding of genotype–phenotype correlations leading to new gene-based disease classification systems, and the development of new treatment options.

This chapter discusses genes, genotypes, and phenotypes of some of the more common congenital eye disorders causing severe visual impairment and implications for clinical management and practice.

GENES, GENOTYPES, AND PHENOTYPES OF CONGENITAL EYE DISORDERS

Genes and Genomics

Genes are the basic functional unit of inheritance and are located on chromosomes. Humans have 46 chromosomes in total (22 autosomes and two sex chromosomes). Each

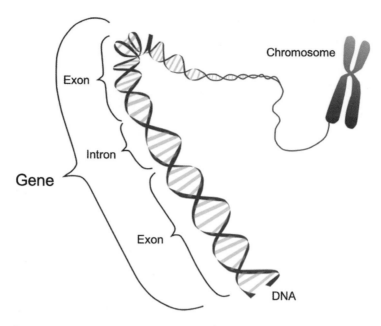

Figure 3.1 Gene structure. Adapted from Smedlib (Wikimedia Commons). This figure is licensed under the Creative Commons Attribution-Share Alike 4.0 International license (https://creative-commons.org/licenses/by-sa/4.0/deed.en).

person has between 20 000 and 25 000 genes, with two copies of each, one inherited from each parent. A gene is composed of DNA and made up of subunits called exons and introns. Exons hold the instructions for making proteins (the coding regions), whereas introns are interspacing non-coding DNA, which can hold regulatory units controlling gene function (Fig. 3.1). A genome is an individual's complete set of DNA and comprises more than 3 billion nucleotides. The exome is all the exons combined together. Protein coding genes form only 1% of the total, the other 99% being non-coding (Seaby et al. 2016). Panel testing is based on whole exome sequencing (testing of all of the exons in an individual) and involves analysis of several specific genes linked to a specific condition. In inherited retinal disorders, this can comprise over 250 genes. In the near future, whole genome sequencing will overtake the use of exome based tests: this will screen all 20 000 genes, covering both exons and introns.

Only 0.2% of human DNA differs between individuals. Most variations are healthy variations but some are disease-causing, and this is the basis of genetic disease. An alteration in the nucleotide sequence is called a mutation. Some genetic mutations can be inherited from parents (germline mutations – present in all cells including the eggs and sperm). These can be passed down to their offspring through different patterns of inheritance: autosomal dominant (one parent carries the dominant gene), autosomal recessive (both parents carry the recessive gene) and X-linked (males affected because they have a single copy of the X chromosome that carries the mutation).

Some mutations (somatic) are acquired by a cell and can occur very early on in the developing embryo itself or later in life and are present in certain cells only. Hence, unless the gametes (eggs and sperm) are affected, these mutations are not passed to the next generation. In de novo (new) mutations parents are unaffected and do not carry that mutation, however future generations may be affected.

EMBRYOLOGY AND EYE DISORDER GENES

Human eye development starts at 3 weeks' gestation and continues through pregnancy and after birth, but much of the development occurs in the first trimester. Therefore, genetic aberrations at this time usually contribute to significant structural congenital globe anomalies. By day 27 of gestation the optic vesicles are established from the neuroectoderm, which invaginates to form the optic cup and future retina. The surface ectoderm forms the anterior segment of each eye including the lens and cornea. The optic fissure forms on the inferior surface of the optic vesicle from week 5, allowing blood vessels and nutrients to enter. The optic fissure fuses by week 7 to form each intact globe.

See Fig. 3.2 for embryonic lens development. There are over 500 genes that are known to contribute to genetic eye disorders and overall the diagnostic rate for patients is 25% (Patel et al. 2019). Many more genes are likely to be discovered through future studies. Eye-related genes often play a role in the development of other body organs. For example, *USH2A* is expressed in the developing hair cells of the inner ear and in retinal photoreceptors. Mutations in this gene therefore can lead to congenital sensorineural hearing loss and retinitis pigmentosa, constituting type 2 Usher syndrome. A significant proportion of patients with developmental eye disorders have features affecting other organs of the body (Harding and Moosajee 2019), necessitating a multidisciplinary approach to management.

Structural Globe Anomalies

MICROPHTHALMIA, ANOPHTHALMIA, AND OCULAR COLOBOMA (MAC)

Microphthalmia, anophthalmia, and coloboma (MAC) lie on a clinical spectrum. Microphthalmia is defined by eye length (less than 19mm at 12 months). Anophthalmia is defined as absence of the eye, optic nerve, and chiasm; presence of a cystic remnant may be called clinical anophthalmia. Ocular coloboma is incomplete fusion of the optic fissure, leaving a cleft involving one or more structures (iris, ciliary body, retina, choroid, and optic nerve). These conditions can occur unilaterally or bilaterally, in isolation or in combination with other eye anomalies. In a prospective study conducted in the UK the overall incidence of MAC by 16 years was reported to be 11.9 per 100 000 (Shah et al. 2011). This study also demonstrated that colobomatous defects are an important part of the whole spectrum, though are less likely to result in severe visual impairment than microphthalmia/anophthalmia. Furthermore, of 135 new MAC cases reported over 18 months, almost 60% of children had systemic abnormalities, with the risk of these being greater in those with bilateral abnormalities (Shah et al. 2012).

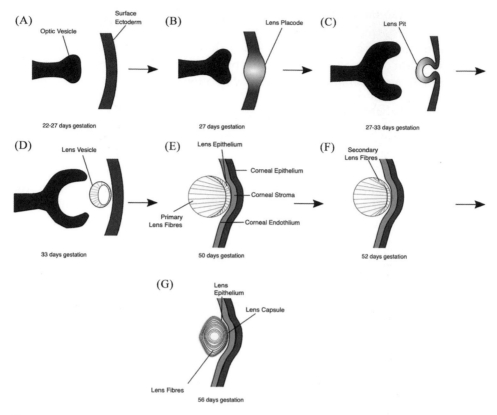

Figure 3.2 The stages of human lens development. Reused from Bell et al. (2020). This figure is licensed under the Creative Commons Attribution 4.0 International license (https://creativecommons.org/licenses/by/4.0/). (A colour version of this figure can be seen in the colour plate section)

There are currently 86 genes currently known to be associated with MAC. Unfortunately, diagnostic rates remain low at less than 10% overall, though these may be higher for severe bilateral microphthalmia/anophthalmia (Williamson and FitzPatrick 2014). The most common mutations identified are *SOX2*, *PAX6*, *OTX2*, *STRA6*, and *GDF6*. All forms of inheritance are noted.

The most common syndromic presentation of coloboma is CHARGE syndrome, which is caused by mutations in the *CDH7* gene. Infants presenting with coloboma therefore require careful systemic evaluation and investigation.

ANTERIOR SEGMENT DYSGENESIS, ANIRIDIA, AND GLAUCOMA

Anterior segment dysgenesis is a spectrum of conditions in which the anterior chamber has failed to fully develop. Over 50% of patients develop associated glaucoma. The main features of syndromic presentations are summarised in Table 3.1.

Table 3.1 Syndromes associated with anterior segment dysgenesis

Condition	Incidence	Inheritance pattern and causative genes	Ocular features may include	Systemic features
WAGR syndrome	1:500 000–1:1 000 000	Sporadic deletions of WT1 and PAX6 genes at 11p13 locus	Partial or full iris hypoplasia, foveal hypoplasia, nystagmus, cataracts, glaucoma corneal keratopathy, optic nerve hypoplasia	Wilms tumour, genitourinary abnormalities, intellectual difficulties, hearing impairment
Axenfeld-Reiger syndrome	1:200 000	PITX2 FOXC1 PAX6 PITX3 FOXE3 CYP1B1 CPAMD8	Corneal opacities, posterior embryotoxon, corectopia (ectopically displaced pupil), iris hypoplasia, cataracts, glaucoma	Maxillary hypoplasia, dental abnormalities, redundant periumbilical skin, cardiac defects, hydrocephalus
Peters anomaly and Peters plus syndrome	4:100 000	AR and AD FOXC1, PAX6, PITX2, CYPB1B1	Corneal opacit es, corectopia, anterior synechiae, iris hypoplasia, cataracts, glaucoma	Distinctive facial features, cleft lip +/– cleft palate Clinodactyly of the 5th finger, short stature, shortened limbs

AD, autosomal dominant; AR, autosomal recessive.

Aniridia is a pan-ocular condition with a prevalence of 1:40 000 to 100 000. Inheritance is usually autosomal dominant but de novo sporadic cases occur. It is characterised by partial or full iris hypoplasia and foveal hypoplasia, nystagmus, corneal keratopathy, cataracts, glaucoma, and optic nerve hypoplasia. In most cases it is associated with mutations of the *PAX6* gene. It may be isolated or occur as part of Wilms tumour-aniridia-genital anomalies-retardation (WAGR) syndrome. WAGR syndrome is associated with deletion of contiguous genes on the short arm of chromosome 11 (11p13 locus) and always includes deletion of *PAX6* and *WT1* (Wilms tumour gene) genes. *WT1* deletion is associated with a high risk (up to 90% by 4 years) of developing Wilms tumour (kidney tumour). Early involvement of a paediatrician is therefore key, requiring regular renal surveillance via ultrasound, until 8 years of age and annually thereafter. *PAX6 deletion* in isolation (without WT1) is not associated with renal tumours.

Primary congenital glaucoma is a severe form of glaucoma occurring when structural anomalies in the anterior chamber angle obstruct aqueous humour (fluid) drainage. A highly variable incidence between different ethnic groups – 1:18 500 UK, and 1:1250 Slovak Romany (Sarfarazi and Stoilov 2000) – indicates a likely genetic aetiology. Cases may be familial or sporadic. Inheritance is autosomal recessive with mutations of *CYP1B1, LTBP2, MYOC, FOXC1*, and *TEK* (Yu-Wai-Man et al. 2018). Affected children will require lifelong monitoring to ensure control of intraocular pressure and the mainstay of treatment is surgery.

Congenital Cataracts and Other Lens Disorders

Congenital cataracts are defined as any lens opacification present at birth or in early childhood, with an incidence rate of 4 to 24 per 10 000 births. One or both eyes may be affected and there may be additional eye abnormalities or systemic features. Early surgical intervention is required to avoid amblyopia (see Chapter 2). Although worldwide maternal infections are an important cause (see Chapter 2), approximately 50% to 90% of bilateral cases are caused by genetic mutations. Over 100 disease-causing genes are known; for bilateral cataracts, genetic diagnostic rates approach 90% (Bell et al. 2020; Bell et al. 2021).

A thorough systemic evaluation by a paediatrician is necessary to rule out systemic associations and syndromes (see Table 3.2). There are other very rare conditions with known mutations in which cataracts may occur.

Inherited Retinal Disorders

Inherited retinal disorders (IRDs) encompass many clinically and genetically heterogeneous conditions including early-onset severe retinal dystrophy (EOSRD) (previously, Leber congenital amaurosis), retinitis pigmentosa, cone, cone/rod, rod/cone, macular dystrophies, achromatopsia, and congenital stationary night blindness. All forms of

Table 3.2 Syndromes associated with cataracts

	Incidence	Clinical features	Inheritance	Gene groups
Cataracts	4–24 per 10 000	Lens opacities with various patterns. Please note if presence of microcephaly, deafness, and brain calcification suggest congenital infection as an underlying cause	All forms of inheritance possible	Crystallin (CRYAA, CRYBA1) Connexins (GJA3 and GJA8) Transcription factors (MAF)
Sticklers syndrome I–VI	1:7500–9000	High myopia, retinal detachment, sensorineural hearing loss, cleft palate, Pierre Robin sequence, musculoskeletal abnormalities	Autosomal recessive	1p21.1 COL2A1 COL9A1 COL9A2 COL9A3 COL11A2
Smith–Lemli-Opitz syndrome	1:20 000–60 000	Syndactyly, distinctive facial features, microcephaly, intellectual disability, and behavioural difficulties	Autosomal recessive	11q13.4 DHCR7
Zellwegers syndrome	1:50 000	Life-limiting hypotonia, seizures, feeding difficulties, hearing loss, skeletal abnormalities, profound developmental impairment, liver, heart, and renal problems	Autosomal recessive	PEX1
Lowes syndrome (oculocerebral syndrome)	Prevalence 1:100 000 males	Neonatal hypotonia, developmental impairment, and abnormal renal function	X-linked	OCRL1 (Xp26.1)

inheritance patterns exist and over 250 genes are known to cause diseases within this spectrum. Exome gene panel testing leads to diagnosis in 60% to 70% cases (Whelan et al. 2020). Varying phenotypic presentations and emerging gene-based therapies are enabling gene-based classification systems, e.g. *RPE65*-retinopathy. A UK prospective incidence study reported an annual incidence of IRDs of 1.4/100 000 children (aged 0–15 years) and the cumulative incidence by age 16 years was 22.3/100 000 (Hamblion et al. 2012). IRDs can be found in isolation (simplex), with other ocular features (complex), and in association with systemic features (syndromic).

EOSRD has the most severe functional outcome, due to the infancy onset of severe visual impairment. At presentation the fundus can appear normal (abnormalities may appear later) and an electroretinogram is necessary to confirm abnormal rod/cone function. EOSRD has a birth prevalence of 1:30 000 to 80 000, and so far, 25 genes account for 70% to 80% of cases (Kumaran et al. 2017). Stargardt macular dystrophy is the most common inherited macular dystrophy and the most common age of onset is the teenage years. Presentation is with loss of central vision, colour vision disturbance, and photophobia, and as the macula atrophies progressive vision loss occurs. Rods as well as cones may be affected. Stargardt is commonly due to mutations in the *ABCA4* gene, and is autosomal recessive in nature (Rahman et al. 2020). X-linked retinoschisis, most commonly caused by mutations in *RS1*, results in visual impairment, which is usually identified at school age but may be identified earlier in some children.

Syndromic inherited retinal disorders must be considered in childhood such as Joubert syndrome (eye movement abnormalities, structural abnormalities in the cerebellum), neuronal ceroid-lipofuscinoses, Alström syndrome, Bardet-Biedl syndrome, and disorders of intracellular cobalamin metabolism. Systemic features may manifest before retinal signs: in Usher syndrome, children are born with sensorineural hearing loss, and retinitis pigmentosa develops early in childhood or in adolescence. Batten disease is the common name for a broad class of rare, neurodegenerative, autosomal recessively inherited disorders of the nervous system also known as neuronal ceroid lipofuscinoses. Several subtypes of this disease are described according to the causative genetic mutations in the *CLN* gene, CLN 1, 2, and 3 being the most common (Mole and Cotman 2015).

Visual loss, seizures, and regression of cognitive and motor skills are common features, though the order of presentation differs between different genetic subtypes. Delay in diagnosis is not uncommon, particularly when visual loss is the initial presenting symptom; alterations in behaviour, faltering school progress, and rapid progression of visual loss should alert professionals to the possibility of a systemic diagnosis (Wright et al. 2020). Research into new treatments to slow or halt progression of symptoms adds further urgency to the need for early diagnosis; cerliponase alfa (Brineura) has been authorised in Europe and the USA for treatment of CLN2 (Johnson et al. 2019).

Retinoblastoma is the most common ocular tumour of childhood, this usually presents in children before the age of 3 years and may affect one or both eyes. Mutations in the *RB1* gene are responsible, either inherited from parents or occurring as a new mutation. Rarely, a deletion on the long arm of chromosome 13 may include the *RB1* gene and children with this 13q monosomy may have additional symptoms (McEvoy and Dyer 2015).

Inherited Vitreoretinopathies

Inherited retinovascular disorders are a heterogeneous group of rare diseases. They are characterised by abnormal retinal development, often affecting blood vessels, causing a range of retinal abnormalities including retinal detachment. Those presenting with severe visual impairment in childhood include Norrie disease, familial exudative vitreoretinopathy, and persistent foetal vasculature syndrome. Key causative genes are *FZD4*, *LRP5*, and *NDP*. *NDP* mutations, which can cause Norrie disease, affect males only as the gene is on the X chromosome. Norrie disease is also associated with progressive sensorineural deafness, with onset usually in the second decade of life. FEVR may be autosomal dominant or recessive, and disease severity varies considerably within the same family (Gilmour 2015).

Optic Nerve Anomalies

Optic nerve anomalies include optic nerve hypoplasia, diagnosed on the basis of an abnormally small optic nerve on fundoscopy. It can be found as part of septo-optic dysplasia, a disorder of early brain development characterised by abnormal formation of midline brain structures including the pituitary and the septum pellucidum. Most cases are sporadic but autosomal recessive and dominant inheritance has been reported (Webb and Dattani 2010; Chen et al. 2017).

Leber's hereditary optic neuropathy is a mitochondrial disorder in which progressive degeneration of the optic nerve occurs, causing painless vision loss. Whilst the most common age of onset is during adolescence, earlier and later presentations do occur. Rarely there are additional systemic manifestations. Common mutations include *MTND4* and *MTND6*.

Albinism

Albinism is a pigmentary disorder in which there is reduced melanin production affecting retina and iris, foveal hypoplasia, and chiasmal misrouting in the visual pathway. Albinism may affect the eye only (ocular albinism) or the eye, hair, and skin (oculocutaneous albinism). Ocular examination shows iris translucency and fundal hypopigmentation, and crossed asymmetry is evident on visual evoked potentials. Foveal hypoplasia causes reduction of visual acuity, which ranges from moderate to severe. Photophobia is common. Ocular albinism type 1 is X linked and due to mutations in the *GPR143* gene. Several subtypes of oculocutaneous albinism are described and inheritance is usually autosomal recessive. Mutations in the *TYR* and *OCA* genes are common. Increased exposure to harmful UV rays is an important cause of morbidity worldwide and social exclusion occurs in some countries (Chan et al. 2021).

PRACTICE AND MANAGEMENT

Early identification of an eye condition is crucial to enable early referrals for developmental and family support. Management of congenital eye disorders requires a multidisciplinary approach including ophthalmology, paediatrics, and other paediatric specialities, including genetics, according to need. Input from teachers, psychologists, and therapists will optimise the child's developmental progress.

Congenital eye disorders are rare and families will require information about the condition and its consequences. Professionals should acknowledge the impact of the diagnosis on the families and ensure that medical, developmental, and educational input and advice is available and that families are signposted to relevant support groups. Early management of severe visual impairment is crucial given its significant impact on infant and childhood vision, as well as broader aspects of development (see Chapters 4 and 8).

Initial Examination and Diagnosis

The initial assessment of a child with congenital ocular abnormalities includes a full history in order to ascertain aetiology and possible co-occurring disorders. Specific details in the history are highlighted in Table 3.3.

Most children with a congenital eye disorder causing severe visual impairment will present at birth or soon after with obvious ocular abnormality or signs of poor vision (see Chapter 2). Physical examination should include measurement of height, weight, and head circumference, and inspection for unusual facial, dental, or skeletal abnormalities. Consideration of the child's developmental status is also useful, though this may also reflect the impact of severe visual impairment (see Chapter 8). Ophthalmic examination will include retinoscopy to examine the fundus (back of the eye), slit lamp to examine the anterior structures (see Fig. 2.2, Chapter 2), measurement of refractive error and visual acuity, and examination of eye movements. Specialist centres may further evaluate with ultrasound, anterior segment and retinal optical coherence tomography, fundus autofluorescence, electrophysiological examination, and photographs of the anterior and posterior chambers. Magnetic resonance imaging (MRI) of the orbits may help to characterise ocular abnormalities.

Confirmation of the ocular diagnosis will help determine whether a genetic cause may be identified and examination of other family members for the presence of asymptomatic

Table 3.3 Guide to clinical history taking for congenital ocular disorders

Antenatal history	Maternal age
	Planned pregnancy, folic acid supplementation, history of miscarriages
	Infection or other illness
	Exposure to alcohol or substances (including medications) that could affect foetal development
Family history	Consanguinity
	Genogram of family members (at least three generations if known) and medical history including childhood deaths and other illnesses
Developmental history	Gestational age
	Birth weight and neonatal history
	Developmental concerns
Vision	First concerns about vision, and current visual skills
	Findings from previous eye examinations
	Current vision assessment findings
Systems enquiry	Hearing impairment, learning difficulties, development delay
	Any unusual body structures, e.g. extra digits (polydactyly), unusual facial features
	Growth
	General health status

related abnormalities may be informative. If a genetic cause is possible, genetic testing will be required to confirm this and results guide genetic counselling and family decision-making (Méjécase et al. 2020). Other investigations will be guided by the likelihood of syndromic diagnoses or to identify systemic features of a confirmed diagnosis.

Neuroimaging

Congenital eye disorders may have associated structural brain malformations, and brain MRI imaging is often a key diagnostic investigation. Images should ideally be reported by paediatric neuro-radiologists as some abnormalities may be subtle. Pituitary views should be requested where optic nerve hypoplasia is under consideration. Other non-midline radiological abnormalities such as cortical malformations or abnormal neural migration may be seen, highlighting the potential increased risk of epilepsy or developmental impairment.

Visual Electrophysiology

The electroretinogram provides information about retinal function and is crucial for diagnosis of retinal dystrophy. It can distinguish between cone and rod abnormalities, and repeat testing can indicate whether a condition is progressive. Flash and pattern visual evoked potentials give information about the pathway from optic nerve to visual cortex and can identify chiasmal misrouting (found in albinism) and hemifield defects (Robson et al. 2018).

Genetic Testing and Genetic Counselling

When genetic testing is required, a genetic counsellor should meet the child and family before and after testing. They can present complex information about genetic inheritance in an accessible way, enabling families to make informed decisions about testing. Information on advocacy and support groups is also crucial. Establishing a diagnosis can have significant implications for the child and family both in terms of emerging treatments and reproductive options. Prenatal testing, which may be invasive (amniocentesis or chorionic villus sampling) or non-invasive (extraction of foetal cells and DNA from maternal blood samples), may be available and help with family decision-making (Méjécase et al. 2020).

The clinical diagnosis will guide decisions about what type of genetic testing will be helpful. For some clinical diagnoses single gene analysis can be requested but for other conditions gene panel testing is more appropriate.

In 2012, the 100 000 Genome Project was launched to sequence the whole genome of patients in England focussing on rare diseases and cancer. Over 5 years, almost 85 000 adults and children were tested and the infrastructure to introduce genomic medicine into the NHS was established. Large-scale studies such as this have increased diagnostic rates for patients by an extra 40% through identifying novel variants and genes.

IMPLICATIONS FOR RESEARCH AND PRACTICE

In December 2017, the first ocular gene therapy, known as Luxturna (or voretigene neparovec), was approved for clinical use by the Food and Drug Administration (FDA) in the USA for the treatment of autosomal recessive *RPE65*-retinopathy. Gene therapy involves delivering the *RPE65* gene within an adeno-associated viral vector to the retina through a sub-retinal injection (Russell et al. 2017; Trapani and Auricchio 2019). Immunosuppressant therapy is required pre- and post-operatively to reduce the risk of inflammatory/immune response. Luxturna was approved in 2019 by the National Institute for Health and Care Excellence (NICE) in the UK and is available at other European and international centres.

As several other clinical trials of genetic therapies are underway, accurate genetic diagnosis should form an important part of clinical management. In addition to the conventional gene replacement therapies using viral vectors, researchers are developing the use of small molecule drugs to target particular types of mutations such as nonsense and splice site variants. This is known as nonsense suppression therapy and antisense oligonucle-otide therapy, respectively. For some patients who remain undiagnosed or whose gene is not under gene therapy development, common disease pathways are being targeted so more therapies with a wider application can be offered – this may be targeted to reducing cell death or oxidative stress, or increasing glucose uptake and metabolism in photoreceptor cells.

Gene therapy cannot restore vision where photoreceptors are lost, but can stabilise and slow further degeneration. Patients who have received Luxturna have maintained navi-gational vision based on a mobility maze test. Ongoing research is needed to improve diagnostic rates, to understand the molecular mechanisms of genetic eye disease and aid therapeutic target development, and to improve understanding of natural history to establish clinical endpoints and the optimal age of intervention. Non-retinal conditions such as MAC and anterior segment dysgenesis pose greater challenges for intervention given the early stage of disordered eye development.

SUMMARY

This chapter considers the range of congenital eye disorders affecting children. Whilst underlying genetic causes are present in the majority, diagnostic rates can be low with only 25% receiving a genetic diagnosis. Diagnostic yield varies between conditions (<10% for structural globe anomalies but up to 90% for bilateral congenital cataracts), reflecting the complexity of the condition and scientific investment in identifying candidate genes. Emerging next generation sequencing technologies, such as whole genome sequencing, have the capacity to read the entire genome of every individual, and identify possible disease-causing variants in coding and non-coding regions. Advances in research have led to the first approved ocular gene therapy with more in clinical trials. An era of per-sonalised medicine has begun, and it is hoped that within the next decade children and families will be able to receive a molecular diagnosis, and be offered targeted genetic therapy to prevent or minimise sight loss where possible.

Key Points

✓ A detailed clinical history, including antenatal, birth, and family history, is important when considering the cause of a congenital eye disorder, and will help to identify additional systemic features and inheritance patterns.

✓ Many conditions have a genetic basis and genetic testing should be undertaken to aid genetic counselling, family planning, and enable future access to therapeutics.

✓ Overall genetic diagnosis rates are low but are improving with the advent of whole genome sequencing.

✓ Multidisciplinary management with ophthalmologists working closely with paediatricians and other disciplines will ensure the best clinical outcomes for each child.

REFERENCES

Bell SJ, Harding P, Oluonye N, Moosajee M (2020) Congenital cataract: a guide to genetic and clinical management. *Ther Adv Rare Dis* **22**(1): 1–22. doi.org/10.1177/2633004020938061.

Bell S, Malka S, Lloyd IC, Moosajee M (2021) Clinical spectrum and genetic diagnosis of 54 consecutive patients aged 0-25 with bilateral cataracts. *Genes* **12**(2): 131. doi: 10.3390/genes12020131.

Chan HW, Schiff ER, Tailor VK et al. (2021) Prospective study of the phenotypic and mutational spectrum of ocular albinism and oculocutaneous albinism. *Gene* **12**(4): 508. doi: 10.3390/genes12040508.

Chen CA, Yin J, Lewis RA, Schaaf CP (2017) Genetic causes of optic nerve hypoplasia. *J Med Genet* **54**(7): 441–449.

Hamblion EL, Moore AT, Rahi JS, British Childhood Onset Hereditary Retinal Disorders Network (2012) Incidence and patterns of detection and management of childhood-onset hereditary retinal disorders in the UK. *Br J Ophthalmol* **96**(3): 360–365.

Harding P, Moosajee M (2019) The molecular basis of human anophthalmia and microphthalmia. *J Dev Biol* **14**;7(3): E16. doi: 10.3390/jdb7030016.

Johnson TB, Cain JT, White KA, Ramirez-Montealegre D, Pearce DA, Weimer JM (2019) Therapeutic landscape for Batten disease: current treatments and future prospects. *Nat Rev Neurol* **15**(3): 161–178.

Kumaran N, Moore AT, Weleber RG, Michaelides M (2017) Leber congenital amaurosis/early-onset severe retinal dystrophy: clinical features, molecular genetics and therapeutic interventions. *Br J Ophthalmol* **101**(9): 1147–1154.

McEvoy JD, Dyer MA (2015) Genetic and epigenetic discoveries in human retinoblastoma. *Crit Rev Oncog* **20**(3–4): 217–225.

Méjécase C, Malka S, Guan Z, Slater A, Arno G, Moosajee M (2020) Practical guide to genetic screening for inherited eye diseases. *Ther Adv Ophthalmol* **12**: 2515841420954592. doi: 10.1177/2515841420954592.

Mole SE and Cotman SL (2015) Genetics of the neuronal ceroid lipofuscinoses (Batten disease). *Biochim Biophys Acta* **1852**: 2237–2241. doi: 10.1016/j.bbadis.2015.05.011.

Patel A, Hayward JD, Tailor V et al. (2019) The Oculome panel test: next-generation sequencing to diagnose a diverse range of genetic developmental eye disorders. *Ophthalmology* **126**(6): 888–907. doi: 10.1016/j.ophtha.2018.12.050.

Rahman N, Georgiou M, Khan KN, Michaelides M (2020) Macular dystrophies: clinical and imaging features, molecular genetics and therapeutic options. *Br J Ophthalmol* **104**(4): 451–460.

Russell S, Bennett J, Wellman JA et al. (2017) Efficacy and safety of voretigene neparvovec (AAV2-hRPE65v2) in patients with RPE65-mediated inherited retinal dystrophy: a randomised, controlled, open-label, phase 3 trial. *Lancet* **390**(10097): 849–860. doi: 10.1016/S0140-6736(17)31868-8.

Robson AG, Nilsson J, Shiying L et al. (2018) ISCEV guide to visual electrodiagnostic procedures. *Doc Ophthalmol* **136**: 1–26.

Sarfarazi M, Stoilov I (2000) Molecular genetics of primary congenital glaucoma. *Eye* **14**: 422–428.

Seaby EG, Pengelly RJ, Ennis S (2016) Exome sequencing explained: a practical guide to its clinical application. *Brief Funct Genomics* **15**(5): 374–384.

Shah SP, Taylor AE, Sowden JC et al. (2011) Anophthalmos, microphthalmos and typical coloboma in the United Kingdom: a prospective study of incidence and risk. *Invest Ophthal Vis Sci* **52**: 558–564. https://doi.org/10.1167/iovs.10-5263.

Shah SP, Taylor AE, Sowden JC et al. (2012) Anophthalmos, microphthalmos, and coloboma in the United Kingdom: clinical features, results of investigations, and early management. *Ophthalmol* **119**: 362–368. https://doi.org/10.1016/j.ophtha.2011.07.039.

Trapani I and Auricchio A (2019) Has retinal gene therapy come of age? From bench to bedside and back to bench. *Human Molecular Genetics* **28**(R1): 108–118.

Webb EA, Dattani MT (2010) Septo-optic dysplasia. *European Journal of Human Genetics* **18**(4): 393–397.

Whelan L, Dockery A, Wynne N et al. (2020) Findings from a genotyping study of over 1000 people with inherited retinal disorders in Ireland. *Genes* **16;11**(1): E105. doi: 10.3390/genes11010105.

Williamson KA, FitzPatrick DR (2014) The genetic architecture of microphthalmia, anophthalmia and coloboma. *Eur J Med Genet* **57**(8): 369–380.

Wright GA, Georgiou M, Robson AG et al. (2020) Juvenile Batten disease (CLN3): detailed ocular phenotype, novel observations, delayed diagnosis, masquerades, and prospects for therapy. *Ophthalmol Retina* **4**(4): 433–445.

Yu-Wai-Man C, Arno G, Brookes J, Garcia-Feijoo J, Khaw PT, Moosajee M (2018) Primary congenital glaucoma including next-generation sequencing-based approaches: clinical utility gene card. *Eur J Hum Genet* **26**(11): 1713–1718.

CHAPTER 4

Assessment and Habilitation of Vision in Infants and Young Children

Alison Salt and Jenefer Sargent

INTRODUCTION

Vision matures rapidly in typically developing children in the first years of life. In infants and young children with vision impairment, maturation may also occur, though from a lower baseline and with a less certain trajectory and outcome. Given the critical importance of vision in early development, the focus of vision habilitation must be on enhancing any potential for visual development in the early years, thus ensuring the child has the best available vision to reduce developmental vulnerability.

Assessment of vision in children with severe vision impairment provides a detailed understanding of the child's current vision level and its impact on development and learning. It is the essential framework for planning vision habilitation, guiding adaptation of tasks and the environment for optimal interaction and learning.

This chapter describes the early development of vision, and evidence and methods for vision assessment and habilitation in the early years of life for infants and young children with severe vision impairment.

ASSESSMENT AND HABILITATION OF VISION

Development of Vision

Vision is a complex construct encompassing multiple functions, including clarity of vision (acuity), eye movement control (binocularity, saccades, and smooth pursuit), understanding what is seen, and ability to focus attention on visual targets (see Chapter 2). These functions develop from birth through the early years with maturation seen in ocular structures and evolving brain connectivity in visual pathways and association areas. Rapid maturation and development of cortical circuits of relevance to visual function are seen in the first months of life (Kostović and Judaš 2007).

Infant visual development has been studied extensively (Braddick and Atkinson 2011). With the exception of the most severe structural anomalies (e.g. bilateral anophthalmia), children with severe vision impairment due to congenital disorders of the primary visual system (ocular and anterior pathway disorders) have potential for improvement in visual acuity especially in the first and second year of life (Sonksen et al. 1991; Weiss and Kelly 2007; Salt et al. 2020). In children with cerebral visual impairment, improvement has also been reported in a high proportion (up to 50%) of the children studied (Matsuba and Jan 2006). Improvement in vision tends to follow a similar trajectory but at a lower level and more slowly than in children with no visual difficulties. Final visual outcomes, however, are unpredictable and limited by the constraints of the particular vision disorder.

The mechanisms for this improvement have not been thoroughly investigated or understood, but a combination of maturation of retinal receptors and visual pathways combined with increasing cognitive interest in poorly formed visual images are likely to be involved. In addition, there is evidence that reorganisation of visual pathways occurs (Guzzetta et al. 2010; see Chapter 7).

Given the critical role of vision in early development (see Chapter 8), understanding that the visual system can develop despite no or very low levels of vision in the early months underpins the imperative for very early habilitation. There is evidence that without targeted habilitation during the time of greatest brain plasticity, vision development may take place more slowly or not at all (Sonksen et al. 1991).

Assessment Approaches

Assessment of children with no or very low levels of vision should target both vision functions (at the level of structure and function, according to the International Classification of Functioning, Disability and Health: Children and Youth [ICF-CY] framework) and functional use of vision (Fig. 4.1).

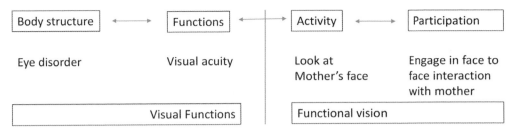

Figure 4.1 ICF-CY framework for vision functions and functional use of vision

Visual Functions

Systematic measurement of vision tends to focus on visual functions (i.e. how the eye and visual pathways function), for example measurement of acuity (Chapter 2). For young children who cannot yet name or match letters (to measure recognition acuity), resolution acuity can be measured with grating cards, displaying black and white lines of decreasing width, using preferential looking methods at 0.5m or less. However, this can be challenging in young children with low vision, as extremely low levels of acuity may not be captured by such tests and behavioural co-operation may be limited. There is also no accepted classification of severity of vision reduction using near measures; internationally recognised classification systems are based on 'distance' measures of recognition acuity (see Chapter 2).

Research from our team has shown that infants with no vision or light perception only, are those who are most at risk developmentally, irrespective of the nature of the peripheral visual system disorder (Dale et al. 2017). A simple functional classification based on presence or absence of 'form' vision (detection of non-light reflecting lures) is therefore highly valuable for clinical, habilitation, and research purposes (Sonksen and Dale 2002). Form vision can be further quantified using the Near Detection Scale (NDS), devised by Sonksen et al. (1991; Salt et al. 2020). This 10-point scale provides a practical measure for identifying the smallest size of single target/lure detected at a standard distance of 30cm.

In a study of 93 infants with congenital disorders of the peripheral visual system and severe vision impairment, only 35% achieved a reliable resolution acuity measure at 13 months of age, but all achieved a score on the NDS (Salt et al. 2020). Detection vision measurement enables identification of lower levels of vision than the grating acuity cards. The NDS is therefore a valuable assessment tool for monitoring developing vision and guiding vision and developmental habilitation advice (Sonksen et al. 1991).

Functional Vision

Functional vision refers to how the child functions when performing tasks meaningful to everyday activity and participation (Fig. 4.1). There are a number of questionnaires designed to estimate this in school-aged children (Khadka et al. 2010; Gothwal et al. 2012; Tadić et al. 2013), but only one includes a short proxy questionnaire for 0 to 4-year-olds (Hatt et al. 2019). When assessing functional vision in very young children with low vision, the interpretation of the child's visual responses must take into account what is expected and appropriate for their age, according to both expected visual behaviours and general development level (Anstice and Thompson 2014; Sonksen 2016). Assessment and classification of functional vision must also map on to but does not replace the systematic measurement of the child's visual functions (see Chapter 5).

Vision Habilitation

As vision in those with severe vision impairment can improve in the first 2 years of life, the aim of vision habilitation is to accelerate this development to provide the best possible level of vision for learning at the earliest age. However, as vision is likely to improve in most children, assessing the effectiveness of an intervention is challenging. There is evidence that vision is 'experience dependent', i.e. use of vision accelerates development of the vision system (Berardi et al. 2003; Celesia 2005; Jandó et al. 2012), and lack of vision causes irreversible constraints. Unilateral vision deprivation studies in kittens show that obstruction to vision input in one eye inhibits development of the associated area of the visual cortex (Wiesel and Hubel 1963). Research also shows that there is a critical period for visual development, with the first year being the time of most rapid change in brain growth and connections (Berardi et al. 2003; Kostović and Judaš 2007; Chapter 7) This evidence suggests that, if a child with vision impairment does not use their vision optimally, full potential may not be achieved effectively due to visual deprivation.

The seminal study by Sonksen et al. (1991) showed that experience drives vision development when habilitation is tailored to the child's vision needs and alerts cognitive interest and attention. This randomised controlled trial of a 'programme of vision development' was undertaken in 58 children under the age of 13 months at baseline with severe visual impairment originating in congenital ocular and cerebral disorders. The children receiving the developmentally based vision programme showed a significant clinically relevant improvement in all nine visual measures in those in the intervention arm compared to controls. Improvement was seen even in 40% of the 29 children with no vision or light perception only at baseline. This benefit also extended to those with severe learning disability. The programme of vision development favourably influenced visual outcome when introduced at any time during the first 13 months of life, although earlier introduction enabled greater benefit to be derived from the improved vision. Therefore it was recommended by the authors that infants are referred to a developmental centre or service for promoting vision development as soon as severe visual impairment is suspected. Since this study, which has yet to be replicated, there has been limited research and thus it remains the main empirical case for vision habilitation with infants with low vision.

Two reviews (one focussed on children with neurodevelopmental disorders or at risk of cerebral palsy) found some limited evidence for effectiveness of visual habilitation (Vervloed et al. 2006; Chorna et al. 2017). Of the studies included, only Sonksen et al. (1991) described the use of a contingent multisensory approach to facilitate the use of vision in everyday tasks in children under the age of 13 months at baseline.

SUPPORT AND MANAGEMENT: ASSESSMENT AND HABILITATION

Assessment of Vision

In young children with severe vision impairment, a multidisciplinary approach, including the ophthalmology team and neurodevelopmental paediatrician, provides the holistic developmental framework for assessing and monitoring vision from the earliest possible age to guide the vision habilitation programme. Parents and the early intervention practitioner will play a key role, bringing expertise and observations from their everyday experience into the early intervention programme.

A full ophthalmological examination is essential not only to provide diagnostic information but also to ensure identification and treatment of any additional impairment. Some ocular disorders are associated with higher rates of refractive error or squint and correction of these may make a critical difference to the child's visual functions and functional use of vision.

The assessment should begin with a detailed history to clarify the ophthalmological diagnosis, any associated risk factors, and to document parents' concerns and observations of their child's eyes and visual behaviours. Some guiding questions can support parents in giving clear descriptions (Box 4.1).

VISUAL FUNCTIONS

Key visual functions to be considered during assessment (Chapter 2) include fixation, eye movements, detection and acuity, contrast sensitivity, stereopsis, visual fields, colour vison, and higher-order visual functions (Chapter 5). Many basic visual functions can be assessed in young children with appropriate choice of materials. However, in those with the lowest levels of vision, assessment may be confined to establishing the level of detection vision.

Box 4.1 Examples of questions to ask parents

What do you notice about what your child can see?

✓ Do they turn towards light/silent objects or faces? At what distance?

✓ Do they reach towards light/silent objects or faces? At what distance?

✓ What is the smallest object or thing that they seem to see? At what distance?

Table 4.1 Development of infant visual skills (adapted from Sonksen 2016)

	Visual behaviour	
Age by which skill established	**Near**	**Distance**
Neonate	Turns to diffuse light	
2–4 weeks	Fixes on parent's face	
4–8 weeks	Fixation shift	
	Follows a face	Watches adult at <1m
3 months	Follows a small object horizontal and vertical *(6.25cm dangling yellow ball)*[a]	
	Watches hands	
4 months	Able to converge	Watches adult at 1.5m
5 months	Fixes on smaller objects *(2.5cm brick)*[a]	
6 months	*(1.25cm lure yellow sweet)*[a]	Watches adult at 3m
9–12 months	*(1mm lure)*[a]	2.5cm ball at 6m
Developmental age in typically sighted	**Developmental skills required for assessing vision**	
Neonate	Preferential looking	
From 15 months	Understanding object labels – where's the cup?	
From 18 months	Naming objects – what's this?	
From 21 months	Naming pictures – what can you see?	
From 30 months	Matching symbols/letters – recognition acuity	

[a]Near Detection Scale lures.

In infants and toddlers, observation of fixation, fixation shifts, and reaching responses are central to vision assessment. Knowledge of the typical sequence of vision and general development is important and will guide the choice of developmentally appropriate assessment materials and interpretation of responses (Table 4.1). As children's visual and general development and skills develop, the repertoire of assessment measures available increases (Table 4.1; see Chapter 2).

The following section describes a systematic approach to assessment of basic visual functions in young children with severe visual impairment (see also Chapter 2). Comprehensive approaches to assessment of vision in newborns and infants at high risk have also been described (Ricci et al. 2010; Rossi et al. 2017). This is considered further in Chapter 5 and Chapter 6.

Eye Structure and Squint
Simple observation of the child's eyes will alert to obvious structural differences such as small eyes, cloudy cornea, squint, or abnormal eye movements including nystagmus.

The ophthalmological assessment will provide full information; prompt referral is always required when ocular abnormality or poor visual responses are suspected.

Detection Vision

The NDS provides a systematic way to assess detection vision. The scale ranges from no light perception through to fixation on a 1mm lure at 30cm (Sonksen et al. 1991; Salt et al. 2020) (Fig. 4.2). After observing the child's spontaneous visual behaviour, a lure to assess fixation and detection vision can be chosen. If the child appears to show vision awareness in a normally lit room, observing fixation on the assessor's face is a good starting point as this is the most socially salient target for a very young infant (Fig. 4.3).

Eye Movements

Lures within the child's level of detection on the NDS and relevant to developmental interest can be selected. Using these, smooth pursuit movements (following) and saccades in both horizontal and vertical directions can be tested.

Visual Acuity and Contrast Sensitivity

Estimates of resolution acuity using preferential looking responses to grating cards (see Chapter 2) can be attempted soon after birth, although many infants with severe visual impairment may have insufficient vision capacity for this. Older children who are able to perform matching/naming tasks may be assessed using a recognition acuity test adapted for children using optotypes or letters. Examples include Lea symbols (Hyvärinen et al.

	Near Detection Scale (NDS)		Profound visual impairment (PVI) / severe visual impairment (SVI)	NDS score	
'in space'	No light perception		PVI	0	
	Light in dark room Light reflecting object	Glowing light Mirror/tinsel ball	PVI	1	
	12.5cm non-light reflecting	Black and yellow ball	SVI	2	
	6.25cm	Yellow ball	SVI	3	
On table top, plain background	6.25cm	Yellow ball	SVI	4	
	2.5cm	Yellow cube	SVI	5	
	1.2cm	Sweet (smartie)	SVI	6	
	0.5cm	Sweetener	SVI	7	
	0.3cm	Sweetener	SVI	8	
	0.1cm	Cake decoration	SVI	9	

Figure 4.2 The Near Detection Scale. (A colour version of this figure can be seen in the colour plate section)

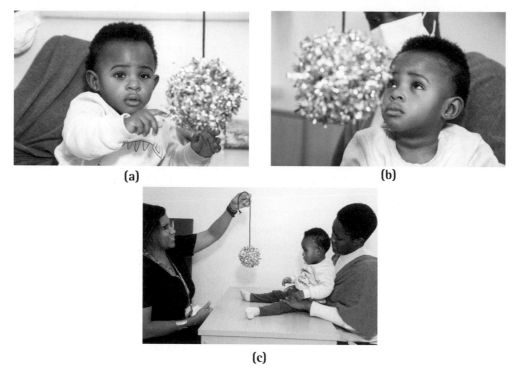

(a) **(b)**

(c)

Figure 4.3 Detection vision assessment. (A colour version of parts a and c of this figure can be seen in the colour plate section)

1980), Kay Pictures (Kay 1993), Sonksen logMAR (Sonksen et al. 2008), and Crowded Keeler logMAR (McGraw and Winn 1993). Note that Kay Pictures may overestimate acuity (Anstice et al. 2017). Contrast sensitivity measurement may not always be feasible in infants and young children with very severe visual impairment. The Hiding Heidi test developed by Lea Hyvärinen (www.lea-test.fi) may be most suitable for use with infants.

Visual Fields

Formal assessment of fields using perimetry is not possible in young children but simple methods based on distraction testing using two observers can be effective (Koenraads et al. 2015). A frame or wand can help guide the lure into the child's visual field (www.lea-test.fi). Gross reduction in visual fields can be identified by encouraging fixation on a central target, followed by introduction of a lure (that must be within the child's detection range) from behind the child into the lateral, upper, and lower visual fields, and estimating the angle from the midline when the child alerts to the lure.

FUNCTIONAL VISION

To complement the objective measurement of visual functions, consideration of a child's functional use of vision in everyday activities is also important for planning vision habilitation. However, care must be taken in interpreting observations as the child with vision impairment may use tactile and auditory cues and familiarity to support recognition of everyday objects. For example, a child may reach for a bottle using an auditory cue or recognise a familiar toy or picture using colour and shape clues.

Consider the following questions when enquiring about the child's functional vision: What do they look at (sustained fixation)? Does colour or luminance alter the response? At what distance do they lose interest? Do they show recognition (e.g. smiling when seeing a parent's silent face or favourite toy, showing excitement when seeing a silent bottle)? For older preschool children, do they show interest in and recognition of photos or pictures, and if so, how does the quality or familiarity of the picture (colour contrast, outline) alter their response?

The Record of Developing Vision in the Developmental Journal for babies and young children with visual impairment (DJVI) developed by Patricia Sonksen allows parents to record their observations of their young child's everyday vision function in partnership with their early intervention practitioner (Salt and Dale 2017; see Chapter 8).

Vision Habilitation

Sonksen et al.'s study (1991) was pioneering in incorporating many of the elements of early intervention now recommended (Sukkar et al. 2016). Their approach targeted gaining the best possible vision for optimum development as early as possible. Key components include: (1) day-to-day intervention to be parent-delivered in the everyday home environment, (2) supported by guidance by the practitioner, (3) incremental, goal-directed activities within a structured developmental vision framework, (4) providing sufficient challenge for current vision function skill level. Until more research evidence is available, this approach continues as 'recommended best practice'.

Two key elements of intervention can be identified, namely (1) promotion of the child's visual development, (2) adaptation of learning materials and environment to ensure that the child is able to use currently available vision to its maximum to support learning. These elements should be fully integrated into the developmental habilitation programme.

VISION PROMOTION

The vision habilitation programme developed by Sonksen et al. (1991) is provided in modified form for parents and practitioners in the Vision materials of the DJVI to support early intervention at home (Salt and Dale 2017).

The sequence of the intervention is as follows:

1. Ensure the tasks are at the appropriate level for the child's developmental stage and interests.

2. Identify the child's level of visual function and ascertain the lure, toy, or object of which the child shows awareness.

3. Introduce strategies that increase the child's cognitive interest and motivation in 'looking' through multisensory approaches, e.g. use of touch of object when looking at it. Sound will also increase the child's attention to the lure.

4. When each goal is achieved, increase the challenge, e.g. increase distance or reduce size or luminance or contrast.

5. Once fixation has been gained reliably, tasks can be introduced that support the development of smooth pursuit movements (following at close range) and tracking at a distance.

In the appropriate sequence, goals will be aimed at each of the visual functions described above. As vision matures through infancy and into the second year of life for the majority of conditions causing visual impairment in childhood, regular monitoring of vision level is needed (Sonksen et al. 1991; Salt et al. 2020). The DJVI provides a framework for setting goals for vision progress using the Vision Activity Cards to guide habilitation (Salt and Dale 2017).

Adapting the Environment for Learning

As vision plays a crucial role in learning and development, everyday routines, interaction, and play should be carried out in optimal visual conditions. The findings of the vision assessment will be essential to support this adaptation.

Once the infant/child's level of vision is established, everyday objects, play, and the environment must be adapted to support the best use of vision. All targets should be made optimally visible by altering luminance, size, separation, and contrast with an ideally uniform background, minimising overlap and clutter. The Vision Environment and Visual Materials cards (DJVI) provide a method for parents, working with their practitioner, to identify the child's current level of vision, plan adaptations of the visual environment, and integrate with their general developmental habilitation goals and activities (Salt and Dale 2017 and Chapter 8).

Two examples of vision promotion and adaptation of the environment are given in Table 4.2. As vision continues to develop in the early years, tracking of vision levels is essential so that vision habilitation tasks can be updated (Salt et al. 2020). In children with progressive vision loss it is also important to ensure understanding of the level of vision as it deteriorates so that support required is provided in a timely way. There are also children who have deteriorating vision in whom treatment may be successful in restoring vision. These children also require appropriate support and adaptation for their vision needs during the period of vision reduction to ensure that their learning continues unabated and quality of life is maintained.

Table 4.2 Vision habilitation activities

Visual promotion	Example 1	Example 2
1. Developmental age and interests	Social and emotional development: in the early months parent–infant interaction (face-to-face play if sufficient vision)	Play and learning: infants begin to learn to reach for a toy (*in infants with typical sight from around 4 months' developmental age*)
2. Visual assessment	Shows some awareness of large form at 20cm but not yet sustained fixation (NDS point 3)	Shows fixation on a light in a dark room and brief fixation on a light-reflecting large form at 30cm (NDS point 1)
3. Visual goal	To increase sustained fixation on large form especially parent's face	To sustain fixation on a light-reflecting or producing toy at close range
4. Lure (visual target)	Parent's face at 20cm in well-illuminated room	A toy that glows in the dark or is light-reflecting in a well-illuminated room or with light directed onto the lure
5. Everyday activity	In face-to-face interaction talk to the infant and guide their hand to parent's face to encourage visual interest through touch and sound (parent talking to infant)	During play time encourage the infant to fixate on and reach to explore a toy. If reach is not spontaneous, guide arm so that hand touches the toy, to alert cognitive interest
Adapting the environment	Direct light on parent's face; mother could wear lipstick or make-up to increase the contrast of her facial features	During play time and learning to reach, either dim the lights and use toys that light up/glow or well-lit toys that are light-reflecting and feel interesting to explore once touched

NDS, Near Detection Scale.

IMPLICATIONS FOR RESEARCH AND PRACTICE

Research on the most effective approaches for early visual habilitation has not advanced significantly since Sonksen et al.'s 1991 study. Replication of the methodology, combined with new neurophysiological measurements now available, is needed. Randomised clinical trials exploring other methodologies, building on similar principles, would help advance the field and identify the most effective methods for promotion and habilitation of vision function and development.

Given the critical stage of neuroplasticity and potential for rapid visual development in the first year of life, early identification of children with severe visual impairment and referral to appropriate health and early intervention services for vision and developmental habilitation should be at the earliest possible opportunity once a vision impairment is identified. This should be ideally starting at 4 to 6 months of age if not earlier. A combined health-education strategy brings together the most effective team for supporting early vision development and learning.

SUMMARY

The aim of vision habilitation is to ensure that vision is maximised as early as possible. Although limited, research evidence for the best vision habilitation approach in infancy is based on recommended practice principles in early intervention and the active use of vision, engaging cognitive interest and motivation through multisensory approaches. Assessment of vision underpins any vision and developmental habilitation advice; a systematic approach will be enabled by close collaboration between ophthalmologists, paediatricians, and practitioners delivering early intervention with parents as key partners.

Key Points

- ✓ Infants and young children with severe vision impairment have the potential for improving vision, especially in the first years of life.
- ✓ Vision habilitation should be started as early as possible in order to optimise visual potential at the time of greatest neuroplasticity.
- ✓ Assessment of early vision should include assessment of vision functions and functional use of vision and underpins the vision habilitation programme.
- ✓ Vision habilitation should use multisensory methods to enhance the infant's cognitive interest for using vision and be undertaken within a structured developmental framework covering vision development.
- ✓ The infant and young child's environment, toys, and other everyday objects need to be adapted to the child's current level of vision, to maximise use of available vision for learning.
- ✓ Early developmental and vision habilitation should be provided in an integrated structured programme integrating general development and vision development.

REFERENCES

Anstice NS, Jacobs RJ, Simkin SK, Thomson M, Thompson B, Collins AV (2017) Do picture-based charts overestimate visual acuity? Comparison of Kay Pictures, Lea Symbols, HOTV and Keeler logMAR charts with Sloan letters in adults and children. *PLoS One* **12**(2): e0170839.

Anstice NS, Thompson B (2014) The measurement of visual acuity in children: an evidence-based update. *Clinical and Experimental Optometry* **97**: 3–11.

Berardi N, Pizzorusso T, Ratto GM, Maffei L (2003) Molecular basis of plasticity in the visual cortex. *Trends in Neurosciences* **26**: 369–378. doi:10.1016/S0166-2236(03)00168-1.

Braddick O, Atkinson J (2011) Development of human visual function. *Vision Research* **51**: 1588–1609. doi:10.1016/j.visres.2011.02.018.

Celesia GG (2005). Visual plasticity and its clinical applications. *J Physiol Anthropol Appl Human Sci* **24**: 23–27.

Chorna OD, Guzzetta A, Maitre NL (2017) Vision assessments and interventions for infants 0–2 years at high risk for cerebral palsy: a systematic review. *Ped Neurol* **76**: 3–13. doi: 10.1111/j.1469-8749.2010.03710.x.

Dale N, Sakkalou E, O'Reilly M, Springall C, De Haan M, Salt A (2017) Functional vision and cognition in infants with congenital disorders of the peripheral visual system. *Dev Med Child Neurol* **59**: 725–731. doi: 10.1111/dmcn.13429.

Gothwal VK, Sumalini R, Bharani S et al. (2012) The second version of the L. V. Prasad-functional vision questionnaire. *Optom Vis Sci* **89**: 1601–1610. doi: 10.1097/OPX.0b013e31826ca291.

Guzzetta A, D'acunto GII, Rose S et al. (2010) Plasticity of the visual system after early brain damage. *Developmental Medicine & Child Neurology* **52**: 891–900.

Hatt SR, Leske DA, Castañeda YS et al. (2019) Development of pediatric eye question-naires for children with eye conditions. *Am J Ophthalmol* **200**: 201–217. doi: 10.1016/j.ajo.2019.01.001.

Hyvärinen L, Nasanen R, Laurinen P (1980) New visual acuity test for pre-school children. *Acta Ophthalmol (Copenh)* **58**: 507–511.

Jandó G, Mikó-Baráth E, Markó K, Hollódy K, Török B, Kovacs I (2012) Early-onset binocularity in preterm infants reveals experience-dependent visual development in humans. *Proceedings of the National Academy of Sciences* **109**: 11049–11052.

Kay HA (1983) New method of assessing visual acuity with pictures. *British Journal of Ophthalmology* **67**: 131–133.

Khadka J, Ryan B, Margrain TH et al. (2010) Development of the 25-item Cardiff Visual Ability Questionnaire for Children (CVAQC). *Br J Ophthalmol* **94**: 730–755. doi: 10.1136/bjo.2009.171181.

Koenraads Y, Braun KP, Van Der Linden DC et al. (2015) Perimetry in young and neurologically impaired children: the Behavioral Visual Field (BEFIE) screening test revisited. *JAMA Ophthalmology* **133**: 319–325.

Kostović I, Judaš M (2007) Transient patterns of cortical lamination during prenatal life: do they have implications for treatment? *Neuroscience & Biobehavioral Reviews.* **31**(8): 1157–1168. doi: 10.1016/j.neubiorev.2007.04.018.

McGraw PV, Winn B (1993) Glasgow Acuity Cards: a new test for the measurement of letter acuity in children. *Ophthalmic Physiol Opt* **13**: 400–104.

Matsuba C, Jan JE (2006) Long-term outcome of children with cortical visual impairment. *Dev Med Child Neurol* **48**: 508–512.

Rossi A, Gnesi M, Montomoli C, Chirico G, Malerba L, Merabet LB (2017) NAVEG Study Group, Fazzi E. Neonatal Assessment Visual European Grid (NAVEG): unveiling neurological risk. *Infant Behav Dev* **49**: 21–30.

Ricci D, Romeo DM, Serrao F et al. (2010) Early assessment of visual function in pre-term infants: how early is early? *Early Human Development* **86**: 29–33. doi: 10.1016/j.earlhumdev.2009.11.004.

Salt AT, O'Reilly MA, Sakkalou E, Dale NJ (2020) Detection vision development in infants and toddlers with congenital vision disorders and profound-severe visual impairment. *Dev Med Child Neurol* **62**(8): 962–968.

Salt A, Dale N (2017) *Developmental Journal for Babies and Young Children with Visual Impairment,* 2nd Edition. London: Great Ormond Street Hospital for Children. Available from https://xip.uclb.com/i/healthcare_tools/DJVI_professional.html.

Sonksen PM (2016) *Developmental Assessment: Theory, Practice and Application to Neurodisability.* London: Mac Keith Press.

Sonksen PM, Wade AM, Proffitt R, Heavens S, Salt AT (2008) The Sonksen logMAR test of visual acuity: II. Age norms from 2 years 9 months to 8 years. *JAAPOS* **12**: 18–22.

Sonksen PM, Dale N (2002) Visual impairment in infancy: impact on neurodevelopmental and neurobiological processes. *Dev Med Child Neurol* **44**: 782–791.

Sonksen P, Petrie A, Drew K (1991) Promotion of visual development of severely visually impaired babies: evaluation of a developmentally based programme. *Dev Med Child Neurol* **33**: 320–335.

Sukkar H, Dunst CJ, Kirkby J (2016) *Early Childhood Intervention: Working with Families of Young Children with Special Needs.* London: Routledge.

Tadić V, Cooper A, Cumberland P, Lewando-Hundt G, Rahi JS (2013) Development of the functional vision questionnaire for children and young people with visual impairment: the FVQ_CYP. *Ophthalmology* **120**: 2725–2732. doi: 10.1016/j.ophtha.2013.07.055.

Vervloed MP, Janssen N, Knoors H (2006) Visual rehabilitation of children with visual impairments. *Journal of Developmental & Behavioral Pediatrics* **27**: 493–506.

Weiss AH, Kelly JP (2007). Acuity development in infantile nystagmus. *Invest Ophthalmol Vis Sci* **48**: 4093–4099.

Wiesel TN, Hubel DH (1963). Single-cell responses in striate cortex of kittens deprived of vision in one eye. *Journal of Neurophysiology* **26**: 1003–1017.

CHAPTER 5

Cerebral Visual Impairment

Naomi Dale, Els Ortibus, Jenefer Sargent, and Richard Bowman

INTRODUCTION

Cerebral visual impairment (CVI) refers to a range of vision dysfunctions that originate from brain injury and disorders of cerebral visual pathways. These include reduction of visual acuity, impaired contrast sensitivity, visual field deficits, and disorders of higher-order vision processing. As the brain is a highly inter-connecting system of neural networks, the condition and its manifestations often coexist with other aspects of developmental disorder, but they can also occur in isolation. A systematic multidisciplinary approach should underpin the identification of CVI, taking into account ophthalmological, neurological, and neurodevelopmental dimensions. A developmental perspective is crucial to assist the interpretation of the child's vision and their total learning profile and to update and review progress. This chapter describes research and evidence-led clinical approaches to the identification, assessment, and management of CVI.

CEREBRAL VISUAL IMPAIRMENT

Definition of Issues

The cerebral visual system is extensive and complex, leading from the optic chiasm and posterior central pathways including the optic radiations, to the primary visual (or occipital) cortex, and from there to the higher visual association areas in the temporal and parietal lobes, and the frontal areas (see Fig. 5.1 and Fig. 7.1 for the visual networks of the brain). Definitions of CVI in the scientific literature commonly refer to visual impairment caused by damage to the retro-chiasmatic central vision pathways with normal or near normal eye health (Sakki et al. 2018). The authors propose that a more pragmatic definition of CVI for assessment and diagnostic

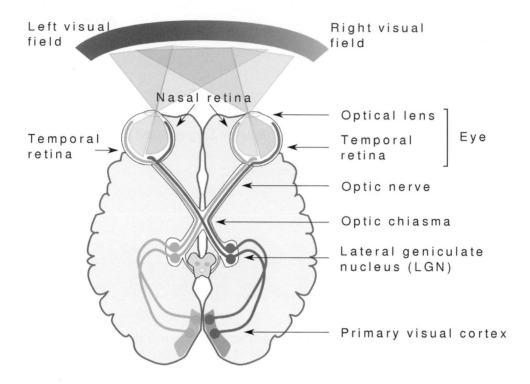

Figure 5.1 Diagram of the optic pathways. Reused from Miquel Perello Nieto (Wikimedia Commons). This figure is licensed under the Creative Commons Attribution-Share Alike 4.0 International license (https://creativecommons.org/licenses/by-sa/4.0/deed.en). (A colour version of this figure can be seen in the colour plate section)

purposes is a *verifiable* visual dysfunction which cannot be attributed to disorders of the anterior visual pathways or any potentially co-occurring ocular impairment (Sakki et al. 2018).

Due to changing definitions and measurement of CVI, prevalence rates vary but many studies report it as a major cause of childhood visual impairment in high-income countries (see Chapter 2). Broad population estimates may include very young children where the differentiation of vision and other neurological impairments is less reliable (Rahi and Cable 2003; see also Chapter 2). The rate may also be increasing globally with improved neonatal and paediatric care and increased survival of those born preterm or who suffer perinatal insult such as hypoxic-ischemic encephalopathy (Rahi and Cable 2003; Pehere et al. 2018). In addition to preterm birth and hypoxic-ischemic encephalopathy, other risk factors in the pre-, peri-, or early postnatal period include infection, hydrocephalus, intra-cerebral haemorrhage, structural malformation, seizures, and hypoglycaemia (Fazzi et al. 2007; Khetpal and Donahue 2007; Chong et al. 2014). Some are idiopathic; chromosomal aberrations have been found in 7% (Bosch et al. 2014). Late onset causes include traumatic/acquired head injury, cerebro-vascular accident, infection, and brain tumours (Kozeis 2010).

The most frequently reported brain pathology is damage to the visual cortex and white matter, including periventricular white matter disease (or periventricular leukomalacia), reflecting its higher prevalence in children born preterm and/or with cerebral palsy (Ortibus et al. 2011a). CVI as a 'disorder of widespread white matter connectivity' has been shown in terms of dramatic reduction in structure, volume, and network integrity of the inferior longitudinal fasciculus and the superior longitudinal fasciculus, according to magnetic resonance imaging (MRI) or diffusion tensor imaging (DTI), leading to associated impairments in specific vision functions (Ortibus et al. 2012; Bauer et al. 2014). For more information on the structural architecture and function of the brain and its potential for plasticity and restitution of visual function in congenital and acquired CVI, including hemianopia (where vision is impaired in half of the visual field), see Chapter 7.

Features of CVI

Vision functions that may be affected include visual acuity, contrast sensitivity, stereopsis (binocularity disparity and 3D vision), and visual fields. Treatable ophthalmic conditions such as refractive error, accommodative insufficiency, and cataract may be present (Pehere et al. 2018). Other features include disordered eye movement control and anterior visual pathway dysfunction, such as optic atrophy (van Genderen et al. 2012; Philip and Dutton 2014).

Higher-order vision functions at risk include object recognition, face recognition (prosopagnosia), depth and visuo-spatial perception, visuo-motor integration, motion perception, and visual attention. Some of these dysfunctions manifest as difficulties detecting a target against a complex background or when a target is surrounded by competing peripheral targets or 'crowding' (with severe forms being referred to as simultanagnosia, which is the inability to perceive more than a single object at a time) (Dutton et al. 2006).

CVI is a multidimensional set of disorders of visual function, with different combinations and severity in individual children. The need for greater classification or subtyping of different individual profiles is advocated (Philip and Dutton 2014). One approach has divided vision into two functional visual processing streams: 'ventral' ('what' or object recognition vision) and 'dorsal' ('how and where' or action vision), derived from evidence from non-human primates and adult lesion studies (Goodale and Milner 1992). Subsequent imaging studies have been able to link both functional streams to separate structures in the brain with integrity of the inferior longitudinal fasciculus associated with impaired object recognition ('ventral' stream) and the superior longitudinal fasciculus associated with the 'dorsal' stream in children (Ortibus et al. 2012;

Martín et al. 2016). Evidence of impaired directional motion or 'global motion' processing in neurodevelopmental disorders, such as Williams syndrome, fragile X syndrome, or infants born very preterm, suggests a 'dorsal stream vulnerability' (Taylor et al. 2009; Braddick et al. 2011).

A complementary approach is to identify subtyping of the individual children's profiles (and in the longer term develop a classification system) that is empirical and objective using a data-driven approach (Sakki et al. 2021). In this study of school-aged children aged 5 to 15 years with an ophthalmological diagnosis or high suspicion of CVI, standard assessment scores of basic and higher-order vision (visual perception, visuo-motor integration) were collected (Sakki et al. 2021). Three groups were established through statistical cluster analysis and group comparisons, showing a spectrum of symptom clusters and severity, with Group A1 including normal or near-normal visual acuity and selective difficulties in higher-order vision, Group A2 having difficulties in basic and higher-order vision, and Group B having greater reduction of basic vision including vision acuity (moderate to severe reduction). Groups A1, A2, and B also differed significantly according to frequency and severity of intellectual disability, cerebral palsy (including Gross Motor Function Classification System level), and ophthalmological disorders (strabismus, nystagmus). These co-occurring disorders followed a similar spectrum of severity, with absence or mild severity in Group A1 through to high proportion and severity in Group B, with A2 intermediate.

ASSESSMENT AND MANAGEMENT

The Multidisciplinary Team

The research literature and clinical experience highlight the necessity for an integrated multidimensional assessment by a multidisciplinary paediatric team. The team required to undertake comprehensive assessment and reach clinical diagnosis and identification of needs includes paediatric ophthalmology expertise (with optometry and orthoptics) and child development/neurodisability skills (including neurodevelopmental paediatrics, clinical neuropsychology, physiotherapy, and occupational therapy). The child, parent, education, and habilitation specialists are key partners in this ongoing process and for future management of care. The trend is towards use of scientifically established assessment methods with practitioners trained to undertake these measures in an integrated multidisciplinary framework (Ortibus et al. 2019). Neurology, neuroradiology, neuro-ophthalmology, and neuropsychology will be involved in the diagnosis, care, and management of children with acquired brain injury and head trauma including loss of visual function.

See Table 5.1 for comprehensive multidisciplinary assessment of CVI-related concerns, including contributors, areas of assessment and results.

Table 5.1 Comprehensive multidisciplinary assessment of CVI-related concerns

Contributor	Area of assessment	Results
Parent and caregiver/ community health and paediatrics/education	Screening for and identifying children at risk Parent and referrer concerns	Observations in the everyday environment Developmental and school attainment test results
Ophthalmology, including optometry/ orthoptists	History-taking: medical history and current visual concerns Eye examination	Documentation of visual difficulties
	Basic vision	Detection Acuity Fields Refraction Accommodation Contrast sensitivity Ocular movements Strabismus Stereovision
Neurodisability: multidisciplinary including neuropsychology, occupational therapy and physiotherapy/ neurology, paediatrics	History taking: detailed medical history, developmental history, current visual concerns	Documentation of neurodevelopmental history and current functioning with relevant medical background Documentation of visual difficulties Neurological examination to identify abnormalities of relevance to medical history and reported visual concerns
	Basic vision in infants and very young children or those who are low functioning or complex neurodisability	Detection vision, acuity, field, ocular movements
	Cognitive assessment Higher vision including neuropsychological, visual perception, and visuomotor	Developmental, cognitive, and attainment tests Visuo-spatial perception and other neuropsychological Visuo-motor integration and motor coordination
Neuroimaging	Clinical brain scan if indicated	Classification and description of possible lesions

Screening and Identification of Early Concerns

Children at risk of, or with identified congenital and early brain injury and neurodevelopmental disorders and an abnormal pre- or perinatal medical history including those born preterm, are at greatest risk of CVI (van Genderen et al. 2012). They should be screened and closely monitored for vision disorders. If concerns, these children should be referred for further multidisciplinary assessment (van Genderen et al. 2012).

Early vision-related developmental milestones, such as fixating on the parent's face, fixating and following a moving target in near distance, smiling at the parent's face, and fixating on a favourite toy or reaching out to grasp, need to be monitored at community child health level. Any significant delay and concern regarding poor vision, or obvious associated defects (e.g. squint, cataract), should be followed up with referral to the children's eye clinic.

Although not yet empirically applied to infancy or preschool level, children in Group B (Sakki et al. 2021) are more likely to raise early concern regarding poor vision. This is supported further by the Andhra Pradesh India study, where 124 children diagnosed with CVI had been referred for concerns regarding poor vision (76%) or squint, with the majority presenting under 2 years old (44%) with profound visual impairment (88%) (Pehere et al. 2018).

In addition to those presenting early, as a child goes through the preschool or school years the caregiver or teacher may notice certain difficulties that appear vision-related. Reported behaviours may include difficulty finding targets against cluttered backgrounds, inaccurate visually directed reach, difficulty with managing level floor boundaries, recognizing objects or faces, following moving targets, or making judgements about the location of fast-moving objects and whether they can be seen or not (Dutton et al. 2006). Education-related difficulties such as problems with reading, spelling, and handwriting and spatial aspects of mathematics and related subjects may also be reported.

Scientifically developed parent-rated questionnaires, such as the CVI Inventory (Macintyre-Beon et al. 2013) and the CVI Questionnaire (Ortibus et al. 2011b) have shown validity, internal consistency, and reliable factor structure and may be a potentially useful supplement for capturing ecologically relevant everyday functional behaviours. They are not, however, diagnostic and do not replace direct vision assessments that need to be undertaken. Moreover, they may lead to too many false positives if used in isolation (van Genderen et al. 2012) or with children whose characteristics do not match those of the original test population.

Diagnostic assessment should include structured clinical history-taking to document the medical and developmental history and should seek past and current visual concerns and their potential impact on child functioning. Standard structural brain imaging may be informative and contribute to the overall explanatory picture in some but not all cases. For example, in a heterogeneous sample of 63 children with definite and suspected CVI, half of the sample had signs of periventricular leukomalacia (29%) and intraventricular haemorrhage (21%) on their clinically collected brain scans (Sakki et al. 2021).

Advanced neuroimaging techniques like diffusion MRI (DTI) for white matter connectivity are still in their early days for clinical application (Merabet et al. 2017).

Systematic assessment of vision and related developmental functions is required. Methods should cover the full spectrum of presentations, including basic and higher-order vision, while accommodating the full range of developmental, cognitive, and motor abilities. All test results need to be interpreted within the context of the child's overall developmental profile. See Chapter 6 for assessment of vision in the context of complex neurodisability profiles including significant motor and intellectual disability.

Assessment of Basic Vision

The first stage includes assessment of visual acuity and related visual functions and ophthalmological disorders, including eye movements, visual fields, refraction, and assessment of accommodation (see further Chapter 2). Detection of basic visual dysfunction in infancy can be undertaken systematically by an ophthalmologist or paediatrician with appropriate training (Ricci et al. 2010; see Chapter 4).

Visual acuity reduction is an important aspect of CVI and needs immediate attention. Possible co-occurring cognitive or movement disorders, which may affect functional responses, should be considered and developmental assessment is important for considering the child holistically.

Assessment of Higher-Order Vision

The second stage of assessment includes assessment of higher-order vision processing if the child has sufficient acuity falling within the mild-moderate visual impairment range or better. A number of scientifically validated tools have been developed for this purpose and according to different chronological and developmental age ranges. These may cover vision perception, visuo-motor coordination, and other visuo-cognitive abilities such as object or face recognition. The Children's Visual Impairment Test for 3- to 6-year-olds (or equivalent developmental age) has been shown to have sound psychometric properties for assessing four factors of visual perceptual abilities. These include local–global (where local refers to details and parts and global to the whole picture), object and scene recognition, motion perception, and degraded object perception (where limited visual information is available) (Vancleef et al. 2019).

In the typically developing child, performance on visuo-cognitive test tasks, such as visual perception, is closely associated with the child's overall cognitive level as a reflection of the latent construct of 'intelligence' or 'reasoning'. Therefore for any testing of visuo-cognitive deficits it may be necessary to establish whether the child's performance includes a significantly greater reduction from their verbal cognitive level, suggestive of a specific non-verbal visuo-cognitive difficulty (Sakki et al. 2021). This can be viably addressed by the assessment input of a neuropsychologist who is sufficiently experienced in visual impairment and cognition to establish this (see further Chapter 12).

As described earlier in this chapter, Sakki et al. (2021) have validated a standard clinical assessment battery for assessment of the broad spectrum of CVI in school-aged children. For the higher functioning group of children with acuity in the mild-moderate visual impairment or normal-near normal range, children were tested on basic vision functions (acuity, contrast sensitivity, stereopsis, field) and higher-order vision functions (standardised measures of visual perception and visual motor integration including separating motor-free visual perception and motor coordination). Individual profile analysis was undertaken and showed that even at the milder end of the spectrum (Group A1) specific subtests, such as those of figure-ground or form constancy, were often in the clinically relevant range compared to age norms and verbal comprehension cognitive index. Using this 'core' assessment battery provided a potentially robust method for identifying specific areas of vision dysfunction and dividing the children into different subtypes. Further clinical validation to consider its applicability in the formulation and identification of CVI and differentiation from other neurodevelopmental disorders is in progress.

Supplementary tests used by the neuropsychologist could include tests of selective visual attention, line of orientation judgement, facial recognition and memory, object and scene recognition, and complex visuo-spatial organization and memory. Standardised attainment testing of reading, spelling, writing fluency, handwriting, and numeracy can be valuable, as well as assessment of gross motor and fine motor abilities.

All information from the comprehensive assessment, as well as observations in the preschool or school environment if necessary, are integrated. These provide a complete diagnostic profile enabling identification of CVI if appropriate and accompanying functional needs. By being made easy to understand and cater for, the explanation and reporting of the assessment findings will help the parent and health and education practitioners reach shared understanding, establish eligibility for specialised habilitation and educational support, and jointly plan appropriate educational modifications and needs. Regular review is valuable as the child develops from the early years and through school years, as each child's profile and needs may change. For instance, visual acuity may improve over time in very young children (see further brain and vision plasticity, Chapters 4 and 7). In contrast, certain areas of difficulty, such as specific problems with reading, may become more apparent as the child matures and educational demands increase.

For acquired brain injury, the child or young person and their family may need sensitive and skilled counselling and integrated rehabilitative assistance to help the child adjust to their vision impairment and learn compensatory skills. The age and severity of vision loss and other brain functions affected will be relevant to the period of emotional adjustment and additional mental health considerations needed (see Chapter 18).

From Assessment to Intervention and Habilitation

Infants with severe acuity reduction need urgent referral for early effective vision habilitation and developmental intervention, along the same principles for infants with congenital disorders of the anterior visual system (see further details in Chapters 4 and 8). Early comprehensive developmental enrichment is recommended for all children with identified neurodevelopmental disorders who are at risk of CVI. However, these infants are more likely to have complex co-occurring disorders, such as cerebral palsy, and their developmental programmes will need to be considered within the framework of multidisciplinary assessment and a coordinated care pathway.

Functional Vision

As part of the comprehensive assessment at preschool and school level, functional vision (i.e. use of vision in developmentally appropriate everyday tasks and situations) will need to be considered. The child's functioning in different contexts, visual environments, and learning scenarios merits consideration to establish current needs and the required modifications that will help them move forward to achieve their potential and to support increased participation in everyday life. Information can be gained through parent-reported and teacher-reported questionnaires, and with older children through self-reported questionnaires; these need cautious interpretation and do not replace direct child assessment. The Visual Function Classification System (VFCS) has been developed for children with cerebral palsy (Baranello et al. 2019). For older children with significant vision impairment in the moderate or more severe range, the psychometrically robust self-report Functional Vision Questionnaire for Children and Young People (FVQ-CYP) captures the functional impact of visual disability from their perspective (Tadić et al. 2013).

Children with higher functioning visuo-cognitive deficits (e.g. Groups A1 and A2 in Sakki et al. 2021) are at risk of having their needs underestimated or misinterpreted or neglected, which may lead to increased risk for developing behaviour problems, mental health needs and school failure. Sakki et al. (2021) found that parent-reported paediatric quality of life was adversely affected across all three CVI groups. The impact of CVI and the functional vision problems on classroom learning (including reading and writing), communication and social relations, orientation and mobility, daily life activities, and sustained near vision tasks must be addressed as part of the child's habilitation. Children with social communication disorders/autism may be at higher risk of co-occurring CVI; differential diagnosis is therefore required so that all needs can be addressed (Philip and Dutton 2014; also see Chapter 11).

There are few scientifically evaluated habilitative interventions for CVI, as shown in a systematic database scoping review (Williams et al. 2014). The only limited evidence is that if children also have refractive errors there is a strong case for provision of spectacles. Because of the high incidence of refractive errors in children with CVI and cerebral palsy, this is a useful reminder to clinicians not to forget this and to ensure this is checked for. However, there are no other habilitation recommendations specific to CVI at the current time.

Identification of specific areas of dysfunction and difficulty will ensure that appropriate intervention is provided in a timely way. The systematic clinical assessment provides the basis for assessment-led guidance and goal-directed intervention, based on the detailed assessment and understanding of the individual profile of visual and developmental needs. This intervention must be motivational, developmentally appropriate and adapted to or compensating for the child's vision needs (Williams et al. 2014). Most interventions focus on environmental or educational modifications to accommodate the child's vision-related needs in everyday life by ensuring that reading, educational and play materials are all accessible (Philip and Dutton 2014). Detailed understanding of the child's visual perceptual problems may lead to specific habilitational strategies (e.g. the reduction of vision crowding). For instance, specific habilitational strategies have been suggested in response to specific questions in the CVI inventory. This approach has recently been shown to improve quality of life in children aged under 12 in an uncontrolled before and after study (Tsirka et al. 2020). The use of multisensory approaches, including verbal and kinaesthetic scripts to help the child copy a complex figure or learn to write a new letter, may compensate for degraded vision processing ability. The approach needs to be individualised and practical, with recognition of the child's adaptive strategies, what can or cannot be easily remedied, and a problem-solving approach for compensatory or augmentative methods. In rare cases a child cannot discern written symbols at all and may need to learn braille, for instance. Additional examination time in secondary school or college may be needed for slow vision processing of text and written response, which are common.

IMPLICATIONS FOR RESEARCH AND PRACTICE

There is now a drive towards achieving internationally accepted consensus in relation to evidence-based clinical guidelines and standards for screening, definition, diagnosis, assessment, and classification of CVI; a European consensus group project is in progress (Ortibus et al. 2019). This will aim to provide the accepted clinical standards to guide research and clinical and educational practice, including consensus over diagnosis and diagnostic thresholds, clarification of who is eligible for services and trials, and systematic outcome measures and benchmarking. Further scientific assessment tools are in development, including those for the toddler age range in Ortibus' team. At the milder end of the spectrum (what would be referred to as the A1 end of the spectrum in Sakki et al. 2021), it can be difficult to differentiate whether the child has sufficient level of difficulties, including their functional impact which may be quite task-specific, to warrant a diagnosis of CVI or whether an alternative or additional special educational needs diagnosis is appropriate such as dyslexia or dyspraxia. This requires further clinical consideration, systematic research, and consensus to set clinical diagnostic thresholds as it has relevance for the type and eligibility of support provision.

The high variability of CVI has made research advances challenging and few intervention trials have been performed. More information is needed on effective habilitative programmes to promote improved function and environmental modifications to facilitate engagement of children with their surroundings (Williams et al. 2014). New scientific insights such as the involvement of parents in coaching, the use of technology and the value of focussing on participation and quality of life will be important for future trials. Further trials of promotion of infant vision in at risk infants is advocated (see Chapter 4).

Novel neuroscience projects such as those focussing on functional subtyping (Sakki et al. 2021) or those on underlying white matter connectivity (Bauer et al. 2014) are providing greater insights into the functional organisation of the human visual system, paving the way for more systematic habilitation trials. An objective data-driven analysis into resting-state functional MRI data of 470 individuals has revealed three dissociated areas on the dorsal, ventral, and lateral surfaces of the occipital lobe, suggestive of three visual cortical pathways (Haak and Beckmann 2020).

Insights from vision restitution in adults who have lost vision as a result of stroke may possibly be applied to children with CVI, including those with late acquired brain injury, though this is currently only speculative. Improvement has been shown with targeted basic vision perceptual training or action video gaming, such as location in the visual field or enhanced attention across the visual scene (Green et al. 2010; Sagi 2011; Herzog et al. 2017). Technological advances like virtual reality can provide novel objective and ecologically valid measurements of performance, which may in the future improve vision assessments and provide the basis for neural investigations and habilitation interventions (Bennett et al. 2019).

SUMMARY

Understanding and meeting the needs of children with CVI is advancing with research and practice focussing on developing validated methods of screening, detection, diagnosis, assessment, and classification. There is wide variation of individual profile patterns involving diverse basic and higher visual functions across a spectrum of severity. Children with CVI frequently have additional difficulties; their needs and strengths change over time and across environments. Strategies should support better opportunities for children and young people with CVI, including identification of needs as early as possible and habilitative and possibly restitutive interventions and support to ensure their optimal inclusion and participation in society.

Key Points

✓ A multidisciplinary integrated team approach is key for assessment and diagnosis of CVI and identification of needs.

✓ Identification and assessment should commence with 'at risk' and clinical-presenting populations at birth and in the early years and continue as required throughout childhood.

✓ Basic and higher vision functions must be assessed through evidence-based standard assessment protocols appropriate to the child's chronological and developmental age and motor capabilities.

✓ Habilitation is to be individualised and goal-directed and based on clinical assessment and assessment of functional vision and everyday needs.

✓ Consensus on definition, screening, diagnosis, assessment, and classification of CVI will lead to improved research, clarity of diagnosis and outcomes, and evidence-based habilitation including participatory outcomes.

REFERENCES

Baranello G, Signorini S, Tinelli F et al. (2019) Visual Function Classification System for children with cerebral palsy: development and validation. *Dev Med Child Neurol* **62**(1): 104–110.

Bauer CM, Heidary G, Koo BB, Killiany RJ, Bex P, Merabet LB (2014) Abnormal white matter tractography of visual pathways detected by high-angular-resolution diffusion imaging (HARDI) corresponds to visual dysfunction in cortical/cerebral visual impairment. *J AAPOS* **18**(4): 398–401.

Bennett CR, Bex PJ, Bauer CM, Merabet LB (2019) The assessment of visual function and functional vision. *Semin Pediatr Neurol* **31**: 30–40.

Bosch DGM, Boonstra FN, Reijnders MRF, Pfundt R, Cremers FPM, De Vries BBA (2014) Chromosomal aberrations in cerebral visual impairment. *Eur J Paediatr Neurol* **18**(6): 677–684.

Braddick O, Atkinson J, Wattam-Bell J (2011) VERP and brain imaging for identifying levels of visual dorsal and ventral stream function in typical and preterm infants. *Prog Brain Res* **189**: 95–111.

Chong CF, McGhee CN, Dai S (2014) A cross-sectional study of prevalence and etiology of childhood visual impairment in Auckland, New Zealand. *Asia Pac J Ophthalmol* **3**: 337–342.

Dutton GN, McKillop EC, Saidkasimova S (2006) Visual problems as a result of brain damage in children. *Br J Ophthalmol* **90**(8): 932–933.

Fazzi E, Signorini SG, Bova SM et al. (2007) Spectrum of visual disorders in children with cerebral visual impairment. *J Child Neurol* **22**: 294–301.

Goodale MA, Milner AD (1992) Separate visual pathways for perception and action. *Trends Neurosci* **15**(1): 20–25.

Green CS, Li R, Bavelier D (2010) Perceptual learning during action video game playing. *Top Cogn Sci* **2**(2): 202–216.

Haak KV, Beckmann CF (2020) Understanding brain organisation in the face of functional heterogeneity and functional multiplicity. *Neuroimage*. Available at: <https://pubmed.ncbi.nlm.nih.gov/32574808/ doi: 10.1016/j.neuroimage.2020.117061>.

Hannula D, Simons D, Cohen N (2005) Imaging implicit perception: promise and pitfalls. *Nat Rev Neurosci* **6**: 247–255. https://doi.org/10.1038/nrn1630.

Herzog MH, Cretenoud AF, Grzeczkowski L (2017) What is new in perceptual learning? *J Vis* **17**(1): 23.

Khetpal V, Donahue SP (2007) Cortical visual impairment: etiology, associated findings, and prognosis in a tertiary care setting. *J AAPOS* **11**(3): 235–239.

Kozeis N (2010) Brain visual impairment in childhood, a mini review. *Hippokratia* **14**(4): 249–251.

Macintyre-Beon C, Young D, Dutton GN et al. (2013) Cerebral visual dysfunction in prematurely born children attending mainstream school. *Doc Ophthalmol* **127**(2): 89–102.

Martín MB, Santos-Lozano A, Martín-Hernández J et al. (2016) Cerebral versus ocular visual impairment: the impact on developmental neuroplasticity. *Front Psychol* **26**(7). 1958. doi: 10.3389/fpsyg.2016.01958.

Merabet LB, Mayer L, Bauer CM, Wright D, Kran BS (2017) Disentangling how the brain is 'wired' in cortical/cerebral visual impairment (CVI). *Semin Paediatr Neurol* **24**(2): 83–91.

Ortibus EL, De Cock PP, Lagae LG (2011a) Visual perception in preterm children: what are we currently measuring? *Ped Neurol* **45**(1): 1–10.

Ortibus E, Laenen A, Verhoeven J et al. (2011b) Screening for cerebral visual impairment: Value of a CVI questionnaire. *Neuropediatrics* **42**(4): 138–147.

Ortibus E, Verhoeven J, Sunaert S, Casteels I, de Cock P, Lagae L (2012) Integrity of the inferior longitudinal fasciculus and impaired object recognition in children: a diffusion tensor imaging study. *Dev Med Child Neurol* **54**(1): 38–43.

Ortibus EL, Fazzi E, Dale NJ (2019) Cerebral visual impairment and clinical assessment: the European perspective. *Semin Pediatr Neurol* **31**: 15–24.

Pehere N, Chougule P, Dutton GN (2018) Cerebral visual impairment in children: causes and associated ophthalmological problems. *Indian J Ophthalmol* **66**: 812–815.

Philip SS, Dutton GN (2014) Identifying and characterising cerebral visual impairment in children: a review. *Clin Exp Optom* **97**(3): 196–208.

Rahi JS, Cable N (2003) Severe visual impairment and blindness in children in the UK. *Lancet* **362**: 1359–1365.

Ricci D, Cesarini L, Gallini F et al. (2010) Cortical visual function in preterm infants in the first year. *J Pediatr* **156**(4): 550–555.

Sagi D (2011) Perceptual learning in vision research. *Vis Res* **51**(13): 1552–1566.

Sakki HEA, Dale NJ, Sargent J, Perez-Roche T, Bowman R (2018) Is there consensus in defining childhood cerebral visual impairment? A systematic review of terminology and definitions. *Br J Ophthalmol* **102**: 424–432.

Sakki H, Bowman R, Sargent J, Kukadia R, Dale NJ (2021) Visual function subtyping in children with early-onset cerebral visual impairment. *Dev Med Child Neurol* **63**(3): 303–312.

Tadić V, Cooper A, Cumberland P, Lewando-Hundt G, Rahi JS (2013) Development of the functional vision questionnaire for children and young people with visual impairment: the FVQ-CYP. *Ophthalmology* **120**(12): 2725–2732.

Taylor NM, Jakobson LS, Maurer D, Lewis TL (2009) Differential vulnerability of global motion, global form, and biological motion processing in full-term and preterm children. *Neuropsychologia* **47**(13): 2766–2778.

Tsirka A, Liasis A, Kuczynski A et al. (2020) Clinical use of the Insight Inventory in cerebral visual impairment and the effectiveness of tailored habilitational strategies. *Dev Med Child Neurol* **62**(11): 1324–1330.

Van Genderen M, Dekker M, Pilon F, Bals I (2012) Diagnosing cerebral visual impairment in children with good visual acuity. *Strabismus* **20**(2): 78–83.

Vancleef K, Janssens E, Petre Y, Wagemans J, Ortibus E (2019) Assessment tool for visual perception deficits in cerebral visual impairment: development and normative data of typically developing children. *Dev Med Child Neurol* **62**(1): 111–117.

Williams C, Northstone K, Borwick C et al. (2014) How to help children with neurodevelopmental and visual problems: a scoping review. *British Journal of Ophthalmology* **98**: 6–12.

CHAPTER 6

Vision Assessment of Children with Complex Neurodisability

Jenefer Sargent, Alison Salt, and Elisa Fazzi

INTRODUCTION

Children with neurodevelopmental disability can have multiple co-occurring conditions including cerebral palsy, epilepsy, cognitive impairment, behavioural challenges, social communication difficulties, and sensory disorders, and may be described as having 'complex' neurodisability. As described in Chapter 5 these children are at higher risk of both cerebral visual impairment and disorders affecting eye structure and function (Salt and Sargent 2014). This chapter considers the epidemiology of vision disorders in this high-risk population, practical aspects of vision assessment in affected children, and current research and practice issues.

Children with developmental delays and disabilities are at greater risk of suboptimal health, educational attainment, and wellbeing than are children without such disabilities, and therefore early identification of visual impairment and appropriate support are essential (Global Research on Developmental Disabilities Collaborators 2018). Vision assessment in children with complex neurodisability must be adapted to take into account co-occurring impairments, including the child's level of development and physical limitations.

VISION DISORDERS AND COMPLEX NEURODEVELOPMENTAL DISABILITY

Complex neurodevelopmental disabilities are a heterogenous group of conditions resulting from impairments that affect a child's physical, learning, or behavioural functioning. These children have a higher risk of visual disorders related to the underlying causes of their disability, which include pre-, peri-, or postnatal brain injury, preterm birth, genetic disorders with brain involvement, or other developmental brain anomalies.

Large-scale epidemiological studies of eye abnormalities and visual impairment in children with complex neurodisability are scarce. However, studies of children attending specialised schools in the UK reported that 12% to 33% had reduced acuity sufficient to meet the World Health Organization criteria for visual impairment (logMAR 0.5 or worse) (Das et al. 2010; Woodhouse et al. 2013; Pilling and Outhwaite 2017; Donaldson et al. 2019). Similar studies in Nepal (Puri et al. 2015) and Nigeria (Ezeh et al. 2018) found reduced acuity in 25% and 12% respectively of children examined. Visual acuity reduction is also found in studies of children with specific conditions, including cerebral palsy (Fazzi et al. 2012) and Down syndrome (Watt et al. 2015).

Uncorrected refractive errors (often newly identified) have been found in a significant proportion (28–59%) of children with special educational needs in low- and middle income countries (Vora et al. 2010; Gogate et al. 2011; Abu Bakar et al. 2012; Limburg et al. 2012; Puri et al. 2015) and in a high-income country – the UK (Das et al. 2010; Woodhouse et al. 2013; Pilling and Outhwaite 2017; Donaldson et al. 2019). This suggests that lack of identification of refractive errors in these children is widespread and occurs irrespective of country income level.

Oculomotor (eye movement) abnormalities, accommodation difficulties, and strabismus are also more common in children with neurodisability. Fazzi et al. (2012) found significant neuro-ophthalmological abnormalities in 129 children with cerebral palsy, with specific profiles related to the distribution of the movement disorder. Children with cerebral palsy affecting all limbs ($n=61$) had the most difficulties with reduced visual acuity (98%), squint (68%), reduced contrast sensitivity (56%), and abnormalities of rapid eye movement (100%). By contrast, children with predominant lower limb involvement ($n=51$) showed reduced visual acuity (82%), squint (88%), reduced contrast sensitivity (90%), and abnormalities of rapid eye movement (78%).

See Table 6.1 for an overview of eye abnormalities and impairments in basic visual functions in children with complex neurodisability compared to the general population. Impairments of higher-order visual processing are also commonly associated with complex neurodisability (see Chapter 5).

Table 6.1 Impairments of eye structure and basic visual function in children with complex neurodisability (see also Salt and Sargent 2014[a])

Neurodisability disorder/risk factor	Ocular impairments (%)	Reduced acuity (%)	Refractive error (%)	Other
Down syndrome	Cataract (14) Squint (25)[a]	Reduced corrected acuity >2 years compared to normal population By age 6–19 years mean acuity of logMAR 0.33 +/– 0.18[b]	ANY (55–80)[b] Hyperopia >+2.0 D (57) Myopia <–0.75 (13) Astigmatism <–1.0 (37)	Accommodation difficulties common[b]
Preterm birth	Optic disc dysplasia Squint (13.5 11)	log MAR <1.0 (0.8) logMAR <0.6 (2.5)	ANY (19) Hyperopia >+3.0 D (4–6) Myopia <0.0 (10–19) Astigmatism <–1.0 (13)	
Cerebral palsy	Optic disc pallor[c] Squint (59) Oculomotor abnormalities – affecting smooth pursuit movements and saccades[c] (varies according to distribution of cerebral palsy)	logMAR <1.0 (9–11)	ANY (60) Hyperopia >+2.0 D (10) Myopia (<0.0) (46) Astigmatism >–1.0 (20)	Field defects[c] Accommodation difficulties Contrast sensitivity[c]
Autism[d]	Squint (9–15) Oculomotor abnormalities	Usually not reduced	Hyperopia >+2.0 D (17) Astigmatism >–1.0 (12–25)	Accommodation and convergence difficulties reported in some
Learning difficulty IQ <80	Squint (27)	logMAR <1.0 (3.8)	ANY (44) Hyperopia >+2.0 D (24) Hyperopia >+3.0 (15) Myopia <–0.5 (11) Astigmatism <–1.0 (20)	

(Continued)

Table 6.1 Impairments of eye structure and basic visual function in children with complex neurodisability (see also Salt and Sargent 2014[a]) (Continued)

Neurodisability disorder/risk factor	Ocular impairments (%)	Reduced acuity (%)	Refractive error (%)	Other
Intellectual disability IQ <50		logMAR <1.0 (22.4)	ANY (44) Hyperopia >+3.0 D (22) Myopia <0.0 (16) Astigmatism <−1.0 (35)	
General population	Squint (4–7.5)	logMAR <1.0 (0.06)	ANY (3-5) Hyperopia >+2.0 D (3) [e]Myopia <−0.5 (1.6–6.7) Astigmatism <−1.0 (4–7)	

ANY = any refractive error. For quoted % see references in Salt and Sargent (2014) unless specified. [a]Haargaard and Fledelius (2006), [b]Watt et al. (2015), [c]Fazzi et al. (2012), [d]Little (2018). [e]Varies with ethnicity and age – lowest proportion for white age 5 and 10 years respectively, Rudnicka et al. (2016).

PRACTICAL ASPECTS OF VISION ASSESSMENT IN COMPLEX NEURODISABILITY

Assessment Objectives

Given the increased rate of eye and vision disorders in children with neurodisability, a primary objective of assessment is to identify disorders that impact on vision (such as refractive error or squint) that can be medically treated and managed. Establishing the degree of any acuity reduction or presence of other impairments will also inform the necessary adaptations to minimise these additional barriers to developmental progress and support participation.

Visual difficulties may be present without obvious behavioural signs or symptoms and their identification may be overshadowed when more prominent features such as epilepsy or movement disorders or nutritional needs demand medical, family, and therapy attention.

Severe visual impairment due to eye abnormalities usually manifests with overt signs such as nystagmus or abnormal visual fixation (see Chapter 2) and therefore assessment of acuity/vision is an integral part of the diagnostic assessment. Such signs may be absent or harder to detect in children with complex neurodisability. Vision assessment of children with complex neurodisability may also be more challenging and not undertaken or not possible in a busy clinic setting (Donaldson et al. 2019). Therefore, report of a normal eye examination should not lead to the assumption that vision function/acuity is normal. Parents may not appreciate that a normal eye examination can co-exist with reduced vision and may assume that previous consultations with the eye care team for specific concerns (e.g. squint) is reassurance that all vision function is normal. It is crucial that arrangements are made to actively assess all visual functions in children with complex neurodisability using methods appropriately adapted for each child.

For children with severe physical impairment, vision is a critical sense for learning and sometimes provides the only behavioural response method for everyday communication or access method when using augmentative communication materials (Sargent et al. 2013). Therefore, a thorough understanding, not only of what the child is able to see (capacity for processing visual information input) but also of how the child can actively fixate during interactions (capacity to use visual responses for expressive communicative output), will be crucial for adaptation of assessment and for supporting the child at home and at school (Fleming et al. 2010; Brady et al. 2012; Sargent et al. 2013).

Assessment of vision in children with complex neurodisability must take account of the child's neurodevelopmental profile. Therefore, a coordinated multidisciplinary or interdisciplinary approach to assessment is needed. This will include eye examination and assessment of basic visual functions including refraction, acuity, eye movements, and visual fields by eye clinic staff (involving ophthalmology, optometry, and orthoptists) with the paediatric neurodisability/neurodevelopmental team providing valuable information about the child's developmental status and disabilities as well as assessment of visual function and functional use of vision (Lundy et al. 2011). It is also necessary to provide interpretation of these results, making the findings accessible to those providing intervention in order to guide adaptation of learning materials, for example acuity measures could be described in terms of line thickness and width of gaps between items (see below).

Early Identification

Infants with risk factors for brain injury or malformation are those at high risk of vision difficulties. Assessment of basic visual functions in infancy can be undertaken systematically by a paediatrician with appropriate training (Ricci et al. 2010). Early vision milestones, such as fixating on the parent's face, fixating on a near object and following its movement, smiling to a parent's face, and visually directed reach, need to be monitored and any significant delay and concern followed up with referral to an eye clinic/ophthalmology service.

Several assessments such as the Neonatal Assessment Visual European Grid (NAVEG) (Rossi et al. 2017) and that described by Ricci (Ricci et al. 2010) have been developed and validated for early paediatric screening of visual function and can be administered in infants born preterm and full-term from the first days of life. Atypical responses on the NAVEG may be the earliest indicator of more widespread brain injury identified through brain imaging (Rossi et al. 2017).

These early assessments can identify abnormal fixation responses to the assessment materials and obtain systematic information on acuity and eye movements. Infants with no or very low levels of vision identified in the early months need rapid referral to early intervention support for monitoring and habilitation advice encompassing both vision and developmental promotion (see Chapters 4 and 8).

A Developmental Approach to Vision Assessment in Young and Older Children

A systematic and objective developmental approach is required for assessment of children with complex neurodisability of all ages (Salt and Sargent 2017). Age, physical impairment, and developmental level may limit the child's responses. Therefore, a comprehensive assessment requires a holistic multidisciplinary consideration of the child's profile, including cognition, language, behaviour, social relating, and attention as well as visual functions. However, in some complex children, the precise contributions of visual or developmental difficulty may not be conclusive necessitating review over time as the child's skills develop. Assessment will often be reliant on repeated observation of the child's visual behaviour and responses.

Children with complex neurodisability may show differences in visual performance that reflect developmental weaknesses or co-occurring difficulties rather than problems with the visual system. Conversely, these difficulties may also obscure problems in the visual system. A child may show a lack of or unusual vision responses for a number of reasons. First, the assessment task presented may be too complex for the child's level of visual development, and therefore it is important to understand expected visual responses and vision milestones according to the child's developmental age. Chapter 4 gives some guidance on maturation of the visual system and vision function measures at different ages. Second, the child may not comprehend the assessment task because their cognitive level does not reach the level required by the test, for example to understand a matching task. Third, social communication difficulties/autism in the child may lead to lack of interest in the tasks presented or in behavioural co-operation with the assessor and examination. Fourth, children with neurodisability may take time to process new information and effect motor responses and therefore giving the child sufficient time to respond is necessary.

Furthermore, failure to establish or maintain reliable fixation on visual tasks may reflect a child's level of general attention control, which may be too immature for the demands of the task. Failure to recognise these issues and challenges to testing can lead to a premature diagnosis of visual impairment and an inappropriate interpretation of the child's visual responses. Children with developmental difficulties may also be at higher risk of slower visual maturation making it essential to monitor the child's visual development over time.

Identifying a Reliable Test Response

Before embarking on vision function assessment, it is necessary to understand what kinds of reliable, repeatable responses a child is able to make to presented vision materials. Can the child speak with sufficient clarity to name objects, pictures, or letters? Can the child understand spoken language and follow instructions, and perform matching tasks? Can the child point or reach reliably to indicate an object, picture, or letter, using finger/hand or other body movements? If pointing/reaching are physically challenging, does the child have a reliable 'yes/no' response for use if the assessor adapts task presentation by selecting one option and asking a closed question (e.g. 'is this the one that's the same' or 'is this the one you chose?'). If the child has limited or unreliable body movements, does the child have sufficient eye movement and visual attention to use fixation as a response method? (Fleming et al. 2010). Clarke et al. (2020) have developed an eye pointing classification scale, which provides a practical guide to description and recognition of a child's eye pointing ability. This highlights to practitioners and parents the need to distinguish between simple looking, and looking-to-point which is deliberately communicative. For children with non-verbal response methods that need reliable interpretation, use of a second observer who is unaware of the location of visual targets and who can make judgements of the child's visual and other responses can be useful. Always consider whether the responses observed are consistent and reliable, and occurring in response to a specific stimulus. Repetition is important to be sure observations are not affected by chance responses. Understanding the individual child's response method and skills must be an integral part of the vision assessment.

Consideration of Eye Movement Difficulty

When a child's only response method for testing vision is fixation, it is crucial to understand the nature of the child's eye movements; the increased risk of eye movement disorders in children with complex neurodisability creates additional assessment challenges. If a squint is present, it is important to establish which eye is the fixating eye. Are smooth eye movements seen as the child holds fixation on a moving target? In preferential looking tasks does the child have the ability to move the eyes rapidly (saccades) to a new target? The child may need more time to establish fixation and may need to use head movements to overcome any eye movement limitations.

Lack of eye movements may also be explained by very low visual acuity, grossly restricted visual fields, and in some cases by an inability to pay visual attention to more than one object at a time (sometimes referred to as simultanagnosia). These possibilities should also be considered.

PREPARING FOR AND UNDERTAKING THE VISION ASSESSMENT

Children with the most severe motor impairments will produce their best visual performance when they are comfortable and have optimal postural support. Visual attention will also be optimised in a low distraction environment (see Box 6.1).

The practical elements of the vision assessment (assessment of vision functions and functional vision) are described further in Chapters 2 and 4. However, adaptations are likely to be required in order to match the child's level of ability and response methods with the assessment materials chosen.

As ophthalmological disorders are so common in this at risk population, all children with complex neurodisability should routinely have an ophthalmological assessment by a specialist eye team. These assessments can be undertaken in special education school settings (Black et al. 2019; Donaldson et al. 2019).

ELECTROPHYSIOLOGICAL ASSESSMENT

Visual evoked potentials (VEP), a bioelectrical signal generated in the visual cortex of the brain in response to visual stimulation, can provide a measure of the integrity of the visual pathway and visual cortex. Combined with electroretinograms, they can distinguish whether pathology is retinal or post-retinal. Stimuli can include flash VEP (a repeated flash of light), pattern onset VEP (pattern onset – checkerboard or gratings, presented repetitively from a luminance matched grey background), or pattern reversal VEP (a phase alternated pattern). Testing is not, however, available outside of specialist centres. The correspondence between VEPs and visual acuity measures may not be clear-cut as some children may have relatively intact VEPs but fail to make any apparent behavioural response to vision stimulus; thus interpretation in the clinical situation must be cautious.

NEUROIMAGING

Magnetic resonance imaging (MRI) of the brain may indicate an increased risk of visual dysfunction when specific areas of the visual cortex and visual pathways are damaged, especially in infants born preterm or in infants with stroke or hypoxic-ischaemic

> **Box 6.2** Questions to elicit parent descriptions of child's fixation, recognition, and use of vision during everyday interactions
>
> ✓ Does your child look directly at a toy/object when this is placed directly in front of them?
>
> ✓ Does your child need an additional prompt to look at the object or toy? (Please tell us what: e.g. sound, movement)
>
> ✓ If two or more objects are in front of your child, do they look at each toy in turn, inspecting each toy? This is sometimes called shifting gaze.
>
> ✓ If there are two or more objects in front of your child, is it easy to tell which object your child is looking at?
>
> ✓ Does your child shift gaze between an object and a person (that is, does your child look at an object and then look at a person, or the other way round)?
>
> ✓ Does your child look directly at a familiar person who is seated opposite them?

encephalopathy (Guzzetta et al. 2001). Therefore, review of the MRI brain scan may help to identify those who require more careful vision monitoring (see Chapters 5 and 7).

Parent-Reported Vision Behaviours

When systematically asked about vision-related behaviours, parents of children with complex neurodisability can provide helpful information about their child's everyday visual performance and challenges. Other developmental issues such as cognition, school attainment, and motor abilities can also be explored. More precise descriptions of fixation skills can be useful particularly for children with extreme movement limitations; some useful starter questions are given in Box 6.2, in addition to those given in Chapter 4.

Assessment of Functional Vision

As described in Chapter 4 assessment of vision includes assessment of vision functions and functional vision for everyday tasks. Both aspects will be critical in supporting the child's learning, communication, and participation. Consideration must be given to the child's level of functioning and everyday tasks of relevance to them. To complement clinical history taking, some tools have been developed to explore functional visual skills as reported by parents.

Validated questionnaires can be useful. The Preverbal Visual Assessment is a reliable validated questionnaire that aims to evaluate infants' visual cognitive abilities (visual attention, visual processing, visual communication, and visuo-motor coordination) from birth to 24 months and has been shown to accurately differentiate normal and abnormal visual maturation against ophthalmological evaluation in a high risk group presenting to an eye/ophthalmology clinic (Garcia-Ormaechea et al. 2014). However, on some items of this questionnaire, difficulties may be explained by general cognitive delay rather than specific visual difficulties.

The Visual Skills Inventory (McCulloch et al. 2007) (validated in children aged 7 months to 16 years with neurological impairment) has been shown to confirm good visual function, as measured using behavioural tests, with high sensitivity but low specificity. In the children reported to lack visual skills, 19% to 37% had good visual function suggesting that negative responses to the questions may reflect other factors such as motor or cognitive deficits. The Functional Vision Questionnaire (evaluated in children with cerebral palsy and severe to profound motor and intellectual disability) is designed to gather evidence of basic visual function and daily visual performance in areas relating to play and communication (Ferziger et al. 2011). This questionnaire has good interrater reliability and correlates with clinical assessment of visual performance.

A systematic review (Deramore Denver et al. 2016) highlighted the relative lack of suitable instruments for measuring vision function in children with cerebral palsy. Subsequently, Baranello et al. (2019) developed a Visual Function Classification System for describing vision function in children and young people with cerebral palsy. Deramore Denver et al. have reported initial work on the development of a tool to measure use of vision by children with cerebral palsy in everyday activities (Deramore Denver et al. 2021). These tools are designed to describe how vision is used and are not a substitute for detailed assessment of the child's visual functions.

Assessment of Vision Function

The following section considers assessment of vision functions (Box 6.3) in children with complex neurodisability and particularly with significant physical disability.

The following questions should guide assessment, noting carefully the evidence for forming conclusions (e.g. fixation, reach, vocalisation).

- What is this child's most effective response method when presented with a task? Can this be reliably observed? Would a second observer increase objectivity?
- Are there any abnormalities of eye movement, affecting smooth pursuit or saccades or both?
- If evidence of squint, which eye is the child using to fixate?
- Can the child establish, and sustain, fixation (attention) on a target? What is the evidence? Are observations repeatable?
- If weaknesses in fixation/attention are seen, what factors may explain this? (Weaknesses in visual attention, weaknesses in general attention, bodily distractions such as pain or tiredness, developmentally inappropriate materials shown).
- What is the child's visual detection capacity? For what size of object? At what distance?
- What is the child's level of visual acuity (level of detail discriminated)? The testing method and distance should be stated and interpreted according to published norms for age.

Box 6.3 Assessment

Ophthalmological assessment including refraction, eye health, squint:

Vision Functions

✓ Eye movements – pursuit and saccades

✓ Detection
  - Near (Near Detection Scale; see Chapter 4)
  - Distance detection (how far away can a child show fixation)

✓ Acuity
  - Resolution methods using preferential looking methods (grating acuity [Keeler/Teller/Lea grating acuity test, Cardiff Cards])
  - Recognition methods using optotype matching or naming tasks

✓ Visual Fields

Functional Vision

✓ Detection of everyday objects (fix on reliably but no evidence of recognition)

✓ Recognition of familiar people

✓ Recognition of everyday objects

✓ Ability to shift gaze between objects – supports active searching and inspection

✓ Ability to shift gaze between object and person – supports joint attention and communication

✓ Recognition of pictures (note level of contrast, clarity of outline, and complexity)

Environment

✓ Consider lighting conditions, contrast of materials, and background

✓ Consider other potential distractions (sound, movement)

Pitfalls

✓ Abnormal visual behaviour may be misinterpreted as visual impairment, or non-specifically labelled as 'cerebral visual impairment', without specification of precise functional consequences.

✓ Reduced visual experience may not be reported by the child or evident on informal observation and thus may remain unidentified unless actively measured.

✓ Practitioners not experienced in assessment of children with complex needs may over- or under-interpret child's responses.

✓ Visual perceptual difficulties (within the cerebral visual impairment spectrum) may be present but only identified when a standardised assessment is completed (see Chapter 5).

✓ Lower visual acuity does not preclude additional perceptual disorders (if acuity is sufficient), but it can mask them. Both aspects of visual impairment should be assessed if possible in order to optimise management, education, and parenting.

- Can the child recognise what is seen? What factors may influence this (e.g. developmental level)?
- If appropriate, assessment for higher visual difficulties (visuo-cognitive) should proceed according to recommended protocols (see Chapter 5).

Start with standard lighting conditions, proceeding to adaptations of materials and environment if no reliable responses are seen (see Box 6.3). Children may show better visual responses for familiar toys, for example they may show more prolonged fixation or recognition of toys/objects they are familiar with and motivated by. This may be because the child can use clues such as shape and colour and familiarity to support identification. In children with poor visual attention, familiarity and cognitive interest may also help the child to sustain attention.

Habilitation

Understanding of a child's vision following detailed assessment will guide habilitation including positioning of the child for optimal viewing of visual materials (best field of vision, distance to materials), adaptation of the environment including lighting, clutter, and the size, colour, and contrast of objects, pictures, or symbols/letters. This will ensure that visual access does not present an additional obstacle for the child in reaching their full potential. Assessment will also support parents understanding of their child's visual and other disabilities and how these impact on their development and learning. The findings should lead to provision of practical ideas for helping their child to use their vision however limited, and how to adapt materials and the environment for the child's level of vision (see Chapter 8). Pehere and Jacob describe a practical approach to assessment and support of children with vision impairment and additional disabilities, in an Indian context (Pehere and Jacob 2019).

RESEARCH AND PRACTICE IMPLICATIONS

There is a small but growing literature suggesting that treatment and management of the vision needs of the child with complex neurodisability will have wider benefits for their learning and behaviour. Measurable visual and behaviour benefits were shown after children received comprehensive in-school eye examinations, on-site spectacle dispensing, and jargon-free reporting of outcomes to teachers and parents (Black et al. 2019). Providing ophthalmological screening services to special schools has been shown to be practical (Donaldson et al. 2019). Models for vision services for this vulnerable population and systematic assessment methods need further evaluation and development.

SUMMARY

Given the high prevalence of abnormalities of eye and visual function in children with complex disability, the case for ophthalmological and visual assessment in this group is clear. Despite this knowledge, assessment of this group in high-, middle-, and low-income countries is often worryingly incomplete. In some children participation at the most basic level of communication is dependent on understanding of vision needs, making assessment of functional vision critical. Models of assessment and service delivery should be implemented to ensure that the visual needs of children with complex neurodisability are appropriately met.

Key Points

✓ Children with complex neurodisability are at high risk of refractive error, strabismus, eye movement disorder, and reduced acuity.

✓ Unidentified visual difficulties may impact on developmental progress, communication, and behaviour.

✓ Ophthalmological assessment and monitoring to assess eye health and visual functions and correction of refractive error, if present, is required.

✓ Functional visual assessment benefits from a multidisciplinary approach that combines ophthalmological and developmental expertise, and includes careful observation of how the child functions in everyday situations.

✓ Results of assessment and practical implications for optimal adaptation of habilitation approaches should be easily understandable by parents and professionals working with the child and parents.

✓ Regular monitoring is necessary to ensure habilitation approaches remain salient.

✓ Research is beginning to establish the benefits for the child, parents, and teachers of identifying unmet vision needs.

REFERENCES

Abu Bakar NF, Chen Ai-H, Md Noor AR, Goh P-P (2012) Comparison of vision disorders between children in mainstream and special education classes in government primary school in Malaysia. *Singap Med J* **53**: 541–544.

Baranello G, Signorini S, Tinelli F et al. (2019) Visual Function Classification System for children with cerebral palsy: development and validation. *Dev Med Child Neurol* **62**: 104–110. https://doi.org/10.1111/dmcn.14270.

Black SA, McConnell EL, McKerr L et al. (2019) In-school eyecare in special education settings has measurable benefits for children's vision and behaviour. *PloS One* **14**(8): e0220480. doi: 10.1371/journal.pone.0220480.

Brady N, Fleming K, Thiemann-Bourque K, Olswang L, Dowden P, Saunders MD (2012) Development of the Communication Complexity Scale. *Am J Speech-Lang Pat* **21**: 16–28. doi: 10.1044/1058-0360(2011/10-0099).

Clarke MT, Sargent J, Cooper R et al. (2020) Development and testing of the Eye-Pointing Classification Scale for children with cerebral palsy. *Disabil Rehabil* **12**: 1–6. doi: 10.1080/09638288.2020.1800834.

Das M, Spowart K, Crossley S, Dutton G (2010) Evidence that children with special needs all require visual assessment. *Arch Dis Child* **95**: 88–892. doi: 10.1136/adc.2009.159053.

Deramore Denver B, Froude E, Rosenbaum P, Wilkes-Gillan S, Imms C (2016) Measurement of visual ability in children with cerebral palsy: a systematic review. *Dev Med Child Neurol* **58**: 1016–1029. doi: 10.1111/dmcn.13139.

Deramore Denver B, Froude E, Rosenbaum P, Imms C (2021) Measure of early vision use: development of a new assessment tool for children with cerebral palsy. *Disabil Rehabil* **10**: 1–11. doi: 10.1080/09638288.2021.1890241.

Donaldson LA, Karas M, O'Brien D, Woodhouse JM (2019) Findings from an opt-in eye examination service in English special schools. Is vision screening effective for this population? *PLoS One* **14**(3): e0212733. doi: 10.1371/journal.pone.0212733.

Ezeh E, Ibanga A, Duke R (2018) Visual status of special needs children in special education schools in Calabar, Cross River State, Nigeria. *Niger Postgrad Med J* **25**: 161–165. doi: 10.4103/npmj.npmj_46_18.

Fazzi E, Signorini SG, La Piana R et al. (2012) Neuro-ophthalmological disorders in cerebral palsy: ophthalmological, oculomotor, and visual aspects. *Dev Med Child Neurol* **54**: 730–736. doi: 10.1111/j.1469-8749.2012.04324.

Ferziger NB, Nemet P, Brezner A, Feldman R, Galili G, Zivotofsky A (2011) Visual assessment in children with cerebral palsy: implementation of a functional questionnaire. *Dev Med Child Neurol* **53**: 422–428. doi: 10.11/j.1469-8749.2010.03905.x 11.

Fleming CV, Wheeler GM, Cannella-Malone HI, Basbagill AR, Chung YC, Day KG (2010) An evaluation of the use of eye gaze to measure preference of individuals with severe physical and developmental disabilities. *Dev Neurorehabil* **13**: 266–275. doi: 10.3109/17518421003705706.

Garcia-Ormaechea I, Gonzalez I, Dupla M, Andres E, Pueyo V (2014) Validation of the Preverbal Visual Assessment (PreViAs) questionnaire. *Early Hum Dev* **90**: 635–8.

Global Research on Developmental Disabilities Collaborators (2018) Developmental disabilities among children younger than 5 years in 195 countries and territories, 1990–2016: a systematic analysis for the Global Burden of Disease Study 2016. *Lancet Glob Health* **6**(10): e1100–e1121. doi: 10.1016/S2214-109X(18)30309-7.

Gogate P, Soneji FR, Kharat J, Dulera H, Desphande M, Gilbert C (2011) Ocular disorders in children with learning disabilities in special education schools of Pune, India. *Indian J Ophthalmol* **59**: 223–28 doi: 10.4103/0301-4738.81036.

Guzzetta A, Cioni G, Cowan F, Mercuri E (2001) Visual disorders in children with brain lesions: 1. Maturation of visual function in infants with neonatal brain lesions: correlation with neuroimaging. *Eur J Paediatr Neurol* **5**: 107–114. doi: 10.1053/ejpn.2001.0480.

Haargaard B, Fledelius HC (2006) Down's syndrome and early cataract. *Br J Ophthalmol* **90**: 1024–1027. doi: 10.1136/bjo.2006.090639.

Limburg H, Gilbert C, Hon DN, Dung NC, Hoang TH (2012) Prevalence and causes of blindness in children in Vietnam. *Ophthalmology* **119**(2): 355–361. doi: 10.1016/j.ophtha.2011.07.037.

Little JA (2018) Vision in children with autism spectrum disorder: a critical review. *Clin Exp Optom* **101**: 504–513. doi: 10.1111/cxo.12651.

Lundy C, Hill N, Wolsley C et al. (2011) Multidisciplinary assessment of vision in children with neurological disability. *Ulster Med J* **80**: 21–27.

McCulloch DL, Mackie RT, Dutton GN et al. (2007) A visual skills inventory for children with neurological impairments. *Dev Med Child Neurol* **49**: 757–763. doi: 10.1111/j.1469-8749.2007.00757.x.

Pehere NK, Jacob N (2019) Understanding low functioning cerebral visual impairment: an Indian context. *Indian J Ophthalmol* **67**(10): 1536–1543. doi: 10.4103/ijo.IJO_2089_18.

Pilling RF, Outhwaite L (2017) Are all children with special needs known to the Eye clinic? *Br J Ophthalmol* **101**: 472–474. doi: 10.1136/bjophthalmol-2016-308534.

Puri S, Bhattarai D, Adhikari P, Shrestha JB, Paudel N (2015) Burden of ocular and visual disorders among pupils in special schools in Nepal. *Arch Dis Child* **100**: 834–837. doi: 10.1136/archdischild-2014-308131.

Ricci D, Romeo DM, Serrao F et al. (2010) Early assessment of visual function in preterm infants: how early is early? *Early Hum Dev* **86**: 29–33. doi: 10.1016/j.earlhumdev.2009.11.004.

Rossi A, Gnesi M, Montomoli C et al. (2017) Neonatal Assessment Visual European Grid (NAVEG): Unveiling neurological risk. *Infant Behav Dev* **49**: 21–30. doi: 10.1016/j.infbeh.2017.06.002.

Rudnicka AR, Kapetanakis VV, Wathern AK et al. (2016) Global variations and time trends in the prevalence of childhood myopia, a systematic review and quantitative meta-analysis: implications for aetiology and early prevention. *Br J Ophthalmol* **100**: 882–890. doi: 10.1136/bjophthalmol-2015-307724.

Salt A, Sargent J (2014) Common visual problems in children with disability. *Arch Dis Child* **99**(12): 1163–1168. doi: 10.1136/archdischild-2013-305267.

Salt A, Sargent J (2017) Fifteen-minute consultation – the child with a developmental disability: is there an ocular or visual abnormality?. *Arch Dis Child – Education and Practice* **102**(6): 304–309. doi: 10.1136/archdischild-2016-311252.

Sargent J, Clarke M, Price K, Griffiths T, Swettenham J (2013) Use of eye-pointing by children with cerebral palsy: what are we looking at? *Int J Lang Commun Disord* **48**: 477–485. doi: 10.1111/1460-6984.12026.

Vora U, Khandekar R, Al-Harami K (2010) Refractive error and visual functions in children with special needs compared with first grade school students in Oman. *Middle East Afr J of Ophthalmol* **17**: 297–302 doi: 10.4103/0974-9233.71590.

Watt T, Robertson K, Jacobs RJ (2015) Refractive error, binocular vision and accommodation of children with Down syndrome. *Clin Exp Optom* **98**: 3–11. doi: 10.1111/cxo.12232.

Woodhouse JM, Davies N, McAvinchey A, Ryan B (2013) Ocular and visual status among children in special schools in Wales: the burden of unrecognised visual impairment. *Arch Dis Child* **99**: 500–504. doi: 10.1136/archdischild-2013-304866.

CHAPTER 7

Brain Development and Plasticity

Francesca Tinelli and Andrea Guzzetta

INTRODUCTION

Humans are highly dependent on their sense of vision in order to interact with their surrounding world. The lack of visual function associated with blindness and visual impairment has a dramatic impact on an individual's quality of life and independence (Dagnelie 2013). Compensatory behaviours may be intimately related to underlying changes in the overall structural and functional organisation of the brain resulting from profound vision impairment (Voss et al. 2014). The ability of the brain to reorganise itself in the process of learning a task distinguishes the nervous system from all other tissues. This ability, called 'plasticity', appears to be greatest during infancy, at a time when many of the neural pathways are still in a phase of maturation. The neural changes associated with learning in the human brain generally involve neural networks that are designed for a given function: for instance, the visual cortex for vision function. However, it is now well known that the brain can also transfer functions outside the traditional areas when it is forced to compensate for neuronal damage or deficiency and this phenomenon is called 'adaptive plasticity'. This chapter explores the different ways in which lack of vision may impact on brain development and some of the risks associated, such as autistic-related behaviours, pragmatic language deficits, peer relationship, and emotional problems (Bathelt et al. 2017) and also how the brain may adapt through plasticity mechanisms.

BRAIN CHANGES FROM VISION DISORDERS

Adaptive Plasticity of the Visual System

Lack of vision impacts on the development of the visual system from the retina to the primary visual cortex (see Fig. 7.1, Chapter 5). Incoming vision stimuli through the retina have a corresponding retino-topographic location in the occipital or visual cortex. If one eye is deprived of vision during early life there is a corresponding lack of development of the retino-topographic ocular dominance columns in the visual cortex, a condition known as amblyopia (Hubel et al. 1977). This is due to the presence in early life of a *critical period* for vision development (from 0–5 or 6 years of age) – a time when the quality of visual inputs has the highest effects on brain structural organisation. Amblyopia is a significant clinical disorder (see further Chapter 2) that can be prevented by temporarily occluding the best eye to ensure that the less efficient one (*lazy eye*) is actively used. This, however, holds true only when the intervention is started sufficiently early, and more specifically before the age of 7 years, as after the end of the *critical period* its efficacy is dramatically reduced with only modest improvements of visual acuity thereafter (Fronius et al. 2014).

Scientific evidence has emerged suggesting that the visual cortex retains some neuroplastic properties through childhood and into adulthood and well beyond the closure of the *critical period*. A clear 'plastic' response to short-term visual deprivation has been shown in adults with a fully mature visual cortex after a few hours or a few days of binocular light deprivation, in the form of a modulation of excitability in the primary visual cortex (Boroojerdi et al. 2000). Interestingly, a paradoxical effect was observed when only one eye was deprived for a few hours, consisting of the shifting of the retino-topographic dominance in the visual cortex in favour of the deprived eye (but not the non-deprived one) (Lunghi et al. 2011). This effect has been interpreted as a compensatory reaction of the visual cortex aimed at maintaining the overall visual cortical activity at a constant level, as a form of 'homeostatic plasticity' (Turrigiano 2012). Notably, this property of the adult visual brain has recently been shown in adults and children with amblyopia, both for the non-affected (Lunghi et al. 2016) and for the affected eye (Zhou et al. 2013), with potential consequences for the development of new interventional therapies. Piano and Simmers (2019) have also highlighted that more recent research shows traditional and newer monocular and binocular learning techniques can be effective in older children.

Brain Organisation in Children With Low-Vision or Blindness

What happens to the brain in the case of a total absence (or very low levels) of visual experience from infancy, and how is its structural and functional architecture affected? To address these questions, behavioural, structural, and functional studies have been performed in adults with congenital profound vision impairment. This permits defining and differentiating the plastic changes resulting from the compensatory enhanced utilization of tactile and auditory sensory channels (which is referred to as *cross-modal plasticity*). These studies also explore the development of those networks that are formed irrespective of the visual input in typically sighted, and in congenitally blind individuals, as a result of *supra-modal* organisation (these are networks subserving visual and/or non-visual perception of form, space or movement) (Ricciardi et al. 2014).

Individuals with profound or very severe visual impairment from congenital disorders of the anterior visual system have comparable, and often superior, abilities in the tactile and auditory domains compared with their typically sighted peers (Merabet and Pascual-Leone 2010). It has been shown how these abilities are supported by neuroplasticity in brain areas responsible for the processing of touch, hearing, and smell (Hamilton et al. 2004) but also by the *cross-modal reorganisation* of areas of the brain typically associated with the processing of vision. Neuroimaging studies (predominantly functional magnetic resonance imaging [fMRI]) have demonstrated that individuals with profound or very severe visual impairment show robust activation within the occipital cortex while performing non-visual tasks such as braille reading, sound localisation, odour perception, as well as higher-order cognitive tasks including language processing and verbal memory recall (Merabet and Pascual-Leone 2010). Auditory-to-visual cross modal neuroplasticity within the primary visual cortex has been shown in early and late-blind echolocation experts. Processing of click-echoes was found to recruit brain regions (the calcarine cortex) typically devoted to vision rather than audition (Thaler et al. 2011). Norman and Thaler (2019) also showed that 'stimulus maps for sound in the primary visual cortex are comparable to those for vision in sighted people' and positively relates to echolocation ability. Further evidence of the cross-modal plasticity of the visual cortex is demonstrated by the increase of grey matter volume in the visual cortex following intensive training of braille in typically sighted adults (Bola et al. 2017).

Although our knowledge about the consequences of early vision impairment on development is still limited, a number of studies suggest they are not negligible. A proportion of children with congenital disorders of the peripheral visual system (CDPVS) and no other known brain disorder ('*simple*' CDPVS) may present with severe learning difficulties and developmental setback, for reasons not yet fully understood (Dale et al. 2019; see Chapter 8). Even in cases of average or superior language abilities, children with 'simple CDPVS' may show uneven neuropsychological profiles (see Chapter 12), or difficulties in social communication skills, sometimes consistent with a diagnosis of autism spectrum disorder (Tadic et al. 2009; see Chapter 11). Children (8–12 years) with 'simple CDPVS', severe vision impairment, and average verbal intelligence have shown abnormal event-related responses in a social cognition paradigm ('subject own name'), as compared to age-matched typically developing children, and those with mild to moderate vision impairment at an intermediate level (Bathelt et al. 2017). In the same group, lower white matter integrity was found in tracts of the visual system, including optic radiations, posterior corpus callosum, and lower left thalamus volume, with neuroanatomical differences that were greater in the severe visual impairment group but with no differences being identified between the moderate vision impairment and the typically sighted control group (Bathelt et al. 2020). Structural abnormalities have also been reported in children with mild or no visual impairment and optic nerve hypoplasia, including reduced ventral cingulum, corpus callosum, and optic radiation structural white matter, as compared with typically developing controls (Webb et al. 2013). Interestingly, children with greater reductions of the ventral cingulum showed higher behaviour scores on a behavioural checklist, suggesting that the reported white matter abnormalities might actually have clinical significance.

Brain Changes in Cerebral Vision Impairment

When visual impairment arises from injury to and abnormality of the visual pathways in the brain (cerebral visual impairment [CVI] – see Chapter 5), the structural architecture of the brain can be variably affected, depending on the site and extent of the damage. See Figure 7.1 for the complex pathways involved in the visual system of the

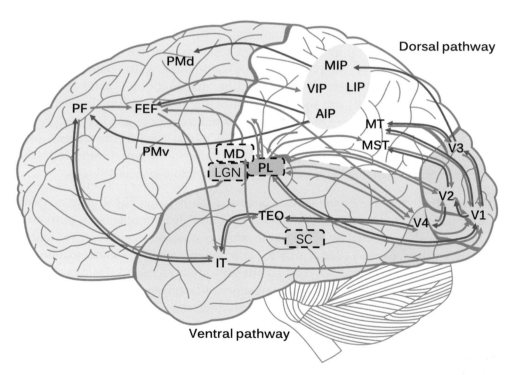

Figure 7.1 Diagram of the visual networks in the brain.

AIP, anterior intraparietal area; FEF, frontal eye fields; IT, inferior temporal area; LGN, lateral geniculate nucleus; LIP, lateral intraparietal area; MD, medial dorsal nucleus of thalamus; MIP, medial intraparietal area; MST, medial superior temporal area; MT, medial temporal area; PF, prefrontal cortex; PL, pulvinar; PMd, dorsal premotor area; PMv, ventral premotor area; SC, superior colliculus; TEO, tectum opticum; V1, primary visual cortex; V2, secondary visual cortex; V3, etrastriate area, V4, extrastriate area; VIP, ventral intraparietal area. (A colour version of this figure can be seen in the colour plate section) brain. Individuals with congenital CVI show greater reductions in volume and fibre numbers of the inferior longitudinal fasciculus, superior longitudinal fasciculus, and inferior fronto-occipital fasciculus, compared with individuals with visual disorders originating in the anterior visual system (Bauer et al. 2014).

While the consequences of early damage to the visual brain are complex and still difficult to predict, increasing evidence suggests that early plasticity occurs in the visual system following similar mechanisms to other systems (e.g. somato-sensory). For instance, a large lesion of the left periventricular white matter involving the optic radiations can be compatible with typical visual fields when occurring at the beginning of the third trimester of gestation, supporting age-specific mechanisms of reorganisation. In a child with such a lesion, MRI tractography has shown how the trajectory of the optic radiations in the affected hemisphere can deviate from the typical course, bypassing the cystic lesion and reaching the final target in the occipital lobe; this is probably due to the specific neuroplastic properties of the brain at the time of the insult (Guzzetta et al. 2010). A similar phenomenon has been previously described in the reorganisation of the somatosensory system following a similar early-third-trimester lesion, suggesting similar mechanisms of reorganisation for the somatosensory and visual systems (Staudt et al. 2006).

Another mechanism that has been observed in the reorganisation of the visual system, as well as in other systems, consists of the persistence of neural connections that in typical conditions would disappear during development as a result of synaptic pruning. Synaptic pruning is the process by which extra neurons and synaptic connections are eliminated during development in order to increase the efficiency of neuronal transmission. This is the case, for example, of a pathway connecting the retina to the pulvinar without involvement of the superior colliculus, which is typically pruned during early development to become a sparse projection by adulthood (Cowey et al. 1994). Warner et al. have shown in an animal model that when a lesion is inflicted to the primary geniculostriate (lateral geniculate nucleus-V1) pathway within the first couple of postnatal weeks, the retinopulvinar-medial temporal (MT) pathway does not show the expected regression and persists into adulthood, as a compensation for the early damage to the visual system (Warner et al. 2015). The pulvinar appears to be responsible for preserved vision following early life V1 lesions in the visual cortex, which suggests that alternative brain structures can compensate. See Figure 7.1 for relevant pathways.

In another study, a patient with a large unilateral lesion of the optic radiations, acquired early in life, was found to have near typical central visual field vision (Mikellidou et al. 2019). The patient underwent surgical removal of a right hemisphere parieto-temporal-occipital atypical choroid plexus papilloma of the right lateral ventricle at 4 months, which presumably altered the visual pathways during in utero development. Both the tumour and surgery severely compromised the optic radiations. Residual vision was tested when the patient was 7 years old; the patient had close to typical visual acuity and contrast sensitivity within the central 25° and a severe impairment in contrast vision in the far periphery (40–50°) of the left visual hemifield. Diffusion tensor imaging revealed the possible reason for this apparent brain–behaviour dissociation: in the lesioned hemisphere a strong connection was observed between an area that responded to motion (putative MT+) and a thalamic region close to the lateral geniculate nucleus. See the pathways in Figure 7.1. The same connection was also present in the intact hemisphere but it was very small, whilst the optic radiations were typically developed. The strong analogy between the thalamic-MT connection in this patient, with the persistence of the retinopulvinar-MT projection in the marmoset with primary visual cortex V1 lesions, suggests that the thalamic-MT connection might arise from the retinopulvinar tract. This might be transient in the typical human developing brain but have become stabilised in this case given the loss of the optic radiation input.

In patients with hemianopia (i.e. where there is less vision or blindness in half of the visual field), typically secondary to stroke, brain tumour, or trauma, the probability that the homonymous scotomata (areas of partial alteration in the vision field of both eyes) recovers during the years following brain injury, correlates strongly with the age of the lesion in adolescent and young patients. In a group of patients who underwent hemispherectomy (i.e. removal of an entire hemisphere) for drug-resistant epilepsy, recovery of visual capabilities was greater when surgery was performed by 7 years, as opposed to later in life (Kiper et al. 2002). A critical role in this type of reorganisation has been attributed to the superior colliculus, as part of a wider anatomical and functional reshaping of neuronal circuitry that allows patients to 'see without perceiving', the phenomenon known as 'blindsight'. Tinelli et al. (2013), compared children with congenital and acquired hemianopia who showed differences in behaviour in daily life. Children with congenital lesions, as opposed to those with acquired brain lesions, were able to navigate the environment without difficulties, to read a text proficiently, and to perform visual search tasks. By using fMRI, it was shown how in these children the lesioned hemisphere could not respond to any visual stimulus, probably due to the profound injury. Yet a massive reorganisation of the visual system had occurred, as shown by the presence of activation at the level of primary visual cortex V1 in the intact hemisphere in response to stimuli in the ipsilateral 'blind' hemifield. Since these children had unilateral damage to one optic radiation, with large cortical and subcortical lesions, it is very difficult to imagine a crossed hemispheric pathway that can relay the signal from the ipsilateral visual field to the primary cortex. A possible explanation is again the strong pulvinar-MT projection, observed in the marmoset and in the patient described above. The ipsilateral visual signals could thus reach the pulvinar through several routes, including via the superior colliculus (see Fig. 7.1).

IMPLICATIONS FOR RESEARCH AND PRACTICE

Further research is needed to consider brain development and function in children with vision impairment in order to understand the underlying mechanisms and to increase the possibilities for interventions that maximise potential in all aspects of development. One area of development that is needed is greater clarity and consensus of classification of the different forms of vision disorder, particularly those involving children with early- and later-onset cerebral vision impairment (see Chapter 5) to ensure that researchers are using matched samples for replicability. The distinct study and comparison of children with 'potentially simple' and 'potentially complex' (i.e. no known or known brain involvement in the diagnosis), congenital disorders of the anterior visual system versus those with cerebral vision impairment, or those with early-onset or acquired brain lesions, will be important for further understanding the developmental processes and implications. Neuropsychological studies that consider the relationship between brain structure and function with functional behaviour and cognition will provide new insights.

Research on brain development and plasticity is still at an early stage, but there are already important lessons to consider for early interventions. The importance of 'environmental enrichment' to enhance neural plasticity has been well demonstrated in animal models, where laboratory-reared animals in more stimulating cages (including sensory, cognitive, motor, and social stimuli) have enhanced neural plasticity in different brain areas (for a review, see Sale 2018). Similar beneficial effects have been shown in animal models of neurodegenerative diseases and brain injury. Of physiological relevance, exposure to environmental enrichment reduced GABAergic inhibition in the visual cortex of enriched animals and a marked recovery of cognitive and visual functions in a mouse model of Down syndrome (Begenisic et al. 2011). Other research is showing promising signs in relation to motor coordination and motor learning, as well as reduced memory deficits and anxiety-related behaviour in a mouse model of Rett syndrome (Lonetti et al. 2010). Different kinds of early multisensory intervention, such as infant massage, have been associated with beneficial effects on the maturation of visual functions in infants with Down syndrome (Purpura et al. 2014). The concept of environmental enrichment has been well accepted in the field of infant vision impairment, though research on neural plasticity has yet to be undertaken.

Early intervention, using a home-based developmental framework designed for infants with vision impairment, using accessible compensatory multisensory approaches and providing matched targeted enrichment at each stage of the infant and young child's development through understandable and accessible guidance to the parent (i.e. the Developmental Journal for babies and young children with visual impairment), has shown acceleration in cognition and expressive language from infancy to 3 years (Dale et al. 2019, see Chapter 8). The importance of multisensory input in a structured vision promotion programme during the first year of life has also shown acceleration in visual development by the second year of life (Sonksen et al. 1991; see Chapter 4). When parents have higher sensitivity to visual impairment needs, their children have shown greater acceleration in verbal comprehension from infancy to 3 years, highlighting that 'environmental enrichment' must take into account the quality of parent–infant inter-actions (Sakkalou et al. 2020, see Chapter 8).

SUMMARY

The loss of visual function associated with profound and severe visual impairment has a dramatic impact on an individual's quality of life and independence, but compensatory behaviours may be intimately related to underlying changes in the overall structural and functional organisation of the brain resulting from impaired vision. The ability of the brain to reorganise itself in the process of learning is known as 'plasticity'. In this chapter, different examples of visual plasticity – adaptive plasticity, homeostatic plasticity, cross-modal, and supramodal plasticity – developmental and neural risks and adaptation, and the importance of environmental enrichment and early intervention to enhance brain growth are explored.

Key Points

✓ The brain visual system has adaptive properties or 'plasticity' for developing at neural and functional vision levels even after damage to its pathways.

✓ Reorganisation of brain visual pathways following early damage and brain surgery has been shown in children, such as in the phenomenon of 'blindsight'.

✓ The importance of infant 'environmental enrichment' to enhance neural plasticity including in the visual system is now recognised.

✓ Research will enhance understanding of the neural mechanisms underlying the positive impact of early vision and developmental interventions, potentially leading to greater enhancement.

REFERENCES

Bathelt J, Dale N, de Haan M (2017) Event-related potential response to auditory social stimuli, parent-reported social communicative deficits and autism risk in school-aged children with congenital visual impairment. *Dev Cogn Neurosci* **27**: 10–18. doi: S1878-9293(17)30020-8.

Bathelt J, Dale NJ, de Haan M, Clark CA (2020) Brain structure in children with congenital visual disorders and visual impairment. *Dev Med Child Neurol* **62**(1): 125–131. doi: 10.1111/dmcn.14322.

Bauer CM, Heidary G, Koo BB, Killiany RJ, Bex P, Merabet LB (2014) Abnormal white matter tractography of visual pathways detected by high-angular-resolution diffusion imaging (HARDI) corresponds to visual dysfunction in cortical/cerebral visual impairment. *J Aapos* **18**(4): 398–401. doi: 10.1016/j.jaapos.2014.03.004.

Begenisic T, Spolidoro M, Braschi C et al. (2011) Environmental enrichment decreases GABAergic inhibition and improves cognitive abilities, synaptic plasticity, and visual functions in a mouse model of Down syndrome. *Front Cell Neurosci* **5**: 29. doi: 10.3389/fncel.2011.00029.

Bola L, Siuda-Krzywicka K, Paplinska M et al. (2017) Structural reorganization of the early visual cortex following Braille training in sighted adults. *Sci Rep* **7**(1): 17448.

Boroojerdi B, Bushara KO, Corwell B (2000) Enhanced excitability of the human visual cortex induced by short-term light deprivation. *Cereb Cortex* **10**(5): 529–534. doi: 10.1093/cercor/10.5.529.

Cowey A, Stoerig P, Bannister M (1994) Retinal ganglion cells labelled from the pulvinar nucleus in macaque monkeys. *Neuroscience* 61(3): 691–705. doi: 0306-4522(94)90445-6.

Dagnelie G (2013) Age-related psychophysical changes and low vision. *Invest Ophthalmol Vis Sci* 54(14): ORSF88–93. doi: 10.1167/iovs.13-12934.

Dale NJ, Sakkalou E, O'Reilly M et al. (2019) Home-based early intervention in infants and young children with visual impairment using the Developmental Journal: longitudinal cohort study. *Dev Med Child Neurol* 61: 697–709.

Fronius M, Cirina L, Ackermann H, Kohnen T, Diehl CM (2014) Efficiency of electronically monitored amblyopia treatment between 5 and 16 years of age: new insight into declining susceptibility of the visual system. *Vision Res* 103: 11–19. doi: 10.1016/j.visres.2014.07.018.

Gilbert CD, Li W (2013) Top-down influences on visual processing. *Nat Rev Neurosci* 14: 350–363.

Guzzetta A, D'Acunto G, Rose S, Tinelli F, Boyd R, Cioni G (2010) Plasticity of the visual system after early brain damage. *Dev Med Child Neurol* 52(10): 891–900. doi: 10.1111/j.1469-8749.2010.03710.x.

Hamilton RH, Pascual-Leone A, Schlaug G (2004) Absolute pitch in blind musicians. *Neuroreport* 15(5): 803–806. doi: 00001756-200404090-00012.

Hubel DH, Wiesel TN, LeVay S (1977) Plasticity of ocular dominance columns in monkey striate cortex. *Philos Trans R Soc Lond B Biol Sci* 278(961): 377–409.

Kiper DC, Zesiger P, Maeder P, Deonna T, Innocenti GM (2002) Vision after early-onset lesions of the occipital cortex: I. Neuropsychological and psychophysical studies. *Neural Plast* 9(1): 1–25. doi: 10.1155/NP.2002.1.

Lonetti G, Angelucci A, Morando L, Boggio EM, Giustetto M, Pizzorusso T (2010) Early environmental enrichment moderates the behavioral and synaptic phenotype of MeCP2 null mice. *Biol Psychiatry* 67(7): 657–665. doi: 10.1016/j.biopsych.2009.12.022.

Lunghi C, Burr DC, Morrone C (2011) Brief periods of monocular deprivation disrupt ocular balance in human adult visual cortex. *Curr Biol* 21(14): R538–539. doi: 10.1016/j.cub.2011.06.004.

Lunghi C, Morrone MC, Secci J, Caputo R (2016) Binocular rivalry measured 2 hours after occlusion therapy predicts the recovery rate of the amblyopic eye in anisometropic children. *Invest Ophthalmol Vis Sci* 57(4): 1537–1546. doi: 10.1167/iovs.15-18419.

Merabet LB, Pascual-Leone A (2010) Neural reorganization following sensory loss: the opportunity of change. *Nat Rev Neurosci* 11(1): 44–52. doi: 10.1038/nrn2758.

Mikellidou K, Arrighi R, Aghakhanyan G et al. (2019) Plasticity of the human visual brain after an early cortical lesion. *Neuropsychologia* 128: 166–177. doi: 10.1016/j.neuropsychologia.2017.10.033.

Norman LJ, Thaler L (2019) Retinotopic-like maps of spatial sound in primary 'visual' cortex of blind human echolocators. *Proc R Soc B* 286: 20191910. http://dx.doi.org/10.1098/rspb.2019.1910.

Piano MEF, Simmers AJ (2019) 'It's too late'. Is it really? Considerations for amblyopia treatment in older children. *Ther Adv Ophthalmol* 11: 1–8. doi: 10.1177/2515841419857379.

Purpura G, Tinelli F, Bargagna S, Bozza M, Bastiani L, Cioni G (2014) Effect of early multisensory massage intervention on visual functions in infants with Down syndrome. *Early Hum Dev* 90(12): 809–813. doi: 10.1016/j.earlhumdev.2014.08.016.

Ricciardi E, Bonino D, Pellegrini S, Pietrini P (2014) Mind the blind brain to understand the sighted one! Is there a supramodal cortical functional architecture? *Neurosci Biobehav Rev* 41: 64–77. doi: 10.1016/j.neubiorev.2013.10.006.

Sakkalou E, O'Reilly MA, Sakki H et al. (2021) Mother.infant interactions with infants with congenital visual impairment and associations with longitudinal outcomes in cognition and language. *J Child Psychol Psychiatry* **62**(6): 742–750.

Sale A (2018) A systematic look at environmental modulation and its impact in brain development. *Trends Neurosci* **41**(1): 4–17. doi: 10.1016/j.tins.2017.10.004.

Sonksen PM, Petrie A, Drew KJ (1991) Promotion of visual development of severely visually impaired babies: evaluation of a developmentally based programme. *Dev Med Child Neurol* **33**(4): 320–335.

Staudt M, Braun C, Gerloff C, Erb M, Grodd W, Krageloh-Mann I (2006) Developing somatosensory projections bypass periventricular brain lesions. *Neurology* **67**(3): 522–525. doi: 10.1212/01.wnl.0000227937.49151.fd.

Tadic V, Pring L, Dale N (2010) Are language and social communication intact in children with congenital visual impairment at school age? *J Child Psychol Psychiatry* **51**(6): 696–705.

Tinelli F, Cicchini GM, Arrighi R, Tosetti M, Cioni G, Morrone MC (2013) Blindsight in children with congenital and acquired cerebral lesions. *Cortex* **49**(6): 1636–1647. doi: 10.1016/j.cortex.2012.07.005.

Thaler L, Arnott SR, Goodale MA (2011) Neural correlates of natural human echolocation in early and late blind echolocation experts. *PLoS One* **6**(5): e20162. doi: 10.1371/journal.pone.0020162.

Turrigiano G (2012) Homeostatic synaptic plasticity: local and global mechanisms for stabilizing neuronal function. *Cold Spring Harb Perspect Biol* **4**(1): a005736. doi: 10.1101/cshperspect.a005736 a005736.

Voss P, Pike BG, Zatorre RJ (2014) Evidence for both compensatory plastic and disuse atrophy-related neuroanatomical changes in the blind. *Brain* **137**(Pt 4): 1224–1240. doi: 10.1093/brain/awu030.

Warner CE, Kwan WC, Wright D, Johnston LA, Egan GF, Bourne JA (2015) Preservation of vision by the pulvinar following early-life primary visual cortex lesions. *Curr Biol* **25**(4): 424–434. doi: 10.1016/j.cub.2014.12.028.

Webb EA, O'Reilly MA, Clayden JD (2013) Reduced ventral cingulum integrity and increased behavioral problems in children with isolated optic nerve hypoplasia and mild to moderate or no visual impairment. *PLoS One* **8**(3): e59048. doi: 10.1371/journal.pone.0059048.

Zhou J, Thompson B, Hess RF (2013) A new form of rapid binocular plasticity in adult with amblyopia. *Sci Rep* **3**: 2638. doi: 10.1038/srep02638.

PART 2

Child Development and Learning from Birth to Older Childhood

CHAPTER 8

Early Years, Early Intervention, and Family Support

Naomi Dale, Elena Sakkalou, and Jackie Osborne

INTRODUCTION

The early years are a critical time for developmental growth and learning in all children. This is the period of rapid brain development, laying down neural pathways and circuits that will underpin all future development and learning. Congenital vision impairment has therefore been described as a 'developmental emergency' (Sonksen 1997) as vision plays such a vital role in early brain development and learning. Infants with vision impairment face significant developmental challenges and delays in the early years. Lack of vision impacts on all areas of development including use of hands, working out where sounds are coming from, being socially responsive to one's parent/caregiver, making vocal sounds, and vision itself. Parents can struggle to understand their infant's cues and to support their infant's learning about the environment. Together the infant and family are in a highly vulnerable period and need urgent help and support. This chapter addresses the risks and needs for the infant and their family during the early years and the importance of early assessment and early intervention to achieve optimal child developmental progress, parental coping, and family support.

EARLY YEARS, FAMILY SUPPORT, AND VISION IMPAIRMENT

Bringing the Senses 'Alive'

In infancy vision is the dominant sense and integrates the input from touch and sound in the typically developing infant (Atkinson 2002). Touch and auditory senses therefore have to be 'brought alive' as early as possible in the absence of vision or degraded vision. Infants face challenges in exploring their environment with their hands; they need to learn to use their hands 'as eyes' but may be wary of touching things or having their hands guided. Although research evidence is lacking about how these sensory processes are first activated in the absence of vision, clinical experience of our group has shown the need to provide anticipatory cues, like placing the object over the back of the infant's hand rather than putting it directly in the child's palm and fingers. This prevents the infant from having a startle reaction and removing their hands quickly, which can turn into longer-term tactile avoidance. The parent's voice has to be introduced carefully without background noise distraction so that the infant can start to listen to and recognise their vocal sounds. Guidance is therefore crucial to show parents and caregivers how to introduce tactile and auditory stimuli in ways that activate the senses without the infant becoming overwhelmed and withdrawn.

Early Development and Risks

In the second year of life young children have to learn that objects have permanence, spatial locations, properties (like motion), and can relate to other objects (such as containers and lids). They need to learn that objects have everyday functions, such as a cup is used for drinking. However, the process of object recognition and concept formation is far more complex without vision. These challenges can potentially lead to significant and cumulative delays in mastering basic milestones of sensorimotor understanding (or non-verbal cognition) (Reynell and Zinkin 1975; Vervloed et al. 2000; Dale et al. 2017). Alongside sensorimotor understanding and cognition, affected infants show challenges and delays in gross and fine motor development and hand skills (see Chapter 9), response to sound and verbal comprehension, as well as expressive language, social interaction, and communication (Dale and Sonksen 2002; Dale and Salt 2007; Mosca et al. 2015; see Chapters 10 and 11).

Auditory and tactile stimuli play a fundamental role in the development of the mental framework and concepts of the very young child with vision impairment. As the child progresses, language also becomes the internal mental framework for understanding the world around them (Galliano and Portalier 2011). Very young children will need to be exposed to language made intelligible to them by initially being directly referenced to their own actions and direct experiences gained through audition and touch (Kekelis and Andersen 1984). There is otherwise a risk that the language input of the parent is based on visually inaccessible information and empty of accessible meaning to the child (Moore and McConachie 1994). The child may develop superficial fluency in expressive language, through using verbal echoing and learned phrases, but the language lacks comprehension and understanding (Dale and Sonksen 2002; see also Chapter 10).

Although there is individual variation, the normative picture is of general developmental delay in all areas compared with young children with typical vision (Vervloed et al. 2000; Dale and Sonksen 2002; Mosca et al. 2015). A considerable proportion have additional neurological impairment (Rahi and Cable 2003) and any accompanying brain disorder impacts further on their rate of learning (Dale et al. 2017). Rates of development are variable in specific domains within and between individual children; time lags can be protracted leading to deceleration in developmental quotients between 10 to16 months and 27 to 54 months in some children (Dale and Sonksen 2002).

Overall, those children with profound vision impairment (no vision, or light perception at best) show the greatest delays and are most at risk (Dale et al. 2017). This was confirmed in a longitudinal study of a national cohort (OPTIMUM) in which the sample included congenital disorders of the peripheral visual system, that is eye globe, retina, and anterior optic nerve (Dale et al. 2019). Those with profound vision impairment lagged behind by an average of 15 developmental quotient points (about 1 year's developmental growth) on Sensorimotor Understanding (Reynell-Zinkin Scales – RZS) when aged between 12 and 36 months, compared with those with severe vision impairment (i.e. having at least basic 'form' vision); the gap was even larger when those children with known brain disorder were included in the analysis. Play is also at risk, with more sensorimotor and stereotypical and less functional play patterns with age-appropriate toys emerging between 12 and 24 months in those with profound visual impairment in the same cohort, compared with those with severe vision impairment.

A high risk of 'developmental setback' has been found especially in those with profound vision impairment (Cass et al. 1994; Dale et al. 2019; Dale and Sonksen 2002). About a third of those with profound vision impairment show plateauing or regression in their second to third year of life, leading to increasing behavioural difficulties and disordered social communication. The complex mechanism for 'developmental setback' is not currently understood, but risk factors include profound vision impairment (light perception at best) and neurological disorders (Dale et al. 2019).

The majority of children with congenital disorders of the peripheral visual system do, however, make progress and gradually reach expected milestones through their early years with the appropriate support (Dale et al. 2019). Some children make excellent steady progress that is in line with or greater than their typically sighted peers, including in language. This points to neuroplasticity in the developmental system with the same macrostructural changes and succession of phase-shifts in language as typically sighted peers but with more protracted phase-shifts and delayed increases of variability in the early phases of development (Peltzer Karpf 2012). The advent of sufficient visual function to see basic form (as in infants with severe vision impairment) and/or language provide a very important means of helping the child access more information and make more sense of their environment, which can accelerate learning (see Chapter 10). Non-verbal and spatial cognition may, however, lag further behind and continue to need careful support (see Chapter 12).

Parent–Child Interactions and Family Resources

A diagnosis of vision impairment causes great shock, distress, anxiety, and worry for parents. Parents have to adapt to their role as a parent of an infant with an uncertain future and reach a greater understanding of their infant's needs. In the OPTIMUM study, mothers showed higher levels of parenting stress than in the community normative population (with one-third in the clinical range) when their infant was 1 year old (Sakkalou et al. 2018). By 2 years of age many parents had started to adapt to their role and no longer showed such elevated stress levels on average, except in those who had an infant who was profoundly visually impaired and perceived as 'difficult' on the Parenting Stress Index (Abidin 1995). There was, however, individual variation in parenting stress levels at both 1 and 2 years. Greater adult anxiety and depression was seen in those mothers with increased parenting stress.

Behavioural problems create an additional challenge and need to be addressed for the child's and the parent's sake. More mothers perceive their child as 'difficult' if their child has profound vision impairment than severe vision impairment at 2 years (Sakkalou et al. 2018). Infants may be initially more passive and quiet in their early months but by the second or third year of life a proportion will become prone to distress and emotional reactivity, frustration, and temper tantrums, or increasing internalising difficulties and withdrawal (Tirosh et al. 1998; Alon et al. 2010; O'Reilly et al. 2017). There may be an underlying brain vulnerability for some infants with a significant association found between EEG measures of 'frontal asymmetry' in the frontal lobes of 1-year-olds with congenital disorders of the peripheral visual system and increased behavioural difficulties at 2 years of age (O'Reilly et al. 2017).

One area of relevance is parental sensitivity and contingency, that is, how the parent responds to the infant and young child's cues, and whether they 'tune into' the child's emotional needs and requirements sensitively, doing this promptly or contingently to the child's cues (van den Broek et al. 2017). In the absence of direct eye contact, establishing positive parent–infant emotional 'attunement' and reciprocal interactions becomes the basis for affective relationship-building, joint attention, and shared learning. Parents vary in their sensitivity and contingency and this may be influenced by their own personal history and make-up and their child's own behavioural repertoire. This early parenting style has been shown to be important in the OPTIMUM national cohort. Mothers rated with greater sensitivity when their infant was 1-year-old had children who made significantly greater progress of 5 developmental quotients (estimated as about 4 developmental months) in their language skills, in particular response to sound and verbal comprehension, from 1 to 3 years of age compared to those with mothers of lower sensitivity. Greater parental contingency was associated with higher sensorimotor developmental quotients at 1 year; this shows the importance of the parent responding to the infant and young child contingently to help build their interest in, manipulation with, and concepts of the object world (Sakkalou et al. 2020).

This research suggests that identification of parenting stress, and targeting positive parenting styles and the behavioural needs of the child, are of clinical and developmental value. There is interest in using video-feedback interventions to promote positive parenting styles, but an initial trial in the Netherlands investigating attachment-based video-feedback for parents of children aged 1 to 5 years was inconclusive with respect to increasing parental sensitivity and parent–child interactions in the treatment condition (Platje et al. 2018).

SUPPORT AND MANAGEMENT

To support the young child and family across the early years, vision impairment needs very prompt early screening and detection and referral to ophthalmology for timely diagnosis and appropriate management. The optimal period for screening for congenital eye defects and for congenital vision impairment is from birth and within the first 4 months to permit early medical treatments for optimal preservation of visual potential (see Chapter 2) and for urgent referral to the early intervention service and paediatric child development service, with implementation of appropriate provision at the earliest opportunity.

Early intervention in the child's home (or the parents' preferred setting) at community level provides the context for delivering the individual child's programme in collaboration with the parent as a shared partner, taking into account the family and their cultural needs and preferences.

Assessment

Regular developmental monitoring and assessment should lead to appropriate guidance with support for the infant and parent to achieve the next developmental steps. Observational and standardised assessment is recommended for the specialist trained clinician in the paediatric child development team or the specialised developmental vision neurodisability service. There is currently only one semi-standardised play-based assessment method, the RZS, for assessing sensorimotor understanding, response to sound, and verbal comprehension and expressive language (structure and vocabulary) between 0 and 5 years (Reynell and Zinkin 1975; see Fig. 8.1). Regular use of the Reynell Zinkin Scales for young children with visual impairment (RZS), across the early years and until school entry age, enables monitoring of progress of the individual child. In addition to goal-setting, it enables the clinician to assess whether the child's progress is steady or uneven across the subscales and also whether the child is progressing according to age expectations for their vision level or whether there is significant developmental delay. Over time, the clinician can judge whether the child has additional developmental needs beyond that expected for vision impairment.

Around a fifth of children with congenital disorders of the peripheral vision system and no known additional brain disorder will show emerging intellectual disability by the

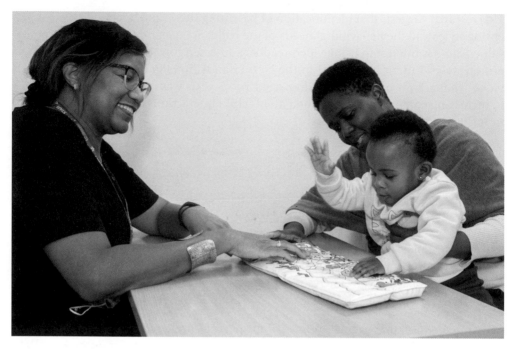

Figure 8.1 Developmental play assessment. (A colour version of this figure can be seen in the colour plate section)

time they are 4 or 5 years old (Dale and Sonksen 2002; Dale et al. 2019). In the national population surveillance (UK) of infants with severe chronic vision impairment, over three-quarters had additional non-ophthalmological impairments and were likely to have more complex neurodisabilities over time (Rahi and Cable 2003), which require early detection and management of needs.

Early Intervention

Due to these developmental risks and vulnerabilities and importance of the parent as the key partner caring for the infant and young child, early intervention is crucial as soon after early diagnosis as possible and in the early months of life (Fazzi et al. 2005).

Different methods of early intervention have been provided in individual countries and also internationally, including the Portage and the Oregon programmes. With the exception of the Developmental Journal (see below) any publicly available materials have not been systematically evaluated for their effectiveness. In 2004 and 2005 the Early Support programme of the UK central government requested that the Developmental Vision team of Great Ormond Street Hospital for Children (London) design and develop a new early intervention programme for young children with vision impairment (0–3 years) based on the principles of the Early Support programme, scientific and clinical developmental

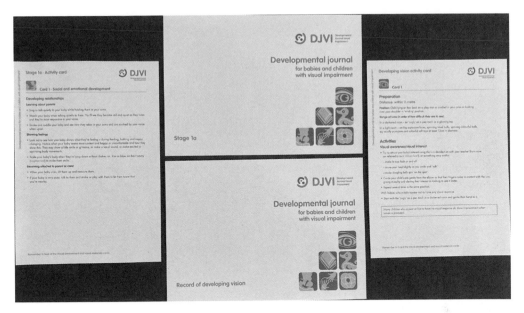

Figure 8.2 Developmental Journal for babies and young children with visual impairment (DJVI, 2nd Edition)

and neuroscience knowledge and expertise for infants and young children with vision impairment and early intervention science with other neurodevelopmental disabilities (Dale and Salt 2007).

The Developmental Journal for babies and young children with visual impairment (DJVI) is a structured developmental and vision developmental framework for tracking and monitoring purposes, and providing activity guidance for goal-setting and achievement (Fig. 8.2; Salt and Dale 2017). It aims to achieve the goals of Box 8.1 and was implemented nationally as a major early intervention programme (Dale and Salt 2007).

The DJVI was designed in partnership with parent and practitioner focus groups. It includes the Developmental Journal, which is a developmental framework for tracking development, and Activity cards, which provide ideas and activities to support the child achieving each step in the Developmental Journal. There is also a Record of Vision, which provides a developmental framework for supporting the development of vision (where possible) and Vision cards to provide guidance for promoting vision (see Chapter 4). The materials are written for parents and are designed to fit into everyday transactions, routines, and practices at home and do not require any special toy materials.

Monitoring of developmental progress in all areas of development (domains of 'Movement and mobility', 'Play and learning' [including Using Hands], 'Social and emotional development', 'Communication, language and meaning', and 'Towards independent self-care') can be undertaken by the practitioner in conjunction with the

> **Box 8.1** Key goals of early intervention
>
> ✓ To track and promote all areas of development and to promote vision development in infants and very young children with vision impairment.
>
> ✓ To mitigate adverse impacts of vision impairment and to prevent cumulative delay and difficulties.
>
> ✓ To enable each child to develop at their optimal rate, taking into account their level of vision and any additional neurological impairments.
>
> ✓ To guide parents in caregiving skills and practices that will support their child's early development and vision and psychological wellbeing, and to enhance parent–child transactions and relating.
>
> ✓ To support partnerships between the parent and practitioner enabling the parent to become involved, informed, and empowered in relation to their child's needs and progress.
>
> ✓ To provide a community framework for supporting families of infants and very young children with vision impairment to support participation and inclusion in society.

parent, encouraging the parent to bring their observations to the planning of the early intervention programme (Dale and Salt 2007).

The parent will need guidance in how to bring the social and physical environment to the infant and very young child through sound and touch, and how to give clear linguistic labelling of the child's early meaningful experiences and emotions. This guidance is given in the area of development, 'Communication, language, and meaning', in the DJVI. Child-centred language of the parent helps linguistic scaffolding of the child's own experiences and ensures that language and communication are linked to the child's own developing understandings of their world.

Another area of higher risk includes 'Social and emotional development'. Themes covered in this area include 'Developing relationships' ('Learning about self and parent/others', 'Showing and understanding feelings', 'Showing "attachment" to parent and familiar others', 'Behaviour and self-regulation'), and 'Social interaction' ('Joining in social interaction', 'Joining in rhyme game', 'Developing early social skills', 'Showing knowledge of social scripts') (see Fig. 8.3).

The booklet 'Getting Stuck' provides a framework and ideas for approaching common problems, including touch sensitivity; sound sensitivity; repetitive behaviours; language concerns/'echolalia' or echoing; resistance to adult direction/tantrums, resistance to change; learning, social, and communication; eating and feeding; and sleeping.

Scientific Evaluation of the Developmental Journal

The first systematic evaluation of early intervention since the 1990s has been an evaluation of the Developmental Journal through a national cohort longitudinal study

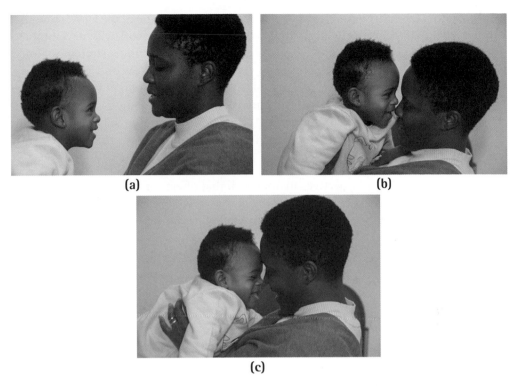

Figure 8.3 Social and emotional development

(OPTIMUM) (Dale et al. 2019). This was undertaken between 2011 and 2016. In 54 infants receiving home-based support from their specialist teacher for the visually impaired, the toatl group receiving intervention with the Developmental Journal made promising higher gains of 5 developmental quotients on average (estimated as about 4 developmental months' gain) in sensorimotor understanding and of 6 developmental quotients on average in structural expressive language on the RZS from aged 1 to 3 years; these are large effect sizes but statistical significance was not reached. In those 34 children with no additional brain disorder, the gains were even higher of 11 developmental quotients on average in structural expressive language in the Developmental Journal group. These gains were evident after controlling for differences in age and level of vision (profound vs severe visual impairment) at the first time point. The group receiving the Developmental Journal also had significantly reduced behaviour withdrawal on the child behavioural questionnaire at final outcome (3 years) compared to those receiving 'other support'. Their mothers reported significantly reduced parenting stress and significantly greater satisfaction with their practitioner including meeting the parent's initial expectations at final outcome. These findings were all in contrast to the 'comparison' group of those receiving 'other forms of support' and not the Developmental Journal.

Key indicators for positive progress and success may be the nature of the Developmental Journal materials including its structured developmental framework with developmental tracking and goal-setting to track and celebrate progress and its strategies aimed to overcome challenges arising from early vision impairment. Second, the participatory-partnership style of the practitioner relationship with the parent to support joint problem-solving and negotiation of the parent's own priorities and personal and cultural style. The intervention materials and strategies appeared to support parents in the process of learning to meet their child's developmental needs through everyday transactions and routines.

From the practitioner's perspective, an approach that offers a 'road map' approach can provide flexibility to create bespoke learning pathways enabling every child to build on their individual strengths and to address areas of vulnerability.

The importance of the integrated vision promotion programme that is embedded in the Developmental Journal is discussed further in Chapter 4.

ENABLING PARTICIPATION

Family-centred care, which is now practised throughout the world by health and education practitioners, has been shown to enhance parental wellbeing, which in turn influences child wellbeing (Dunst and Trivette 2009). Dunst et al. (2014) refer to the foundations of the family capacity-building process and practices including the cycle of introduce and illustrate, engage and support, review and reflect, and new learning opportunities. A key mediating factor is the self-efficacy beliefs of the parent and integral to family-centred care is the need to adopt an empowerment approach to working with the parent (Dale 1995).

The practitioner's knowledge of the impact of vision impairment on early learning is essential in jointly identifying the nuanced approaches that can best support each child and family's individual needs. This sharing of expertise equips families to promote their child's developmental progress and become resilient when facing the challenges that may arise (Dale et al. 2019).

The low incidence of vision impairment leaves many families feeling very isolated and lacking information and guidance to understand their child's visual condition or reinforcing negative emotional reactions regarding opportunities (Lupon et al. 2018). Parents anecdotally report that sharing information, advice, and concerns with those who have similar experiences through personal contact in local or regional family support groups is particularly valuable. Witnessing the progress of other children and families can promote confidence and increase optimism. With the increasing availability of social media, the opportunity to be involved in support networks has been extended to those who may be limited by distance, location, or other circumstances.

The promotion of a positive attitude and focussing on what a child with vision impairment can achieve is important for enabling participation in all developmental and learning situations.

Once the child is attending childcare or a preschool setting, the early intervention programme can be integrated with the mainstream childcare curriculum, as is the case in the context of the Developmental Journal and the Early Years curriculum in England. This alignment offers a favourable means of assisting the child in their first steps in participating in early learning alongside their peers. Using these methods in home and preschool/day care settings provides consistent scaffolding for early learning, avoiding potential contradiction and confusion. From a curriculum perspective, it is important that the preschool centre understands that the very young child with vision impairment is often developing at a slower rate than their typically sighted peers, and needs a high level of one-to-one support and an appropriately adapted programme in order to meet their learning and social and emotional needs. It is valuable for the parent to continue to have access to the early intervention practitioner and receive ongoing guidance in the early years. This is especially so for parents of children with profound vision impairment and with greater developmental needs and behavioural difficulties or emerging social communication difficulties (see Chapter 11), who are most at risk and may need more targeted and longer-term support.

Management of Care in Infancy and Early Years

All infants with confirmed permanent vision impairment should receive early intervention services as soon as possible after diagnosis but ideally starting before 6 months of age and under 12 months. This permits the most effective period for starting developmental promotion of vision (Sonksen et al. 1994; see Chapter 4) and promotion of general development (Dale et al. 2019). These recommendations correspond with the larger scientific literature showing that earlier intervention leads to better outcomes in other disabilities such as at risk of or with autism spectrum disorder (Landa 2018). Evidence also supports regular sustained input with regular visits to the family that continues across the early years for better results (Landa 2018; Dale et al. 2019).

In the early years the optimal integrated management of care for the child and their parent should involve a multidisciplinary health-education network including at least ophthalmology, community child development/paediatric neurodisability, and education as core elements (see Fig. 8.4).

Early intervention is designed to be delivered at community level and can be undertaken by practitioners from a variety of backgrounds including qualified and peripatetic teachers of the visually impaired, habilitation specialists, early years childcare workers, and community health workers. Additional inputs of therapists, such as speech and language therapists, physiotherapists, or occupational therapists, can be integrated with the early intervention programme.

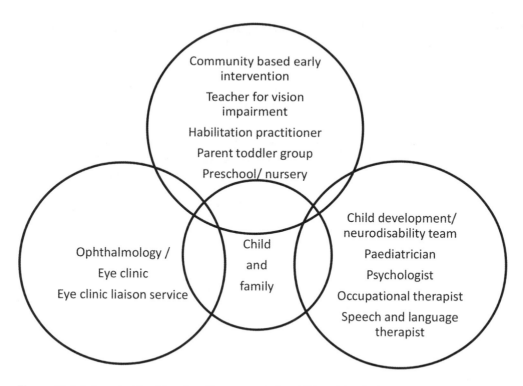

Figure 8.4 Integrated health-education network for child and family in the early years

Training is required in the delivery of early intervention including understanding of the materials and resources as well as in the practice of family-centred care and working with parents in 'partnership'. A set of e-health training materials as part of the Healthy Child Programme (0–5 years) is available for multidisciplinary practitioners providing essential information on supporting infants and young children at neurodevelopmental risk due to disabilities or other challenges to development. The course consists of e-learning sessions including supporting children and young people's development, introducing and using a Developmental Journal, developmental principles of the DJVI, and general developmental principles (e-learning for Health: Healthy Child Programme).

The early interventionist practitioner who knows the child and family well is favourably positioned to act as 'key worker', to integrate liaison and communication between the network, to harmonise early intervention and therapy inputs, and to empower the parents' participation.

Developing Early Intervention in Low-Moderate Income Contexts

As authors in a narrative review point out, studies on early intervention with children at risk of disability and with disabilities in high-income countries have not

Box 8.2 Practice tips for early intervention in low–moderate income countries

✓ Early intervention needs to start as early as possible after the infant's vision impairment has been established.

✓ A practitioner must be allocated to support the infant and family in their community and to provide regular sustained support over the first few years of life.

✓ This can be delivered through a combination of community-based peer group context and individual home visiting, but the effectiveness of each approach is not known.

✓ The practitioner needs experience and expertise in early healthy development of children; they need additional basic training and knowledge of development in infants and young children with vision impairment.

✓ Parents will need practical guidance in how to help promote their child's early vision (if feasible), development, and learning within a structured developmental programme that is adapted to support the infant and young child with vision impairment.

✓ Guidance in responsive caregiving skills should be integrated with the structured developmental programme.

✓ A 'partnership' relationship between the parent and practitioner will help inform and empower the parent, engage in joint problem-solving, and respond to the personal cultural style of the family.

✓ The programme of support must take into account the individual rate of learning of the child; concerns about the rate of progress will need to be followed up by further assessment by a child health service.

been undertaken in a low-moderate income context and more data is needed on the timing of starting early intervention, the dosage or frequency of intervention, and the most effective models in this context (Kohli-Lynch et al. 2019). Emerging evidence supports community-based early intervention with a combination of home visits and community-based groups focussing on peer support, responsive caregiving, and preventing secondary disabling problems. The DJVI has not been formally tested or scientifically evaluated in a moderate-low income country context yet, and it may need tailoring to suit local contexts. However, changing its structure could alter the *fidelity of intervention*, which might reduce its effectiveness (Landa 2018; Dale et al. 2019). See Box 8.2 for some suggested practice tips for supporting infants and families in moderate–low income countries.

IMPLICATIONS FOR RESEARCH AND PRACTICE

The importance of an evidence-based intervention strategy to support the child and family is now established, though the extension of the research to include fathers who play a key role in the family system needs to be undertaken (Huurneman 2018). Future research, including a randomised clinical trial, may seek to further enhance the parental contribution, responsive parenting skills, child-centred communication, and child developmental and behavioural outcomes. Cognitive neuroscience and dynamic systems theory are now starting to model the complex dynamic process between developing neural substrates and environmental experience, such as in specific systems of language acquisition (Pelzer-Karpf 2012). Novel use of functional brain imaging studies could provide further insights into the impact of early experience and early intervention and changes at brain level due to neuroplasticity (see Chapter 7). Future scientific developments of the DJVI, including randomised controlled trials to reach further insights of its mechanism, could include evaluation of its effectiveness in different contexts, including moderate–low income countries, and with different user-friendly formats such as a digital app version for parent-held smartphone or tablet usage.

The value of the RZS for clinical and research purposes is recognised but new norms, further standardisation, and commercial availability would improve its utility in the clinic context and its reliability (Dale and Sonksen 2002; Vervloed et al. 2000). 'Developmental setback' remains a high clinical concern for very young children especially with profound vision impairment; further research is needed to establish the most effective targeted support (Dale et al. 2019).

CONCLUSION

Infants and young children with vision impairment are at risk of delays and challenges to their progress in all areas of development. A multidisciplinary health and education network and community-based early intervention and family support group provision provide the framework of child and family support. Regular assessment and effective early intervention lay the foundation for enhancing the young child's development, meeting additional needs, and empowering parent and family resources and participation.

Key Points

- ✓ Early development across all domains is at high risk of delays and challenges in infants and young children with vision impairment.
- ✓ Parents are at risk of parenting stress in the early years, particularly if their child has profound vision impairment and behaviour challenges.
- ✓ Following timely detection and diagnosis, evidence-based early intervention from the earliest months and through the first years of life is required.
- ✓ Regular clinical assessments and monitoring of development guides early intervention and also detects early signs of additional developmental needs, which need targeted support.
- ✓ Key principles for early intervention are a parent and child-centred structured developmental framework and materials and goal-setting that is designed to support infants and young children with vision impairment, within a participatory practitioner–parent relationship.

REFERENCES

Abidin RR (1995) *Parenting Stress Index,* Third Edition. Odessa FL: Psychological Assessment Resources.

Alon L, Cohen Ophir M, Cohen A, Tirosh E (2010) Regulation disorders among children with visual impairment: a controlled study. *J Dev Phys Disabil* **22**: 57–64.

Cass H, Sonksen P, McConachie H (1994) Developmental setback in severe visual impairment. *Arch Dis Child* **70**: 192–196.

Dale N (1995) *Working with Parents of Children with Special Needs: Partnership and Practice.* London: Routledge.

Dale N, Salt A (2007) Early support developmental journal for children with visual impairment: the case for a new developmental framework for early intervention. *Child Care Hlth Dev* **33**: 684–690.

Dale N, Sonksen P (2002) Developmental outcome, including setback, in young children with severe visual impairment. *Dev Med Child Neurol* **44**: 613–622.

Dale N, Sakkalou E, O'Reilly M, Springall C, De Haan M, Salt A (2017) Functional vision and cognition in infants with congenital disorders of the peripheral visual system. *Dev Med Child Neurol* **59**: 725–731.

Dale NJ, Sakkalou E, O'Reilly M et al. (2019) Home-based early intervention in infants and young children with visual impairment using the Developmental Journal: longitudinal cohort study. *Dev Med Child Neurol* **61**: 697–709.

Dunst CJ, Trivette CM (2009) Meta-analytic structural equation modelling of the influences of family-centered care on parent and child psychological health. *Int J Pediatr,* **2009**: 1–9. doi: 10.1155/2009/576840.

Dunst CJ, Bruder MB, Espe-Sherwindt M (2014) Family capacity-building in early childhood intervention: do context and setting matter? *Sch Comm J* **24**(1): 37–48.

Fazzi E, Signorini SG, Bova SM, Ondei P, Bianchi PE (2005) Early intervention in visually impaired children. *International Congress Series* **1282**: 117–121.

Healthy Child Programme: Early Developmental Support programme (e-learning for health). (2017) https://www.e-lfh.org.uk/programmes/early-developmental-support/ [Accessed July 2021].

Galliano AR, Portalier S (2011) Language and visual impairment: literature review. *Int Psych, Pr Res* **2**: 1–10.

Huurneman B (2018) Heightened parental stress in mothers of children with visual impairment. *Dev Med Child Neurol* **60**: 221.

Kekelis LS, Andersen LS (1984) Family communication styles and language development. *Journal of Visual Impairment and Blindness* **78**(2): 54–65.

Kohli-Lynch M, Tann CJ, Ellis ME (2019) Early intervention for children at high risk of developmental disability in low- and middle-income countries: a narrative review. *Int J Environ Res Public Health* **16**(22): 4449.

Landa R (2018) Efficacy of early interventions for infants and young children with, and at risk, for autism spectrum disorders. *Intern Rev Psychiatry* **30**(1): 25–39.

Lupon M, Armayones M, Cardona G (2018) Quality of life among parents of children with visual impairment: A literature review. *Res Dev Disabil* **83**: 120–131.

Moore V, McConachie H (1994) Communication between blind and severely visually impaired children and their parents. *Brit Journal of Developmental Psychology* **12**: 491–502.

Mosca R, Kritzinger A, Van der Linde J (2015) Language and communication development in preschool children with visual impairment: a systematic review. *S Afr J Commun Disord* **62**: 1–10. doi: 10.4102/sajcd.v62i1.119.

O'Reilly MA, Bathelt J, Sakkalou et al. (2017) Frontal EEG asymmetry and later behavior vulnerability in infants with congenital visual impairment. *Clin Neurophysiol* **128**: 2191–2199.

Peltzer-Karpf A (2012) The dynamic landscape of exceptional language development. *Strabismus* **20**: 69–73.

Platje E, Sterkenburg P, Overbeek M, Kef S, Schuengel C (2018) The efficacy of VIPP-V parenting training for parents of young children with a visual or visual-and-intellectual disability: a randomized controlled trial. *Attach Hum Dev* **20**: 455–472.

Rahi JS, Cable N (2003) Severe visual impairment and blindness in children in the UK. *Lancet* **362**: 1359–1365.

Reynell J, Zinkin P (1975) New procedures for the developmental assessment of young children with severe visual handicaps. *Child Care, Hlth, Dev* **1**: 61–69.

Sakkalou E, O'Reilly MA, Sakki H et al. (2020) Mother-infant interactions with infants with congenital visual impairment and associations with longitudinal outcomes in cognition and language. *J of Child Psych and Psych* **62**(6): 742–750. https://doi.org/10.1111/jcpp.13308.

Sakkalou E, Sakki H, O'Reilly MA, Salt AT, Dale NJ (2018) Parenting stress, anxiety, and depression in mothers with visually impaired infants: a cross-sectional and longitudinal cohort analysis. *Dev Med Child Neurol* **60**: 290–298.

Salt A, Dale N (2017) *Developmental Journal for Babies and Young Children with Visual Impairment (DJVI)*, 2nd Edition (originally Salt A, Dale N, Osborne J, Sonksen P 2005, 1st Edition) https://xip.uclb.com/i/healthcare_tools/DJVI_professional.html [Accessed July 2021].

Sonksen PM (1997) Developmental aspects of visual disorders. *Curr Paediatr* **7**: 18–22.

Tirosh E, Schnitzer M, Davidovitch M, Cohen A (1998) Behavioral problems among visually impaired between 6 months and 5 years. *Int J Rehabil Res* **21**: 63–70.

van den Broek EGC, van Eijden AJPM, Overbeek MM, Kef S, Sterkenburg PS, Schuengel C (2017) A systematic review of the literature on parenting of young children with visual impairments and the adaptions for Video-Feedback Intervention to Promote Positive Parenting (VIPP). *J Dev Phys Disabil* **29**: 503–545. doi: 10.1007/s10882-016-9529-6.

Vervloed MPJ, Hamers JHM, van Mens-Weisz MM, Timmer-van de Vosse H (2000) New age levels of the Reynell-Zinkin developmental scales for young children with visual impairments. *J Visual Impair Blin* **94**: 613–624.

CHAPTER 9

Motor Development and Hand Function

Julia Smyth and Alison Salt

INTRODUCTION

Vision has a powerful influence on motor development, providing necessary feedback for co-ordination of movements and the motivation to move and explore (Sonksen et al. 1984). Children with typical vision use this to guide and refine their gross and fine motor movements, becoming increasingly skilful through the early years (Prechtl et al. 2001; Celeste 2002; Kalagher and Jones 2011; Bakke et al. 2019). Children with severe vision impairment face considerable challenges in the early development of movement, hand function, and proficient functional performance. These essential skills facilitate exploration and navigation, enabling participation in play and self-care activities, and laying the foundations for later independence and autonomy (see Chapter 14; Prechtl et al. 2001; Kalagher and Jones 2011; Haibach et al. 2014). Fine motor skills also enable tactile learning, providing access to the world which is otherwise unseen (Houwen et al. 2009; Withagen et al. 2010).

This chapter reviews evidence concerning the development of functional mobility (use of gross motor skills to navigate the physical environment) and exploratory hand function (use of hands to search for and gather information about an object to enable its purposeful use) in children with severe vision impairment. It considers how these skills may differ from those in peers with typical vision and addresses approaches to assessment and optimisation of engagement and participation.

MOTOR DEVELOPMENT AND VISION IMPAIRMENT

Vision plays a central role in the development of spatial awareness and knowledge. It provides the incentive to move, supporting acquisition of information about the distance and direction of moving objects, allowing anticipation of danger, and supporting the ability to imitate the movements of others (Houwen et al. 2009). Several studies confirm that children with vision impairment are less likely to develop motor skills with the same proficiency, or at the same rate, as their peers with typical vision (Prechtl et al. 2001; Bakke et al. 2019). However, Bakke et al.'s systematic review concluded that there is only limited research (and of moderate quality) that investigates how motor skills develop in children with visual impairment, or how they are used during activities and how they influence participation. The published studies have considerable methodological limitations including small sample sizes. There are, nevertheless, some important themes emerging from the available evidence.

Gross Motor Skills and Functional Mobility

THE EARLY YEARS

Infants and young children with vision impairment show a delay in their acquisition of gross motor skills, compared to children with typical vision (Levtzion-Korach et al. 2000; Celeste 2002). Children with typical neurology and vision impairment demonstrated unusual Fidgety Movements (the spontaneous movements of early infancy seen usually between 9 and 15 weeks post-term), persisting until 8 to 10 months of age (Prechtl et al. 2001). These differences may arise from the absence of vision's modulation on the vestibular and proprioceptive systems (the systems that provide an internal sense of movement, balance, and body position).

Visual–vestibular interactions are responsible for early lateral righting and equilibrium responses in infants, enabling the child to remain balanced and to keep their head in midline during movements. These responses are promoted by the experience of different postures and head positions in physical play, coupled with visual feedback from the environment, for example maintaining an upright position in response to vertical visual information from walls or door frames or reaching out to the floor when sitting. In addition to lacking these visual–vestibular feedbacks, the responses of infants with vision impairment are reduced further by limited motivation for spontaneous postural activities and parental caution during physical play activities.

Some children with vision impairment have low muscle tone (hypotonia) without actual neurological abnormality (Levtzion-Korach et al. 2000), and this impacts on the development of early motor skills. Difficulty with, and slower acquisition of, pre-walking skills such as rolling, sitting, cruising, walking, and stair climbing are found (Celeste 2002). For instance, the infant may be resistant to lying on their front and using their hands to crawl, as this constrains their ability to 'perceive' with their hands.

Lack of vision also limits the child's ability to copy the movements of others. Delays in other aspects of development such as sound localisation and object permanence may impact adversely on motor development, as the young child lacks the understanding and incentive to move towards or explore the object (Fazzi et al. 2002; see Chapter 8).

School Age Years

Early differences in motor function can persist into middle childhood and beyond. Limited visual input to the proprioceptive and vestibular systems contributes to difficulties with skills requiring balance, such as standing on one leg, resulting in a prolonged need to keep both feet on the floor whilst walking and a more hesitant gait (Levtzion-Korach et al. 2000; Hallemans et al 2011). Children who were profoundly visually impaired (mean age 10 years) showed poorer performance in running, jumping, throwing, and object manipulation compared with typically sighted peers (Wagner et al. 2013). In a related study with 100 children aged 6 to 12 years, Haibach et al. (2014) reported more difficulty with movement skills (running, sliding, galloping, leaping, jumping, and hopping) and object control tasks (catching, kicking, striking, dribbling, throwing, and rolling). Skill level was influenced by severity of vision impairment with those who were profoundly visually impaired doing worse, but not according to age. These discrepancies suggest that gross motor skills may emerge differently and the slower skill acquisition is not simply a developmental delay (Haibach et al. 2014; Bakke et al. 2019).

Hallemans et al. (2011) investigated the factors contributing to independent mobility, reporting differences in the gait patterns of children and adults (aged 1–44 years) with vision impairment compared to those with typical vision. The greatest differences were observed in those with little or no vision, with fewer differences observed in those with moderate vision impairment. Those with little or no vision tended to adapt their gait by spending more time with both feet on the ground and by taking shorter steps.

For children with vision impairment with additional disabilities, particularly neuromotor disorders, the acquisition of motor skills is even more challenging. In a study comparing children with cerebral palsy and vision impairment to children with cerebral palsy alone, matched on Gross Motor Function Classification System level and type of cerebral palsy, children with additional vision impairment required a higher level of support from their carers, had reduced functional mobility, and had reduced independence in self-care tasks (Salavati et al. 2014).

Fine Motor Skills and Exploratory Hand Function

Early Years

Hand function emerges differently because reduced vision input creates a higher cognitive demand and memory load, such as perceiving object localisation and permanence, and the properties of objects through sound and touch. A study examined infants aged 9 to 16 months and found that reach to objects and hand use were observed later in infants with vision impairment (Ihsen et al. 2010). Continuous sound-making objects and those that were familiar encouraged reach the most, particularly for children with little or no vision. A previously explored object was considered to reduce the cognitive load of the task, thus making it easier for the child to participate (Ihsen et al. 2010).

Our observational study of children aged 4 to 36 months showed that early hand function was affected by the child's severity of vision impairment and to a lesser extent developmental level (Smyth et al. 2021). Those with profound vision impairment (light perception at best) were the most reluctant to touch objects, at times withdrawing their hands from exploring items. This tactile avoidance reduced opportunities to explore objects actively and therefore to learn from them.

Delays in the development of hand function are likely to be further influenced by gross motor development. For example, a child who is not yet sitting independently has fewer opportunities to reach for objects and to use both hands together for object exploration.

School Age Years

According to experimental research into haptic exploration, Lederman and Klatzky (1987) defined six distinct hand movements (Exploratory Procedures) important for tactile learning: lateral motion, pressure, static contact, unsupported holding, enclosure, and contour-following. Their subsequent research in adults with typical vision found that touch and vision interact when making judgement about object properties, with touch being used more often for judgements about material and vision for judgements about geometric shape (Klatzky et al. 1993). Withagen et al. (2013) found that children aged 7 to 12 years and adults, with and without vision impairment, used the same dominant Exploratory Procedures for judging weight, size, exact shape, and texture as previously described by Lederman and Klatzky (1987). Performance overall was more affected by age than vision status. Limited experience was likely to explain why children demonstrated less efficient exploratory hand function on some tasks (being less accurate and needing more time than adults) and showed wider variation in their Exploratory Procedures (Withagen et al. 2012; Withagen et al. 2013).

Adults with vision impairment were better at judging exact shape and texture than adults with typical vision (Withagen et al. 2012). However, children with vision impairment did not outperform their peers with typical vision and they were slower in exploring for weight. Previously, Withagen et al. (2010) demonstrated that not all haptic skills emerge spontaneously particularly for children with little or no vision. The two areas that may require intervention and habilitative support include searching techniques and recognising objects using touch (Withagen et al. 2010). For children with additional disabilities and neuromotor disorders, spontaneous exploratory hand use may have further challenges and require greater support (McLinden 2004).

SUPPORT AND MANAGEMENT

The Multidisciplinary Team

Supporting motor function requires a multidisciplinary approach. This ideally includes a health-education partnership of paediatricians, occupational therapists, physiotherapists, mobility or habilitation specialists, specialist teachers for vision impairment, sports and recreational clubs, and the child and their parents/carers.

Assessment of Motor Function

Given the challenges to motor skill development in children with vision impairment, careful assessment of the individual child's needs from infancy onwards ensures that risks can be identified and appropriate motor habilitation provided. A key issue for the practitioner is selecting the appropriate assessment methods to guide interventions that support motor function. A systematic review (Bakke et al. 2019) and literature review (Mazella et al. 2014) explored the motor assessments available within the field of vision impairment. Both concluded that there is a lack of tools designed to assess children with vision impairment. The tools for the typically sighted population, even if adapted to accommodate vision impairment, lack reliability and validity for this population.

Bakke et al.'s (2019) systematic review included studies of children with vision impairment (aged 7–10 years) in which standardised assessments were used. They reported that the requirement for task adaptations or exclusions of vision-dependent tasks (such as writing, throwing, catching) in some assessments meant that results could not be considered valid or reliable. Only the Test of Gross Motor Development-2 and Movement Assessment Battery for Children-2 had validity and reliability data for children with low vision. However, the majority of children studied had moderate vision impairment – vision between 6/18 and 6/60 (logMAR 0.5–1.0) – and therefore information on children with lower levels of vision is lacking.

Mazella et al.'s (2014) literature review found that the majority of haptic tests are not suitable for children and reported the Tactual Profile as the only suitable haptic test for children with vision impairment (0–16 years). The assessments reviewed included mostly 3D items, suggesting that there are limited tools to assess the 2D haptic interpretation skills required for braille and tactile images. Another consideration is whether measuring haptic skills in isolation provides accurate information about hand function in daily life.

Early Years

Since assessment tools are limited, practitioners need to rely on systematic observations of the child's motor function and abilities in the early years in order to identify areas of motor strength and difficulty. Making observations of the child's strengths, difficulties, interests, and dislikes during play provides functional information to guide intervention.

For example, focussing gross motor observations on the child's ability to lie prone with the neck extended, roll, walk, cruise, and climb stairs provides information about common challenges to functional mobility in the early years (Levtzion-Korach et al. 2000; Celeste 2002). Similarly, observing the child's Exploratory Procedures, searching techniques, and ability to identify objects by touch provides insights into their exploratory hand use (Lederman and Klatzky 1987; Withagen et al. 2010). The Developmental Journal for babies and young children with visual impairment (DJVI) (Salt and Dale 2017) provides a systematic integrated developmental framework for observing and monitoring progress and identifying appropriate goals, with associated guidance for parents. It covers hand use in 'Play and Learning' (Using Hands) and gross motor skills in 'Movement and Mobility' sections of the Journal (Salt and Dale 2017; see Chapter 8).

School Years

Children with moderate vision impairment or low vision may benefit from assessment using the Movement Assessment Battery for Children-2 or the Test of Gross Motor Development-2. However, these tools should be used cautiously as the validation data comes from two studies only, one with a sample of 40 children and the other with moderate risk of bias (Bakke et al. 2019).

In the absence of more robust assessment tools for children with more severe vision impairment, taking a pragmatic and functional approach to assessment is likely to be most useful. Observing the child complete the task in the environment where it occurs provides detailed information about the challenges facing the individual. Strategies to overcome these barriers can then be addressed.

Motor function, particularly hand use, is associated with cognitive development and may be affected by other neurological conditions, for example children with intellectual disability or multi-disability (including combined vision and hearing impairment) (McLinden 2004). Motor skills need to be considered in the context of the child's overall developmental profile, thus improving the validity and usefulness of observations.

Practical Habilitation

There is little research investigating interventions that support motor function in children with vision impairment, and that take into account the varying levels of severity of vision impairment.

Early Years

Early intervention to address the gross and fine motor needs of children with vision impairment is recommended (Prechtl et al. 2001; Withagen et al. 2012; Haibach et al. 2014). Although evidence is limited, children with more severe vision impairment are likely to benefit from specific support to encourage mobility, hand use and exploration of objects, and to require more time, teaching, environmental modifications, and therapeutic support than children with less severe vision impairment (Haibach et al. 2014; Smyth et al. 2021).

Intervention in the early years should provide children with opportunities to develop postural control and movement play from the early months (Levtzion-Korach et al. 2000; Prechtl et al. 2001). Strategies to encourage development of sound localisation (e.g. reach to sound) are also fundamental to the development of movement (Fazzi et al. 2002). Tactile modelling, physical guidance, and specific teaching are required to help young children to take part in gross motor tasks and activities. They may need many repetitions and extra time to become proficient in novel skills (Haibach et al. 2014).

The evidence to date would suggest that the DJVI (Salt and Dale 2017) as a holistic framework including gross and fine motor skills is the best approach to facilitate these skills. Infants whose parents received the DJVI made clinically relevant longitudinal progress from 1 to 3 years on the Sensorimotor Understanding scale (Reynell-Zinkin Scales) compared to those who did not receive the DJVI (Dale et al. 2019). Success on this scale incorporates fine manipulation of objects including inserting bricks into boxes and putting lids on and off containers, screwing and unscrewing a small bottle, and sorting and manipulating bricks and beads into a container. The holistic developmental programme designed for infants includes everyday techniques described in the DJVI Activity cards to encourage participation in motor activities and development of hand skills. The cards are linked to the appropriate 'Stage' of development in the DJVI, based on observations and tracking, which ensures the child's readiness for each activity. Techniques are specifically designed to include, for example, helping the infant to roll over or to tilt and find the solid base around them to support postural saving reactions or to be encouraged to move towards motivating objects and sound cues.

Play with objects used in everyday life includes exploration of a range of textures and encourages the child's understanding and participation in self-care tasks. For example, play with a hairbrush includes exploration of the bristles, smooth handle, and the object's function. This approach to introducing textural exploration is preferred to introducing textures that are not meaningful to the child. Introducing new textures to the back of a child's hand first, before they begin to explore, may also be more readily tolerated, as the back of the hand is less sensitive than the palm. Guiding the child's hand by gently moving the child's arm from behind the elbow to help them to explore has been well tolerated as advocated in the DJVI (Salt and Dale 2017). Infants often resist when their hand is taken and moved forward to explore. The 'hand-under-hand' approach (adult placing their hand under a child's hand to participate in an activity) to help a child to explore is advocated by some professionals, although there is limited evidence of effectiveness. In this passive, adult-led approach, the child does not have the opportunity to demonstrate initiative, choice, or control over their participation in the task. This approach may, however, provide an opportunity to develop joint attention. Cautious interpretation of the child's level of skill is required when using this approach.

Some children may become particularly avoidant of tactile exploration and ideas to support a systematic approach to this difficulty is set out in the *Getting Stuck* booklet of the DJVI.

MIDDLE CHILDHOOD

In a systematic review of interventions that improve functioning, quality of life, and participation in children with vision impairment including randomised and non-randomised controlled trials, the results suggest that sports camps might be effective in improving functioning and elements of participation and quality of life (Elsman et al. 2019). The results should be interpreted with caution because of moderate to high risk of bias and suboptimal reporting.

Creating environments that promote motor development is an important part of intervention. With school aged children, providing parent education and offering families resources to enable their children's participation in activities, such as sports, was shown to increase the children's physical activity, particularly for males (Robinson and Lieberman 2007). Using tactile graphics workbooks has been shown to be an effective way to support children's interest in reading material and to support their conceptual understanding through actively exploring the images using both hands (Ryles and Bell 2009).

Children with cerebral visual impairments and neuromotor conditions may require more intensive environmental accommodations and parent or caregiver coaching from specialist therapists. Strategies to improve their postural support, manual techniques, and verbal prompting are likely to enhance participation in tasks (Salavati et al. 2014).

IMPLICATIONS FOR RESEARCH AND PRACTICE

There is a need for high-quality studies investigating the gross and fine motor development of children with vision impairment (Bakke et al. 2019). This would enable practitioners and families to identify deviations from expected norms and to provide timely assistance. Assessment tools for children with vision impairment that consider mobility and hand function in the context of overall development are needed (Mazella et al. 2014; Bakke et al. 2019; Smyth et al. 2021). Adaptation and normative referencing of existing motor tools for use with children with vision impairment may be a practicable solution.

Developmental assessments for young children are often reliant on observing the way that the child uses their hands to manipulate play materials (such as in the Reynell-Zinkin Scales). As vision level may have an influence on hand use, this relationship would benefit from further research. Understanding the developmental vulnerability of the subgroup of children with vision impairment who present with a reluctance to touch objects is also needed. As many children with vision impairment have additional disabilities, understanding the impact of vision impairment on motor function in these children would provide breadth to this field.

The evidence to date highlights the importance of supporting infants and young children's fine and gross motor development in the context of a parent-mediated, structured, holistic developmental programme, like the DJVI (Dale et al. 2019). This could be explored further to consider the specific impact of the DJVI on motor functioning and how to ensure best practice of the practitioner facilitators. Further research to support intervention for motor function in older preschool and school-aged children is necessary to guide the provision of habilitation services for children with vision impairment, see Chapter 14. Future studies should focus on those promising interventions for which effectiveness is still unclear (e.g. mobility, social skills), with adequately designed methodology (Elsman et al. 2019).

SUMMARY

Children with severe vision impairment face motor skill challenges that are unique and benefit from support from infancy onwards. Understanding the complex development of motor skills within childhood vision impairment provides a strong rationale for assessment and intervention to support these skills. With the appropriate support, environmental adaptations, habilitation, and mobility guidance, many children will overcome early motor challenges and can become increasingly proficient in motor skills and daily tasks. Some children will continue to have motor challenges, particularly if they also have neuromotor differences, requiring environmental adaptations. There are significant gaps in the scientific knowledge needed to guide assessment and management within the field and a more robust evidence-base is needed.

Key Points

✓ Severity of vision reduction and developmental level both influence early hand use, with profound vision impairment having the greatest challenging impact.

✓ Targeted early intervention that facilitates functional mobility and exploratory hand use within a holistic developmental framework is likely to be the most beneficial.

✓ The scope and nature of interventions offered to children should take into account the child's severity of vision reduction, developmental level, and additional disabilities particularly neuromotor.

✓ As the child progresses, opportunity for participation in sports and physical activities help to improve functioning, participation, and quality of life.

REFERENCES

Bakke HA, Cavalcante WA, Oliveira IS de, Sarinho SW, Cattuzzo MT (2019) Assessment of motor skills in children with visual impairment: a systematic and integrative review. *Clin Med Insights Pediatr* 13: 1–10. doi: 10.1177/1179556519838287.

Celeste M (2002) A survey of motor development for infants and young children with visual impairments. *J Vis Impair Blind* 96: 169–174. doi: 10.4324/9780203440971.

Dale NJ, Sakkalou E, O'Reilly MA et al. (2019) Home-based early intervention in infants and young children with visual impairment using the Developmental Journal: longitudinal cohort study. *Dev Med Child Neurol* **61**: 697–709. doi: 10.1111/dmcn.14081.

Elsman E, Al Baaj M, van Rens GH et al. (2019) Interventions to improve functioning, participation, and quality of life in children with visual impairment: a systematic review. *Surv Ophthalmol* **64**: 512–557. doi: 10.1016/j.survophthal.2019.01.010.

Fazzi E, Josée L, Oreste FG et al. (2002) Gross motor development and reach on sound as critical tools for the development of the blind child. *Brain Dev* **24**: 269–275. doi: 10.1016/s0387-7604(02)00021-9.

Haibach PS, Wagner MO, Lieberman LJ (2014) Determinants of gross motor skill performance in children with visual impairments. *Res Dev Disabil* **35**: 2577–2584. doi: 10.1016/j.ridd.2014.05.030.

Hallemans A, Ortibus E, Truijen S, Meire F (2011) Development of independent locomotion in children with a severe visual impairment. *Res Dev Disabil* **32**: 2069–2074. doi: 10.1016/j.ridd.2011.08.017.

Houwen S, Visscher C, Lemmink KAPM, Hartman E (2009) Motor skill performance of children and adolescents with visual impairments: a review. *Except Child* **75**: 464–492. doi: 10.1177/001440290907500405.

Ihsen E, Troester H, Brambring M (2010) The role of sound in encouraging infants with congenital blindness to reach for objects. *J Vis Impair Blind* **104**: 478–488.

Kalagher H, Jones SS (2011) Developmental change in young children's use of haptic information in a visual task: the role of hand movements. *J Exp Child Psychol* **108**: 293–307. doi: 10.1016/j.jecp.2010.09.004.

Klatzky RL, Lederman SJ, Matula DE (1993) Haptic exploration in the presence of vision. *J Exp Psychol Hum Percept and Perform* **19**(4): 726–743. https://doi.org/10.1037/0096-1523.19.4.726.

Lederman SJ, Klatzky RL (1987) Hand movements: a window into haptic object recognition. *Cogn Psychol* **19**: 342–368.

Levtzion-Korach O, Tennenbaum A, Schnitzer R, Ornoy A (2000) Early motor development of blind children. *J Paediatr Child Health* **36**: 226–229. doi: 10.1046/j.1440-1754.2000.00501.x.

Mazella A, Albaret J-M, Picard D (2014) Haptic tests for use with children and adults with visual impairments: a literature review. *J Vis Impair Blind* **108**: 227–237.

McLinden M (2004) Haptic exploratory strategies and children who are blind and have additional disabilities. *J Vis Impair Blind* **98**: 99–115.

Prechtl HFR, Cioni G, Einspieler C, Bos AF, Ferrari F (2001) Role of vision on early motor development: lessons from the blind. *Dev Med Child Neurol* **43**: 198–201.

Robinson R, Lieberman LJ (2007) Influence of parent resource manual on physical activity levels of children with visual impairments. *RE:view* **39**: 129–139.

Ryles R, Bell E (2009) Participation of parents in the early exploration of tactile graphics by children who are visually impaired. *J Vis Impair Blind* **103**: 625–634.

Salavati M, Rameckers EAA, Steenbergen B, Van Der Schans C (2014) Gross motor function, functional skills and caregiver assistance in children with spastic cerebral palsy (CP) with and without cerebral visual impairment (CVI). *Eur J Physiother* **16**: 159–167. doi: 10.3109/21679169.2014.899392.

Salt A, Dale N (2017) *Developmental Journal for Babies and Young Children with Visual Impairment*, 2nd Edition. London: Great Ormond Street Hospital for Children. Available at: <https://xip.uclb.com/i/healthcare_tools/DJVI_professional.html> [Accessed 28 July 2021].

Smyth J, Richardson J, Salt A (2021) The associations between vision level and early hand use in children aged 6–36 months with visual impairment: a cross-sectional, historical case note review. *Br J Vis Impair*. doi: 10.1177/0264619621994867.

Sonksen PM, Levitt S, Kitzinger M (1984) Identification of constraints acting on motor development in young visually disabled children and principles of remediation. *Child Care Health Dev* **10**: 273–286.

Wagner MO, Haibach PS, Lieberman LJ (2013) Gross motor skill performance in children with and without visual impairments – research to practice. *Res Dev Disabil* **34**: 3246–3252. doi: 10.1016/j.ridd.2013.06.030.

Withagen A, Kappers AML, Vervloed MPJ, Knoors H, Verhoeven L (2012) Haptic object matching by blind and sighted adults and children. *Acta Psychol (Amst)* **139**: 261–271. doi: 10.1016/j.actpsy.2011.11.012.

Withagen A, Kappers AML, Vervloed MPJ, Knoors H, Verhoeven L (2013) The use of exploratory procedures by blind and sighted adults and children. *Atten Percept Psychophys* **75**: 1451–1464. doi: 10.3758/s13414-013-0479-0.

Withagen A, Vervloed MPJ, Janssen NM, Knoors H, Verhoeven L (2010) Tactile functioning in children who are blind: a clinical perspective. *J Vis Impair Blind* **104**: 43–54.

CHAPTER 10

Language and Communication Development

Steve Rose, Kim Bates, and Rebecca Greenaway

INTRODUCTION

Communication connects; language has a distinct role in maintaining relationships, supporting learning, and sharing experiences. Vision supports communication from birth by helping to establish early communication dyads: interest in faces and eye contact steer motivation to vocalise during interaction. As children acquire language, they must integrate this with shared attention and begin to discern patterns in language and linguistic processing. Vision plays a key role in supporting these processes and supports the establishment of shared meaning.

Infants with a vision impairment may be passive and less interested in the world around them. Establishing joint attention through vision is difficult or impossible. This can result in less motivation, fewer means to communicate, and failed attempts at interaction. James and Stojanovik (2007) reported that the impact of vision impairment on communication development has been underestimated in young children.

As the young child's skills develop, their language ability can help compensate for reduced or absent vision and help scaffold experiences and facilitate learning and understanding.

This chapter explores current research relating to language development in children with vision impairment. It addresses the challenges of assessment including the considerations needed to undertake a holistic and meaningful assessment of language abilities. Intervention approaches to support language development and identification of research areas for further study will be discussed.

Table 10.1 The multiple domains of language

Phonology	The sound units and rules of the speech sound system in the language.
Morphology	The rules that determine how the minimal units of language are applied and used to form words in language.
Syntax	The rule-based system of how words are brought together to make sentences.
Semantics	How words and word combinations come together to form meaning.
Pragmatics	The application of words, sentences, and non-verbal features in different contexts to facilitate discourse and conversation.

LANGUAGE DEVELOPMENT

Definition of Issues

Language learning is an ongoing developmental process with rapid learning in the first 5 years of life. In early language learning, vision impairment may affect social interaction, joint attention, non-verbal communication, formation of verbal concepts (meaning – semantics), communication (pragmatics), and linguistic structure itself.

Language comprises multiple domains that create a 'dynamic integrated whole' (Berko Gleason 2005; see Table 10.1). In addition to these domains, Gillon (2004) highlights the importance of 'higher order language skills' including inference, comprehension, self-monitoring ('am I understanding you'), interpretation of complex language, as well as meta-linguistic skills (using language to describe and reflect on language).

There is limited quality research on speech and language skills among children with vision impairment. The prevalence of language difficulties may have been underestimated, since difficulties are often attributed to the child's vision impairment or their social communication deficits, intellectual disability, or other co-occurring conditions. This is highlighted in a systematic review of language and communication development in preschool children with vision impairment (Mosca et al. 2015). This review reported that although communication and language difficulties are common, the specific impact of vision impairment on communication was difficult to disentangle from that of other possible co-occurring conditions. They conclude that difficulties are particularly apparent in the early stages of language development.

CHILDREN WITH VISION IMPAIRMENT

Infancy and Early Years

Difficulties establishing eye contact and detecting facial expression and gestures affect early social reciprocity, a key foundation for language development. These challenges may lead to delays in the early acquisition of word meanings and conceptual understanding until language itself can aid these processes. Initiation of joint tactile attention becomes more effective as language develops in young children with profound vision impairment (Bigelow 2003).

Visual cues also contribute to the developing speech-sound system. Among individuals with typical vision, the additional benefit of seeing the speaker compared to just listening to speech leads to more efficient speech perception (Campbell 2007). This integration of auditory and visual sensory information during speech processing occurs in infancy prior to the development of language. Although research with children with vision impairment is limited, an increased prevalence of speech-sound difficulties was found in children with vision impairment and additional co-occurring conditions (Brouwer et al. 2015).

Studies suggest that language acquisition in children with vision impairment follows the same patterns as children with typical sight, though at a slower rate; language delay relative to peers with typical vision is more evident in the early developmental stages (McConachie and Moore 1994; Dale and Sonksen 2002; Dale et al. 2019).

Differences in early pragmatic aspects of language have been highlighted, including difficulties securing the personal pronouns 'I' and 'me', and an increased use of questions. These pragmatic differences influence how language is applied in social situations and thereby affect the developmental trajectory itself. Given many social cues are visual in nature, it is not surprising that children with vision impairment may have greater difficulty in this area. Indeed, children with vision impairment may regularly hear words that are not meaningfully connected to their current experience because its meaning is visually inaccessible to them.

Echolalia (repeating a word/phrase uttered by another person) is an early stage of typical development that occurs when a child's receptive language outperforms their expressive language. The social desire to communicate in the context of reduced vocabulary or syntactic or semantic skills leads to the child repeating language in order to fulfil their turn in the interaction. This is particularly seen in the enjoyment and participation of social rhymes and vocal routines (Norgate et al. 1998). As expressive language develops, echolalia diminishes. Persistence of echolalia, which is more common in young children with vision impairment, may be an indicator of social communication weakness or a challenge with expressive language development.

Some evidence has been found that the early vocabulary development of children with vision impairment reflects their differing perceptual experience compared to peers with typical vision. For example, young children with profound vision impairment have been found to have a greater proportion of action words compared to object labels and more words relating to non-visual sensory experience (McConachie and Moore 1994). This included more words relating to tactile and movement experiences (e.g. bath and swing) and fewer animal names; the authors suggest young children with vision may be more readily able to learn through experience with picture books.

School-Aged Childhood

A significant proportion of children with vision impairment overcome these early challenges and achieve relatively fluent language by about 5 years. Compared to peers with typical vision, school-aged children with vision impairment may exceed their performance on accessible measures of verbal short-term memory and structural language ability (Tadić et al. 2010).

A possible area of vulnerability in language development is verbal concept development and 'deep word' learning (Vervloed et al. 2014): a child might be able to use the word correctly within a sentence without fully understanding its meaning. Words that pose particular difficulty include concrete words that are outside the child's direct experience and abstract words which do not have a concrete reference. A study of verbal definitions of objects given by children with vision impairment found their descriptions included relatively greater reference to tactile and auditory characteristics (Vinter et al. 2013). As word meaning is argued to be grounded in experience, the authors argue this reflects the differing experiences of children with and without vision impairment.

Relatively more research has explored pragmatic language in school-aged children with vision impairment. Pragmatic language refers to the use and comprehension of language within context. Studies utilising parent-reported measures of everyday language indicate a relative weakness in pragmatic language compared to structural language ability among children with vision impairment (James and Stojanovik 2007; Tadić et al. 2010), including difficulty with initiation and use of context.

Risk Factors and Protective Issues

Studies that have explored language development in children with congenital disorders of the peripheral visual system and no known brain impairment have found that severity of vision impairment is a risk factor for slower language development in the early years (Dale and Sonksen 2002). Having some degree of 'form' vision (see Chapter 4) has been found to be a protective factor and children with profound vision impairment (light perception at best) are at greatest risk of language delay (Reynell and Zinkin 1975; Dale and Sonksen 2002).

Childhood vision impairment can affect parent–child interaction (see Chapter 8). Parents who are attuned to their child's vocal and touch cues are able to compensate for the absence of shared gaze in their interactions (Bigelow 2003). There is evidence for a protective role of parental factors. In the OPTIMUM study, higher parental sensitivity with infants with severe–profound vision impairment predicted a longitudinal acceleration in verbal comprehension with an average increase of five developmental quotient points on the Reynell-Zinkin Scales (Expressive Language: Structure) from 1 to 3 years (Sakkalou et al. 2021).

The co-occurrence of hearing impairment with vision impairment in childhood occurs due to pre- or perinatal factors, genetic conditions (e.g. Usher syndrome, CHARGE), or infection. This dual sensory disability further complicates language acquisition and may increase feelings of isolation and depression (Hersh 2013).

Research into the language abilities of school-aged children with vision impairment without additional needs is sparse, though there is some evidence for relative strengths in aspects of language development such as sentence recall (Tadić et al. 2010). Neuroimaging studies in adults with vision impairment show that the visual circuits of the occipital cortex may be used for processing language involving sentence comprehension tasks; this was found in those adults with early onset blindness (as against later onset) suggesting a 'sensitive period' for plasticity of the neural cortex (Bedny et al. 2012; see Chapter 7).

ASSESSMENT AND PRACTICE

The Multidisciplinary Team

The multidisciplinary team has an important role to play in the assessment and habilitation of language skills, with relevant input from speech and language therapists, neurodisability paediatricians, psychologists, early years practitioners, teachers, habilitation specialists, and specialist teachers for the visually impaired. They need to work closely together with the parents to reach a holistic perspective and to interpret the child's language skills in the context of overall development and needs.

Speech and language therapists can assess multiple aspects of receptive and expressive language skills, advise on language target setting and the communication environment, and may also provide direct intervention. The health team will need to work closely with education to understand the child's language needs and devise an integrated programme of support, in partnership with the parents. Multidisciplinary working is vital to ensure that language is considered alongside other abilities and needs to include vision, cognition, motor, social communication, and overall paediatric status.

Assessment

Pre-language and language skills need to be monitored and enhanced from the first months of life. As part of an early intervention programme, the Developmental Journal for babies and young children with visual impairment (DJVI) (Salt and Dale 2017), there is a structured developmental framework for use with the parent in the home environment (see Chapter 8). It includes a focus on the domain of 'Communication, language, and meaning'. Monitoring of the child's language progress helps identify when a child may be experiencing greater difficulty in language and communication, and can therefore guide referral to specialist language assessment and intervention.

The Reynell-Zinkin Scales for young children with vision impairment are semi-standardised developmental scales that have three relevant subscales for the assessment of early language alongside a subscale assessing sensorimotor understanding for the 0 to 5-year age range (Reynell and Zinkin 1975). The scales have age equivalents based on 'blind' and 'partial sighted' norms, and can help to identify when language development is deviating from normative expectations. Although this is currently the best available developmental scale for young children with vision impairment, it does not meet modern psychometric standards and the norms are in need of updating (Dale et al. 2019). Nevertheless, it remains a very useful clinical tool to monitor progress.

There are no formal language measures designed specifically for school-aged children with vision impairment. Table 10.2 provides examples of assessment tools for assessing language skills that have been used with children with vision impairment from infancy to older school-aged. Standard language assessments typically use picture materials for eliciting language, which make them inaccessible for this population. A further challenge is that standard measures are not validated for use with children with vision impairment. The individual language trajectories of children with vision impairment has elements that are unique to and can vary within this population. Not enough is understood about these factors to rely on assessments standardised on the general child population. Utilising only the subscales that are auditory-verbal in an assessment could provide a limited or even distorted picture of the spectrum of language abilities, with working memory being a key component of sentence recall for instance. Non-verbal domains for eliciting language comprehension or expression are inappropriate for those with insufficient vision. Aspects of processing, categorising, decoding of semantic, morphological, or phonological aspects of language may not be easily assessed.

In the absence of appropriate tools, speech and language therapists have a number of practical options, as follows:

1. to adopt subtests from standardised assessments that rely solely upon auditory presentation;
2. to use language sampling procedures to evaluate speech and language production skills, such as language sample analysis;
3. to modify subtests of standardised assessments or language assessment procedures, e.g. enlargement of pictorial material or production in a tactile medium;
4. to introduce relevant objects to support auditory-verbal stimulus;
5. to use structured developmental or observation checklists and/or use functional assessments of the child's language functions in everyday context.

Table 10.2 Assessment tools for assessing language skills that have been used with children with vision impairment

	Language	Speech	Functional assessment
Infancy and preschool	• Reynell-Zinkin Scales: Developmental Scales for young children with visual impairment (Reynell and Zinkin 1975) • Pre-School Language Scales (Zimmerman et al. 2014) • Language sample	• PACS (Phonology Assessment of Child Speech – toys edition) (Grunwell and Harding 1995) • Speech sample	• Communication Matrix (Rowland 2012) • Developmental Journal for babies and young children with Vision Impairment (Salt and Dale 2017) • The Oregon Project Developmental Checklists (SOESD 2007) • MacArthur-Bates Communicative Development Inventory (Fenson et al. 2007)
School-aged	• Clinical Evaluation of Language Fundamentals (selected subtests) (Semel et al. 2017) • Boehm Test of Basic Concepts (Boehm 2001) • LARSP (Language Assessment, Remediation, and Screening Procedure) (Crystal et al. 1976) • Language sample	• DEAP (Diagnostic Evaluation of Articulation and Phonology) (Dodd et al. 2002) • ALPHA Test of Phonology (Delayed Sentences) • Speech sample	• Communication Matrix • Derbyshire Language Scheme (Knowles and Masidlover 1982)

Taking into consideration the limitations of modified assessment materials, aspects of the 'overall language picture' can be considered using subtests from language assessments that do not require vision and only involve the auditory-verbal mode. This includes tasks based on repetition, auditory comprehension, sentence formulation, and semantic knowledge. This is feasible once conceptual and language level is at a 5- to 6-year developmental age or higher. This language stage is reaching a metalinguistic level (Blank et al. 1978) where there is reflection on, relating to and explaining the language code itself. The speech and language therapist should supplement the language assessment by taking language samples, including word, sentence, narrative, and conversational levels, and utilising language analysis tools to explore the phonetic, semantic, morphological, and linguistic examination as appropriate to need.

Language tasks can be adapted using objects to manipulate, rather than pictures; however, care needs to be taken to ensure that the child has appropriate conceptual understanding

> **Box 10.1** Principles for good practice of assessment and intervention
>
> ✓ Consult the parent, practitioner, and other sources regarding the child's vision and developmental level and establish whether the child is a tactile learner or has low vision.
>
> ✓ Undertake an analysis of the assessment task you are using to tap into the child's language skills. Is it suitable for the child's vision level? Is the task measuring what it purports to measure and what you need to focus on?
>
> ✓ Consider whether visual materials should be adapted to make them accessible, e.g. enlargement, high contrast, or presenting in an auditory or tactile way.
>
> ✓ If using object items, check that the child recognises their conceptual identity before using them in a language test.
>
> ✓ Provide extra time for the child to perceive any visual information presented or to process the auditory language itself (which may be more difficult without visual cues).
>
> ✓ Provide breaks if the child is becoming more distractible and losing concentration.
>
> ✓ Utilise repetition before expecting a response, if the test permits this, to minimise greater load on auditory working memory.

of these. For example a child may be able to distinguish the texture and shape of a 'smooth square' or 'bumpy triangle' but not understand the descriptive language. Given the challenges identified, there is a case for undertaking cumulative functional assessments in a familiar setting, such as home or school, rather than a single time point in the clinic and monitoring the child's progress or needs. This will lead to a fuller and more accurate assessment of the child's ability and needs over time (Hasson and Joffe 2007).

Box 10.1 outlines principles of good practice for designing or undertaking a speech and language assessment with the child with vision impairment.

Identification of Speech and Language Disorder

Although there is a known delay in early language development in children with severe-profound vision impairment (see earlier), it is often assumed that children will 'catch-up' in their language skills once they have acquired basic language skills. However, there remain additional risks such as social communication and pragmatic weakness (see Chapter 11) or semantic challenges due to cognitive and conceptual problems (see Chapter 12).

Some children continue to have language delays greater than other areas of development, unusual use of language or specific problems (e.g. disorganised speech or dysfluency, phonetic problems, word retrieval difficulties) beyond 5 years old. These difficulties are likely to be more entrenched, longstanding, and have greater functional impact and may be an additional impairment not explained by the vision impairment. This will require the consideration of specialist speech and language therapy support. Differential diagnosis of language disorder in the context of possible intellectual disability, attentional disorder, or autism spectrum disorder remains challenging.

HABILITATION AND LANGUAGE FUNCTION

A systematic review highlights the impact of vision impairment on early language and communication development and the need for speech and language therapy intervention (Mosca et al. 2015). The International Classification of Functioning, Disability and Health: Children and Youth (ICF-CY) model is helpful in informing assessment to identify where the strengths and weaknesses are in the child's language profile, including in relation to activity and participation and environmental factors that may be influencing language.

From an intervention perspective, it is important to consider the child's language and communication activity and participation in their everyday contexts, and what is important for the child and family. The American Speech-Language-Hearing Association outlines how the ICF-CY framework can be used to support goal-setting for children with a language disorder and this has been adapted by the authors for children with vision impairment, see Figure 10.1. When using this framework, it will be important to consider

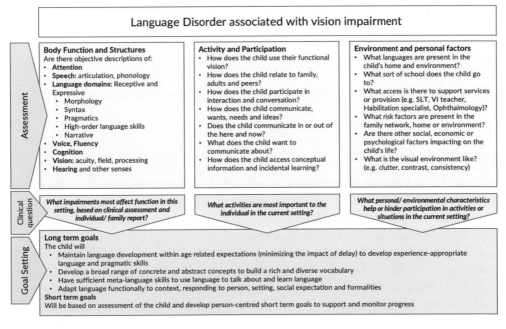

Figure 10.1 Goal setting for children with language disorder within the context of ICF-CY framework, American Speech-Language-Hearing Association case study framework (2020) adapted for children with vision impairment

the child's vision level under Body Function and Structures; how the child uses their functional vision under Activity and Participation; and the layout and modification of the physical or social environment and support services (including habilitation specialist and specialist teacher for vision impairment and other community services) under Environment and Personal factors.

Infancy and Early Years

Promoting language within everyday interactions with parents in the home environment fits within the Activity and Participation domain (ICF-CY) and is integral to early intervention (see Chapter 8). An observational longitudinal evaluation study (OPTIMUM) found clinically relevant gains in expressive language in those receiving home-based intervention with the DJVI, compared to those receiving home-based intervention without the DJVI (Dale et al. 2019). Structured developmental monitoring is combined with activity cards and ideas for everyday activities that can promote language development as well as all other areas of development. This is the first empirical study to show that early intervention can accelerate expressive language development with this population, and highlights the importance of an evidence-based early intervention programme through the vulnerable early years.

As well as supporting early language and communication development, early intervention can help to identify those children who need additional speech and language therapy intervention. For children who meet speech and language therapy intervention criteria, Parent–Child Interaction Therapy (Eyberg and Funderburk 2011) offers an evidence-based approach for children with language delay and disorder with other clinical populations. This is an appropriate intervention for preschool and early primary school aged children with a vision impairment as long as principles of good practice are considered.

School-Aged Children

The speech and language therapist will draw on their clinical skills, expertise, and knowledge of evidence-based language interventions to support areas of need highlighted in the assessment. Most evidence-based language interventions are designed for children with typical vision, see meta-analysis of interventions for children with developmental speech and language delays/disorders (Law et al. 2004). These may be used with caution and adapted for children with vision impairment but their efficacy may not necessarily be in line with the original scientific evaluation. No language intervention programme has been systematically evaluated with children with vision and language impairment to the authors' knowledge.

Intervention aims to support a child's area of need and this can include more than one intervention approach, using the good practice principles (see Box 10.1). As well as working on expressive and comprehension language skills, focussing on the pragmatic and social communicative use of language may be appropriate for older children (see Chapter 11).

Resources such as the Communication Trust's What Works Database review the evidence for and effectiveness of approaches that could be considered. The speech and language therapist should work collaboratively with specialist teachers/primary support worker with expertise in vision impairment to adapt intervention approaches so that they are suitable for the child's level of vision and related needs.

IMPLICATIONS FOR RESEARCH AND CLINICAL PRACTICE

Mosca et al. (2015) highlight the vulnerability of language and communication development, especially at the very early stages of language development. It is recognised that some children with vision impairment show a delay in early language development and there is a risk in assuming all children will 'catch-up' in their language skills. Children with vision impairment are at higher risk of co-occurring neurodevelopmental difficulties including cognition, social communication, autism spectrum disorder, or language difficulties. Therefore, children presenting with early delays in language should be offered early intervention for language and communication as part of their total early intervention programme (see Chapter 8). However, if delays and disorders persist, more targeted assessment and intervention may be required.

There is a great deal that is unknown about language development and protective and risk factors influencing its long-term development in children with vision impairment. Research is needed to investigate interventions to enhance functional activity and participation aspects of language use in everyday environments (including with randomised controlled trials), as argued for other populations with speech impairment according to ICF-CY models (Cunningham et al. 2017). These authors advocate the use of participation-based outcome measures to detect meaningful change in the lives of children and families.

The relative rarity of vision impairment compared to other conditions causing communication difficulties creates difficulty for the individual practitioner to acquire appropriate expertise. Special interest groups can help, as can close working with other practitioners who have experience and expertise with this group of children.

SUMMARY

Although many children with vision impairment reach high levels of fluency and expertise in their language skills, the early years are vulnerable for development in language, speech, and communication. Difficulties can persist in some children, with common vulnerability in pragmatic use of language, and the language domain needs careful monitoring and intervention where difficulties are identified.

Key Points

✓ Language development is vulnerable in the early years, with delays and atypical features.

✓ Later outcomes are variable and those children with no additional co-occurring conditions may develop strong linguistic skills.

✓ Early environmental factors including early intervention and parenting support may accelerate the rate of language development.

✓ Monitoring and assessment of language is recommended in the early years (and later if necessary) with referral to a speech and language therapist where concerns are identified; the challenges of systematic language assessment require a multidisciplinary team and flexible approach.

✓ Identified language disorder requires specialised speech and language therapy support working closely with the parent and other practitioners supporting the child.

✓ Further research into language abilities and interventions is required, including focus on activity and participation at school age.

REFERENCES

American Speech-Language-Hearing Association (2020) *Person-Centered Focus on Function: Language Disorder*. Available at: <https://www.asha.org/uploadedFiles/ICF-Language-Disorder.pdf> [Accessed July 2021].

Bedny M, Pascual-Leone A, Dravida S, Saxe R (2012) A sensitive period for language in the visual cortex: distinct patterns of plasticity in congenitally versus late blind adults. *Brain and Language* **122**(3): 162–170.

Berko Gleason J (2005) *The Development of Language*. Boston, MA: Pearson Education.

Bigelow AE (2003) The development of joint attention in blind infants. *Development and Psychopathology* **15**: 259–275.

Blank M, Rose SA, Berlin LJ (1978) *The Language of Learning: The Preschool Years*. New York: Grune & Stratton.

Boehm AE (2001) *Boehm Test of Basic Concepts-3*. San Antonio, TX: The Psychological Corporation.

Brouwer K, Gordon-Pershey M, Hoffman D, Gunderson E (2015) Speech sound-production deficits in children with visual impairment: a preliminary investigation of the nature and prevalence of coexisting conditions. *Contemporary Issues in Communication Science and Disorders* **42**: 33.

Campbell R (2007) The processing of audio-visual speech: empirical and neural bases. *Philosophical Transactions of the Royal Society B: Biological Sciences* **363**: 1001–1010.

Communication Trust (n.d.) Communication Trust What Works database. Available at: <https://ican.org.uk/intervention-search/> [Accessed July 2021].

Crystal D, Fletcher P, Garman M (1976) *The Grammatical Analysis of Language Disability*. London: Edward Arnold.

Cunningham BJ, Washington KN, Binns A, Rolfe K, Robertson B, Rosenbaum P (2017) Current methods of evaluating speech-language outcomes for preschoolers with communication disorders: a scoping review using the ICF-CY. *Journal of Speech, Language, and Hearing Research* **60**: 447–464.

Dale NJ, Sakkalou E, O'Reilly MA et al. (2019) Home-based early intervention in infants and young children with visual impairment using the Developmental Journal: longitudinal cohort study. *Dev Med Child Neurol* **61**: 697–709.

Dale N, Sonksen P (2002) Developmental outcome, including setback, in young children with severe visual impairment. *Dev Med Child Neurol* **44**: 613–622.

Dodd B, Hua Z, Crosbie S, Holm A, Ozanne A (2002) *Diagnostic Evaluation of Articulation and Phonology (DEAP)*. London: Pearson UK.

Eyberg S, Funderburk B (2011) *Parent-Child Interaction Protocol.* PCIT International Inc.

Fenson L, Marchman VA, Thal D, Dale PS, Reznick JS, Bates E (2007) *The MacArthur-Bates Communicative Development Inventories*. Baltimore: Brookes Publishing UK.

Gillon GT (2004) *Phonological Awareness: From Research to Practice.* New York: Guilford Press.

Grunwell P, Harding A (1995) *Pacs Toys Screening Assessment Manual.* Windsor: NfER Nelson.

Hasson N, Joffe V (2007) The case for dynamic assessment in speech and language therapy. *Child Language Teaching and Therapy* **23**: 9–25.

Hersh M (2013) Deafblind people, communication, independence, and isolation. *Journal of Deaf Studies and Deaf Education* **18**: 446–463.

James DM, Stojanovik V (2007) Communication skills in blind children: a preliminary investigation. *Child: Care, Health and Development* **33**: 4–10.

Knowles W, Masidlover M (1982) *The Derbyshire Language Scheme.* Derby: Derbyshire County Council.

Law J, Garrett Z, Nye C (2004) The efficacy of treatment for children with developmental speech and language delay/disorder. *Journal of Speech, Language, and Hearing Research* **47**: 924–943.

McConachie HR, Moore V (1994) Early expressive language of severely visually impaired children. *Dev Med Child Neurol* **36**: 230–240.

Mosca R, Kritzinger A, van der Linde J (2015) Language and communication development in preschool children with a visual impairment: a systematic review. *South African Journal of Communication Disorders* **62**: 1–10.

Norgate S, Collis GM, Lewis V (1998) The developmental role of rhymes and routines for congenitally blind children. *Cahiers de Psychologie Cognitive* **17**: 451–477.

Reynell J, Zinkin P (1975) New procedures for the developmental assessment of young children with severe visual handicaps. *Child: Care, Health and Development* **1**: 61–69.

Rowland C (2012) *The Communication Matrix Oregon Health & Science University*. Available at: <https://communicationmatrix.org/> [Accessed July 2021].

Sakkalou E, O'Reilly MA, Sakki H et al. (2021) Mother–infant interactions with infants with congenital visual impairment and associations with longitudinal outcomes in cognition and language. *Journal of Child Psychology and Psychiatry* **62**: 712–750.

Salt A, Dale N (2017) *Developmental Journal for Babies and Young Children with Visual Impairment (DJVI)*, 2nd Edition. Available at: <https://xip.uclb.com/i/healthcare_tools/DJVI_professional.html> [Accessed July 2021].

Semel E, Wiig EH, Secord W (2017) *Clinical Evaluation of Language Fundamentals,* 5th Edition. London: Pearson UK/US.

SOESD (2007) *The Oregon Project for Visually Impaired and Blind Preschool Children,* Skills inventory, 6th Edition. Southern Oregon Education Service District.

Tadić V, Pring L, Dale N (2010) Are language and social communication intact in children with congenital visual impairment at school age? *Journal of Child Psychology and Psychiatry* **51**: 696–705.

Vervloed MP, Loijens NE, Waller SE (2014) Teaching the meaning of words to children with visual impairments. *Journal of Visual Impairment & Blindness* **108**(5): 433–438.

Vinter A, Fernandes V, Orlandi O, Morgan P (2013) Verbal definitions of familiar objects in blind children reflect their peculiar perceptual experience. *Child: Care, Health and Development* **39**(6): 856–863.

Zimmerman I, Pond R, Steiner V (2014) *Preschool Language Scales,* UK/US/Aus 5th editions. London: Pearson.

CHAPTER 11

Social Communication and Autism Spectrum Disorder

Naomi Dale and Alison Salt

INTRODUCTION

Early social development depends on vision and non-verbal forms of communication from infancy. The young child with vision impairment and their parent must find other means of social interacting and communicating, such as using voice or touch cues. As the child gets older, they may need extra support to interact with friends, whom they may not recognise nor locate in the playground. With the appropriate support many children can develop excellent social abilities and will develop strong rewarding friendships and relationships as they mature (see Chapter 19).

Children with visual impairment are, however, at higher risk of social communication difficulties and autism spectrum disorder (ASD). This chapter will explore possible reasons for this vulnerability, which range from genetic and neurobiological to experience and learning, along with the impact of vision deprivation. The challenges for identifying social communication difficulties and diagnosing ASD in the context of vision impairment will be considered. Evidence-based strategies for assessment, diagnosis, and intervention will be discussed.

SOCIAL COMMUNICATION RISKS

Definition of Issues

ASD is a heterogeneous class of neurodevelopmental disorder. The diagnostic criteria according to the *Diagnostic and Statistical Manual of Mental Disorders*, 5th Edition (DSM-5)

(American Psychiatric Association 2013) are (1) persistent deficits in social communication and social interaction across multiple contexts and (2) restricted and repetitive patterns of behaviour, interests, or activities. These fall into two factors of Social Affect and Restricted and Repetitive Patterns of Behaviour. The behavioural characteristics range from mild to severe and are not explained by the child's intellectual level, which can vary from intellectual disability to higher intelligence. Every child with ASD is different; some have the full range of described symptoms and some only have a partial presentation. The behavioural signs of ASD in a young child may look different from those in a teenager or adult.

The core features of ASD include impairments in social and behavioural and emotional challenges (Box 11.1). These core features are significantly influenced by the child's developmental level of language acquisition (e.g. pre-symbolic, emerging language, and conversational language) and the severity level of the disorder. In addition to core features, sensory and other challenges such as feeding may be present. There may be other co-occurring conditions such as sleep disorders, neurodevelopmental disorders such as attention-deficit/hyperactivity disorder, epilepsy, gastrointestinal conditions, metabolic conditions, and behavioural and psychiatric disorders.

Lack of vision may lead to similar features, arising from early delays and difficulties in acquiring social, communication, and language skills. In children with vision impairment, there have been longstanding concerns about emotional engagement, social interaction skills, autistic-like features, repetitive and ritualistic behaviours (stereotypies), auditory or tactile sensitivities, and delays and difficulties in communication and language.

Single-channelled attention and difficulty in shifting attention, delays in imaginative play or 'theory of mind' (understanding the other's intentions, beliefs, and points of view), and more restricted interests are common in children with vision impairment (Tadić et al. 2010; Brambring and Asbrock 2010; Pijnacker at al. 2012). More flexible attention-shifting, varied interests, and expanding behavioural repertoires may emerge more slowly and require more support from other developmental trajectories such as language, which, in the absence of sufficient vision, provides a framework for understanding (Tadić et al. 2009). Therefore, a cautious but informed approach is required in considering the nature of the child's social communication and behavioural development and its vulnerabilities from the early years and throughout childhood.

A systematic review using a meta-analysis of studies (1994–2016) found that the overall prevalence of ASD in visual impairment populations was 19% (95% confidence interval 13–25%) and an overall risk-ratio of 31 times compared to the reported ASD prevalence in the general population (Do et al. 2017). Children meeting criteria for ASD range from 12% to 31% in the study samples, with up to 60% having some ASD features (Mukaddes et al. 2007; Parr et al. 2010). The variation in proportions was possibly due to sampling

> **Box 11.1** Abbreviated table of Diagnostic Criteria for Autism Spectrum Disorder (DSM-5) (American Psychiatric Association 2013)
>
> The content has been modified here by the authors for children with vision impairment, including exclusion of deficits in nonverbal communicative behaviours used for social interaction and other details such as number of areas that must have deficits or severity issues.
>
> To meet diagnostic criteria for ASD according to DSM-5, a child must have persistent deficits in areas of social communication and interaction (see A below) plus types of restricted, repetitive behaviours (see B below).
>
> A. Persistent deficits in social communication and social interaction across multiple contexts, as manifested by the following, currently or by history (examples are illustrative, not exhaustive):
>
> 1. Deficits in social-emotional reciprocity, ranging, for example, from abnormal social approach and failure of normal back-and-forth conversation; to reduced sharing of interests, emotions, or affect; to failure to initiate or respond to social interactions.
>
> 2. Deficits in developing, maintaining, and understand relationships, ranging, for example, from difficulties adjusting behaviour to suit various social contexts; to difficulties in sharing imaginative play or in making friends; to absence of interest in peers.
>
> B. Restricted, repetitive patterns of behaviour, interests, or activities, as manifested by the following, currently or by history (examples are illustrative, not exhaustive):
>
> 1. Stereotyped or repetitive motor movements, use of objects, or speech (e.g., simple motor stereotypes, lining up toys or flipping objects, echolalia, idiosyncratic phrases).
>
> 2. Insistence on sameness, inflexible adherence to routines, or ritualised patterns of verbal or nonverbal behaviour (e.g. extreme distress at small changes, difficulties with transitions, rigid thinking patterns, greeting rituals, need to take same route or eat same food every day).
>
> 3. Highly restricted, fixated interests that are abnormal in intensity or focus (e.g. strong attachment to or preoccupation with unusual objects, excessively circumscribed or perseverative interests).
>
> 4. Hyper- or hypo-reactivity to sensory input or unusual interest in sensory aspects of the environment (e.g. apparent indifference to pain/temperature, adverse response to specific sounds or textures, excessive smelling or touching of objects, visual fascination with lights or movement).
>
> C. Symptoms must be present in the early developmental period (but may not become fully manifest until social demands exceed limited capacities, or may be masked by learned strategies in later life).
>
> D. Symptoms cause clinically significant impairment in social, occupational, or other important areas of current functioning.

differences in the causes of the vision impairment and size of samples. Prevalence rates were higher in some studies, in those with the most severe vision impairment and in those with lower developmental quotients. However, ASD was found across all levels of vision impairment and developmental ability.

Another narrative synthesis review (Butchart et al. 2017) on autism and vision impairment reported on studies focussing on specific subpopulations, such as retinopathy of prematurity, optic nerve hypoplasia, septo-optic dysplasia, Leber amaurosis, deaf–blind populations, and genetic disorders associated with vision impairment (e.g. CHARGE). It concluded that autistic traits are evident in children who are congenitally blind in all groups. The authors pointed out that the presence of traits does not necessarily indicate a broad enough range of impairments to warrant an autism diagnosis and that the studies often have methodological limitations, such as smaller screening studies with specific clinical populations. The measures used to define ASD had not been systematically tested on a population with vision impairment. When authors have omitted vision-based items (such as 'eye contact' or 'use of facial expression') in the standardised autism diagnostic measures, this may undermine their validity and reliability.

A similar critique of the methods used in existing studies is given by Molinaro et al. (2020), who draw attention to the current absence of a valid diagnostic methodology of assessing ASD that is adapted for the population with vision impairment. This can lead to unreliable diagnoses based on non-objective clinical impression and inconclusive prevalence data.

Genetic and Neurobiological Causes

While ASD shares characteristic features at the behavioural level, its underlying causes are highly heterogeneous in the general population (Gilbert and Man 2017). Genetic factors are important, with up to 25% of diagnosed individuals having an identifiable genetic variant (Huguet et al. 2013). However, ASD is highly variable in its genetic basis, and includes single gene mutations and associations with copy number variants, with up to 792 genes listed (Butler et al. 2015). Nevertheless, common features at the cellular and molecular levels of the brain are found, with most ASD genes implicated in cortical regulation and patterning, synaptic homeostasis, and neural circuitry (Gilbert and Man 2017). Differences in brain volume, cortical thickness, and connectivity are found in those with ASD compared with those who are typically developing (Pugliese et al. 2009; Hyde et al. 2010).

Many genes associated with congenital disorders of the peripheral vision system (i.e. globe, retina and anterior optic nerve) have been identified (see Chapter 3), and it is conceivable that there is some overlap between eye and ASD-linked genes. Some disorders of the visual pathways are associated with other brain defects, such as optic nerve hypoplasia associated with septo-optic dysplasia including hypothalamic and pituitary defects, which may possibly contribute to the tendency towards higher prevalence of ASD (Parr et al. 2010).

Vision and Experience

Some differences in vision processing, including those associated with the magnocellular and low spatial frequency channels (Greenaway and Plaisted 2005), have been found in children with ASD, suggesting a potential overlap with vision impairment in vulnerable areas of brain development. Functional impairment in visual attention and visual sensorimotor deficits are found in children with ASD, alongside changes in brain development. It is postulated that these impairments along the pathways of the visual system lead to visual sensory deprivation which has an environmental-driven neural effect. As a result input of visual social stimulus such as perceiving facial expressions or subtle social cues may be more limited, leading to the emergence of the social deficits found in ASD (Piven et al. 2017).

There is now evidence that the very early environment of the infant, such as the maternal perinatal environment, can also influence gene expression which in turn may drive brain development (Meaney 2010).

Deprivation of vision stimulus and associated constraint in sensorimotor activity in very young infants with severe vision impairment may possibly limit the development of early social neural networks. A sensory deprivation theory has been proposed by Peter Hobson (2014) who argues that vision impairment limits the development of 'inter-subjectivity' (or joint attention, that is the shared focus of two individuals on an object) between the parent and infant, which has a cumulative impact on the parent–child relationship and relating socially.

Developmental Processes at Risk

The first 2 years of life are a critical stage for rapid synaptic development in the brain and lack of vision will have an impact on early bonding and understanding of 'the other' from the very earliest weeks of life. However, in the first 6 months of life, as in typically developing children, symptoms of difficulties in the social domain may not be evident, although the infant may be more passive and limited in their social responses (Dale et al. 2014).

From 12 months of age the differences may become more marked with reduced opportunities to establish 'inter-subjectivity' and joint attention (Green et al. 2004; Dale et al. 2014). Parents have reported that 10 to 40 months old (mean age 22 months) children with profound vision impairment were less likely to 'share interest in a toy' or 'share interest in an event' than similar age children with severe vision impairment (and basic 'form' vision) or those with typical vision (Dale et al. 2014).

Other areas of vulnerability have been found in attention shifting between two targets, with greater challenges in the subgroup of those who are profoundly visually impaired (light perception at best) in a preschool aged sample of children with congenital disorders of the peripheral visual system (Tadić et al. 2009). When this sample was followed up at primary school age, the subsample, who all had good verbal intelligence, continued to rate significantly lower on a pragmatic measure of communication skills (Children's Communication Checklist) compared to matched typically sighted controls. Nearly half were in the clinical range (Tadić et al. 2010). In another study of the same sample when reaching adolescent age, the young people were doing well cognitively but they continued to show vulnerabilities in the social communicative domain and in adaptive functioning and everyday behavioural executive function (Greenaway et al. 2017).

Differences have also been shown at brain level between different children with congenital disorders of the peripheral visual system, which may reflect a risk. In our OPTIMUM study, infants aged 8 to 15 months with severe–profound vision impairment varied in aspects of their brain activity or 'frontal asymmetry' when undertaking neuro-electrophysiology measures. Frontal asymmetry is an indicator of asymmetric brain activity in the frontal cortex, which refers to asymmetrical activity between the left and right hemispheres. Those who were more 'left leaning' in frontal asymmetry showed greater behaviour problems including emotional reactivity and withdrawal on a behaviour rating scale 1 year later (O'Reilly et al. 2017). At 8 to 12 years of age, children of average-level intelligence with vision impairment and no known brain disorder had less amplitude responses to hearing their own name ('subject's own name' paradigm) than a matched control group with typical vision. They also showed an increased rate of autism-related behaviours, pragmatic language deficits, as well as peer relationships and emotional problems on standardised parent questionnaires (Bathelt et al. 2017). Differences in response to hearing one's own name could be an early biomarker as we also found these differences in infants as young as 8 to 15 months in our OPTIMUM study.

Thus, combinations of genetic and neurobiological variants, visual sensory deprivation, developmental processes at risk and limited opportunities for learning may increase the vulnerability of the developmental processes associated with ASD in children with vision impairment.

Presenting Features of ASD in Children with Vision Impairment

A first sign of concern may be the serious emergence of a 'developmental setback' that is found in 11% to 13% of young children with vision impairment. This is potentially the earliest constellation of features suggesting pre-verbal ASD behaviours. The defining features are plateauing or regression of developmental skills over at least a 12-month period, which first emerge behaviourally at 16 to 27 months and continue in the following year or so. Our team has demonstrated this phenomenon in retrospective clinic studies (Cass et al. 1994; Dale and Sonksen 2002) and in the prospective national OPTIMUM cohort (Dale et al. 2019). Risk factors for setback include severity of vision reduction with a third of those with profound vision impairment (light perception at best) showing setback.

Key features of setback include difficulties in social interaction (e.g. being self-directed, and resistant to social approach), language and communication (e.g. lack of non-verbal communication, echolalia), and behaviour with restricted interests (e.g. tantrums, repetitive behaviours and stereotypies, and limited functional play). These children tend to show continuing long term complex needs including significant intellectual disability and are more likely to be ascribed a later clinical diagnosis of ASD (Dale and Sonksen 2002).

Early signs of ASD in older children need to be distinguished from social communication challenges that we may first see in any younger child with vision impairment (see Chapter 8).

Our group (Dale, Sakkalou, Salt, and colleagues) has recently undertaken the DAiSY project with a representative national cohort of 100 children aged 4 to 8 years with severe–profound vision impairment arising from congenital disorders of the peripheral visual system. The study findings are currently being prepared for scientific publication. The majority of the children had relatively fluent language skills and were in the average range in verbal intelligence. An expert clinician in vision impairment and autism rated videos of the children undergoing structured play and conversation (see details below) and also examined behaviour issues reported by the parent in a structured assessment. The clinician rated each child according to a diagnostic formulation based on DSM-5 for ASD: (1) non-spectrum range, (2) borderline/mild ASD range (not reaching full DSM-5 criteria), and (3) ASD range (reaching full DSM-5 criteria). In this sample the proportions were roughly about a fifth falling into the milder ASD range and about a fifth falling into the full ASD range, with higher rates in the subsample who were profoundly visually impaired (but also had more mixed language ability).

The importance of differentiating autism in individuals with intellectual disability in combination with vision impairments and/or deafblindness has been explored in a preliminary study using a new observational method, the Observation of Autism in people with Sensory and Intellectual Disabilities (OASID) (de Vaan et al. 2018). Sixty individuals participated in the study and the psychometric properties of reliability and concurrent validity of the OASID were found to be promising in this complex clinical population.

SUPPORT AND MANAGEMENT

The Multidisciplinary Team

A dedicated multidisciplinary paediatric team including neurodisability/neurodevelopmental paediatrics, psychology, speech and language therapy, and occupational therapy is needed to undertake a diagnostic assessment. Appropriate training and expertise in the assessment of ASD, and ASD in the context of vision impairment, is recommended. Knowledge of the child's functional vision and of general development of children with vision impairment is vital. The input of the parent and other practitioners who know the child well, including the specialist teacher for visually impaired and class teachers, is also essential.

Later support for the child after diagnosis or assessment of ASD will involve close working between specialists in vision impairment, class teacher, habilitation specialist, speech and language therapist, occupational therapist, educational psychologist, and advisory services for children with ASD in close liaison with the parent and child or young person. Clinical and neuropsychology and mental health services may need to be involved to advise on complex learning profiles, mental health, and behaviour needs. Feeding, sleeping, and anxiety problems are common and may need guidance for parents and child.

A Systematic Approach to Identifying Social Communication Risks and Diagnosing ASD

UNDER 5 YEARS

As every child with vision impairment progresses at a different rate, it is important to take into consideration the child's general development and the current level of vision function and other aspects of their paediatric condition and eye disorder.

Consideration of risks should start in the first years of life, as all areas of development and in particular the social domain are at risk. The Developmental Journal for babies and young children with visual impairment (DJVI) (Salt and Dale 2017) provides a structured developmental framework for tracking all areas of development including the Social Development domain, covering Developing Relationships and Social Interaction (see Chapter 8). Regular developmental monitoring (such as with the Reynell-Zinkin Scales) across the infant and preschool years will provide the means of tracking developmental progress, establishing steady progress, and identifying the emergence of developmental setback or significant developmental delay. The *Getting Stuck* booklet of the DJVI provides guidance on support for those not moving forward, including common problems associated with social interactional and behaviour and sensory sensitivity problems including touch and auditory sensitivity, feeding, and sleeping problems (see Chapter 8).

Some preliminary validated assessment methods have been established with small samples but need further replication in the future such as the Soc-VI interview with parents (Dale et al. 2014; see Box 11.2). The Visual Impairment and Social Communication Schedule (VISS) gives a structured framework for observing the child's social interaction, communication, play, and behaviour in a clinic context (Absoud et al. 2011; see Box 11.3). It enables rating the child's areas of ability that are of concern and if they fit according to the diagnostic criteria for ASD. A threshold rating of less than 35 in children aged 2 to 4 years is an early risk sign for later clinical ASD diagnosis (Absoud et al. 2011). It can also be used as part of an assessment including observations of the child's social interactions and play in older school-aged children who are developmentally under the age of 4 years and have significant intellectual disability (see below).

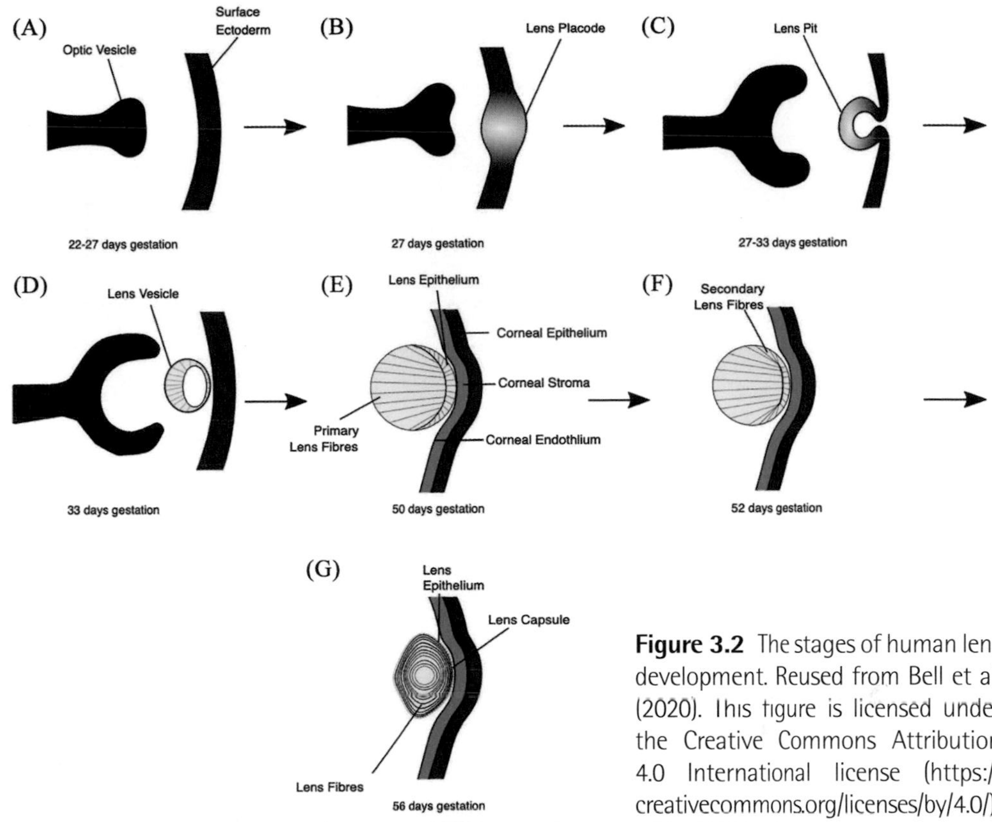

Figure 3.2 The stages of human lens development. Reused from Bell et al. (2020). This figure is licensed under the Creative Commons Attribution 4.0 International license (https://creativecommons.org/licenses/by/4.0/).

	Near Detection Scale (NDS)		Profound visual impairment (PVI) / severe visual impairment (SVI)	NDS score
	No light perception		PVI	0
'in space'	Light in dark room Light reflecting object	Glowing light Mirror/tinsel ball	PVI	1
'in space'	12.5cm non-light reflecting	Black and yellow ball	SVI	2
'in space'	6.25cm	Yellow ball	SVI	3
On table top, plain background	6.25cm	Yellow ball	SVI	4
On table top, plain background	2.5cm	Yellow cube	SVI	5
On table top, plain background	1.2cm	Sweet (smartie)	SVI	6
On table top, plain background	0.5cm	Sweetener	SVI	7
On table top, plain background	0.3cm	Sweetener	SVI	8
On table top, plain background	0.1cm	Cake decoration	SVI	9

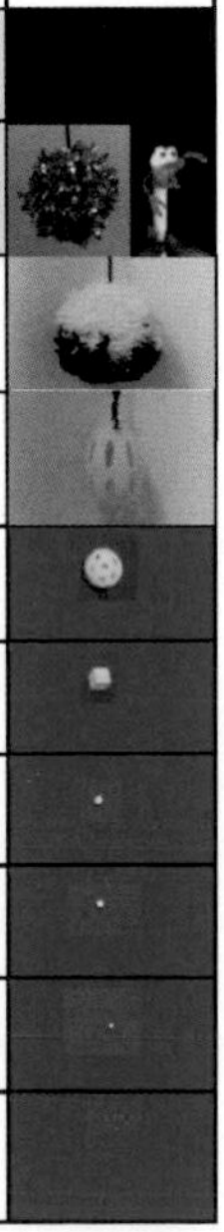

Figure 4.2 The Near Detection Scale

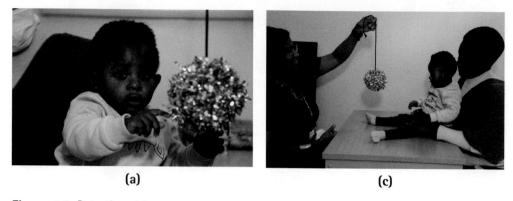

(a)   (c)

Figure 4.3 Detection vision assessment

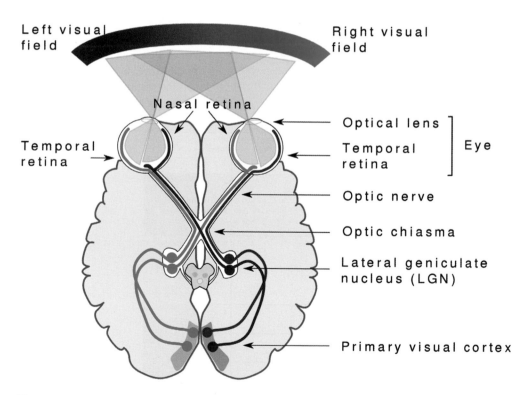

Figure 5.1 Diagram of the optic pathways. Reused from Miquel Perello Nieto (Wikimedia Commons). This figure is licensed under the Creative Commons Attribution-Share Alike 4.0 International license (https://creativecommons.org/licenses/by-sa/4.0/deed.en).

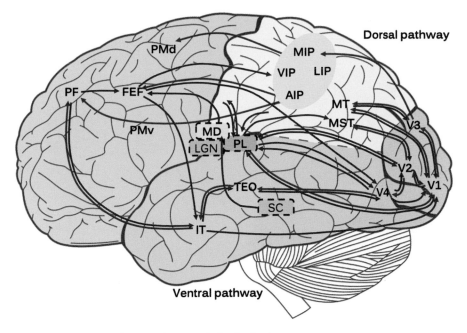

Figure 7.1 Diagram of the visual networks in the brain.

AIP, anterior intraparietal area; FEF, frontal eye fields; IT, inferior temporal area; LGN, lateral geniculate nucleus; LIP, lateral intraparietal area; MD, medial dorsal nucleus of thalamus; MIP, medial intraparietal area; MST, medial superior temporal area; MT, medial temporal area; PF, prefrontal cortex; PL, pulvinar; PMd, dorsal premotor area; PMv, ventral premotor area; SC, superior colliculus; TEO, tectum opticum; V1, primary visual cortex; V2, secondary visual cortex; V3, etrastriate area, V4, extrastriate area; VIP, ventral intraparietal area.

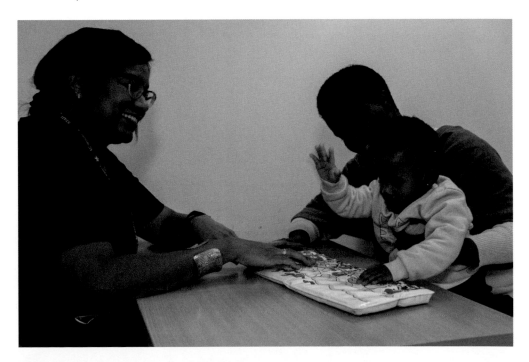

Figure 8.1 Developmental play assessment

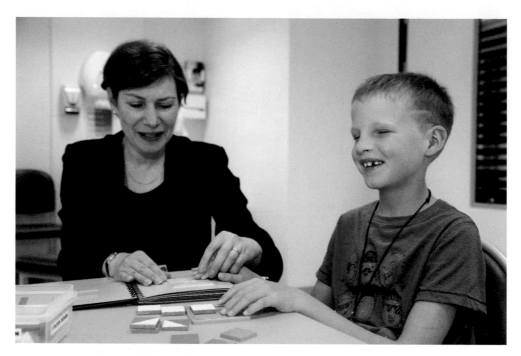

Figure 12.1 Cognitive assessment

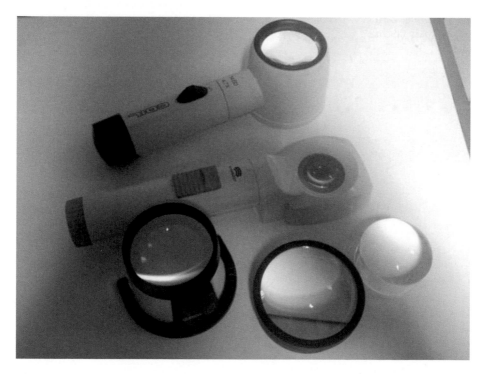

Figure 16.2 Illuminated and non-illuminated stand magnifiers

> **Box 11.2** 13-item Social Communication Interview for Young Children with Visual Impairment (SOC-VI 13) (abbreviated wording of items) (Dale et al. 2014)
>
> 1. Tries to attract your attention
> 2. Indicates wants an action repeated
> 3. Anticipates rhyme game action
> 4. Requests repeat of rhyme game
> 5. Initiates rhyme game
> 6. Social play with favoured object
> 7. Shares experience with toy
> 8. Shares interest in event
> 9. Responds positively if parent joins an activity
> 10. Stops activity when told 'No'
> 11. Indicates 'No'
> 12. Indicates 'Yes'
> 13. Makes requests or show desires

Alternatively, the newly developed Social Communication Scale (Visual Impairment) from our OPTIMUM project, will provide a further way of assessing the child's development of early social communication skills at 2 and 3 years of age and identifying areas of delay and difficulties that may need further targeting for support. This scale is currently under development for clinical use.

It is generally advised that a clinical diagnosis of ASD in children with vision impairment is not reached until a minimum of 4 years 6 months to 5 years even if there are concerns, especially if the child is maintaining steady progress in other areas of development such as language skills. This caution is because of the early general developmental delays, including social, language, and communication delays, associated with significant vision impairment. There is an anticipation that these delays will be overcome with maturing general and language development. However, children showing significant delays or plateauing in the areas of concern, as in developmental setback, should be referred for earlier investigations by the paediatric assessment team and could be referred for additional support from ASD 'early support' services. They can be viewed as 'at high risk of ASD' and should be seen as eligible for targeted early years support. Moreover, if the practitioner has earlier concerns about a child's development in the areas of social communication and behaviour, it is advisable to start monitoring progress and providing additional support as soon as possible.

This section is also relevant to children who are older than 5 years but have significant intellectual disability and are functioning below the 4-year range. As intellectual disability and ASD frequently co-occur, to make a combined diagnosis of ASD and

Box 11.3 Visual Impairment and Social Communication Schedule (abbreviated wording of items) (Absoud et al. 2011)

Social interaction

1. Makes social approach
2. Makes social response
3. Has a social smile
4. Responds to voices
5. Enjoys social touch
6. Positive acceptance of social approach
7. Directs attention of others
8. Directs adult's attention to own activity
9. Joins in activities of others

Communication and language

10. Uses or responds to gestures
11. Communicates need for help by vocalisation or gesture
12. Use of language for social chat
13. Use of language for communication
14. Expresses emotion
15. Uses conventional words and meanings
16. Spontaneous and meaningful use of referential language
17. Appropriate wide range of topics of interest

Play

18. Engage in spontaneous play
19. Engage in functional play
20. Engage in symbolic play
21. Engage in imaginative play

Routines, behaviours, and interests

22. Has appropriately wide repertoire of actions with objects
23. Has range of interests in different objects
24. Uses hands and body in functional manner
25. Willing to be redirected to new activity or focus of attention

intellectual disability the social communication level should be below that expected for the child's general developmental level. It is therefore important throughout the child's early years to consider their general developmental level too (according to visual impairment norms), which can be assessed by, for example the Reynell-Zinkin Scales (see Chapter 8).

FROM 5 YEARS UPWARDS

Ongoing persistence of problems and their interference in the child's everyday function and learning is the most reliable indicator of some underlying difficulties in the domains of social affect and restricted and repetitive behaviours. An assessment can be undertaken at any later age to confirm or explore the possibility of ASD but the age range of 4 years 6 months to 8 years is often valuable if difficulties are persisting during the child's early years at school (Box 11.1).

Children who have more fluent language skills can appear very chatty, attention-seeking, and sociable especially with adult carers, but this may 'mask' underlying difficulties in social understanding and relational abilities. As they get older, their difficulties in peer relationships and other behaviours may become more evident. Repetitive compulsive or obsessional behaviours tend to be seen more at home as they are often embedded in familiar home routines and more spontaneous behaviour such as play, and they may not show up in the structured and more rule-bound and less personal environment of school. The child may be compliant in the classroom but at home be much more prone to emotional outbursts and obsessional rituals.

DIAGNOSIS-GIVING

A key issue in diagnosing ASD is the constellation of features, their persistence over time, and lack of response to sustained attempts to modify and change their trajectories, and their degree of interference in the child's functioning and learning.

There are significant challenges for structured assessment and diagnosis of ASD in children with vision impairment and thus caution is required. The original validated diagnostic assessment tools include the Autism Diagnostic Interview-Revised and the Autism Diagnostic Observational Schedule-2 (ADOS-2) (Lord et al. 2000). The ADOS-2 includes rating indicators that are vision dependent, such as eye contact, facial expression, and non-verbal communication. It also includes 'presses' (i.e. probes or stimuli that tend to bring out some of those behaviours associated with ASD) with visual or pictorial materials (such as bubbles or picture books) during the assessment. These tools as presently constructed are not validated for use with children with vision impairment and should be used with caution without modification. Items that are vision dependent must be excluded in administration and in ratings.

Our group has recently undertaken a scientific validation of the ADOS-2 (Module 3), which is modified for children with vision impairment with the permission of the original author and the test publishers. In the DAiSY project (see above), the children were assessed with modified 'presses' that did not require vision and rated with modified rating scores. The preliminary findings are promising with high inter-rater reliability, internal consistency, and the two factor model. The ratings also point towards sensitivity and specificity with the clinician's independent formulation of the child's ASD status and generating a new diagnostic algorithm for children with vision impairment in the autism spectrum range. The study results are currently being prepared for scientific publication. This preliminary study highlights the importance of using the vision impairment-modified ADOS-2 for children raising concern regarding ASD in this age range as they progress through the early years of school.

Observations of the child in home or school environment are also valuable for giving further insights into the child's social relating and behaviour and these observations can be informed by considering the features of DSM-5 criteria of ASD.

Parent and teacher ratings on standardised behavioural questionnaires of strengths and difficulties, social responsiveness/social communication, and pragmatic language and communication are also informative, though highly vision-dependent items should be omitted and careful interpretation is required as they are not validated for children with vision impairment.

The final decision about whether it is appropriate to give a diagnosis of ASD is based on skilled multidisciplinary clinical judgement, bringing together all forms of knowledge through interview, observations, school visits, and parent and teacher-rated questionnaires. This includes the child's developmental history of difficulties in these areas, current challenges, and patterns of behaviour at home and at school, and other factors that could be affecting their behaviour and development. These might include paediatric illness, hospitalisation, adverse family, and life events including neglect, trauma, and abuse, fostering and adoption, refugee status, and migration.

As there is very little longitudinal knowledge about the longer-term outcomes and prognosis for children with combined vision impairment and ASD, it is useful to explain to parents that the diagnosis and the child's needs can be revisited when the child is older and revised if necessary.

Intervention and Practical Support

From the early months of life infants need support in their social domain and early intervention should include a family-centred structured framework for supporting this area of development. Chapter 8 describes the use of the DJVI and the social domain. Chapter 10 also considers the role of early intervention including the DJVI for tracking and promoting early communication and language.

Table 11.1 highlights some interventions and practices that have been successfully adopted with school-aged children with vision impairment and diagnosed ASD. The best practice advice is to use approaches to management and support for children with vision impairment and ASD that is based on evidence-based or 'criterion standard' strategies for children with ASD in the general population. These may need modification to these strategies so that they are adapted for children with visual impairment according to the child's level of vision.

Table 11.1 Interventions and practices for supporting children with vision impairment and ASD

Daily organisation	Social affect	Language	Behaviour
Regular routines	Enhance social interaction, e.g. familiar joint rhymes, turn-taking for the preverbal child, reciprocal interaction	Keep language simple, clear, and developmentally appropriate and focus on positive actions. Keep language child-centred linking to child's direct experiences	Structured behaviour management support for restricted feeding and sleeping difficulties
Systematic timetable and routines: objects of reference, tactile, braille, or enlarged symbol/print timetable	Build on communication modes, e.g. on-body Makaton, symbol exchange communication, enlarged symbol book	Ensure language is linked to meaning, with multisensory links to child-centred objects, actions, and events. Build on two-way language for reciprocal conversation	Positive consistent handling including clear boundaries where appropriate; reinforcing positive and successful behaviour ('positive parenting' strategies). ABC approaches for behaviour modification, such as 'time out' as a consequence. Emotional regulation and self-calming strategies, e.g. quiet space for relaxing and calming
Prepare for change of activity or routine or introducing novel event	Social skill training and support, e.g. understanding everyday social scenarios, theory of mind and perspective of others including intention, beliefs, and empathy	Avoid language that is abstract or metaphorical and can be misunderstood. Avoid demand/yes/no questions that can lead to demand avoidance	Distraction or limiting of repetitive behaviours and restricted interests, e.g. to certain time of the day or to specific room only
Clear activity sequences – 'first X, then Y'	Structured 'scaffolding' and framework for peer interactions, e.g. buddy system for leisure breaks	Social scripts or narratives and stories to guide regular social situations and appropriate behaviour	Habilitation support and vision impairment extra-curricular activities at school to foster social relationships, adaptive behaviour, independence, and autonomy
Calm quiet orderly environment to avoid sensory overload; child may need a separate room for some study	Opportunities for peer interactions, e.g. school model-making club, sports camp, computer, or drama groups	Provide structuring support to enable peer-to-peer reciprocal conversation, establishing shared topic interests with peers	Good communication between home and school to support parents in similar consistent handling of the child and any sanctions for inappropriate behaviours Monitor child's mental health, e.g. anxiety, and reduce environmental triggers that induce anxiety

These approaches can be successfully integrated with habilitation and visual impairment extra-curriculum support (see Chapter 14). Everyday social and peer opportunities like youth clubs, sports, and summer camps are important for the child who is at risk of becoming isolated and withdrawn (see Chapter 19). Some children with good cognitive ability may struggle in the mainstream school environment, and need extra social and habilitative support and considerations of their social, communicative, and adaptive behaviour needs in the education environment. Other areas of need, such as behavioural executive function (taking initiative, planning and organising, problem-solving, making decisions, and shifting behaviour set), are also important to consider (see Chapter 12).

Children with vision impairment and ASD have increased risk of mental health and behaviour difficulties, including low mood, anxiety disorders, and externalising and challenging behaviours, and may need the supports described in Chapter 18.

IMPLICATIONS FOR RESEARCH AND PRACTICE

Research will lead to next stages in the scientific development and modification of validated assessment tools and approaches for identifying and diagnosing ASD for children and young people with vision impairment. The importance of this has been emphasised in a review of the literature for research directions (Molinaro et al. 2020). Our own group hopes to extend our scientific methodology in the DAiSY project to consider and replicate the development and validation of vision impairment modification of the ADOS-2 and to extend from 8 years old to mid-adolescence. This is being planned in collaboration with the test publishers. These will require clinical feasibility studies to ensure clinically safe and reliable assessment methods. Once these have been established, paediatric teams specialising in developmental assessments including ASD and vision impairment will need diagnostic observational training and reliability updates in the use of these tools so that reliability standards can be maintained. The aim will be to achieve evidence-based clinical guidelines and consensus in the diagnostics of ASD in children with visual impairment, leading to 'benchmark' consistency and quality as has been achieved internationally for the diagnostics of ASD in typically sighted children.

With greater international consensus in assessment and diagnostic methods and tools, research can be undertaken in preventative and intervention practices that may enhance the social communication and behaviour outcomes in children with vision impairment, including those with ASD. Developments in education in mainstream and specialist schools can support the holistic needs of children with ASD and vision impairment to thrive in the school environment, whereas presently many children with these difficulties struggle in the noisy busy classroom and during playground leisure times.

Many areas need greater research insights such as the aetiologies and causation of ASD in children with vision impairment, including potential genetic contributions and possible different ASD phenotypes in different genetic eye disorders. More reliable and better methods for diagnosing ASD will lead to the potential for more reliable population studies of prevalence and identification of service needs and practical support. This includes behavioural guidance for parents and young people, mental health support, and other areas of need. In addition we need much greater research information on longer-term outcomes and needs and the impact on adolescence and transition into adult life and beyond.

SUMMARY

Children with vision impairment are at higher risk of ASD, especially those with profound vision impairment and those with intellectual disability, but also across all levels of vision impairment and cognitive ability. Vulnerability is likely to be due to a complex interaction of factors including genetics, specific eye and vision anomalies, and brain impairments, and the interplay of vision sensory deprivation, development and learning, and environmental factors. There is a need for the child to receive continuing support for the development of social and social communication skills and adaptive behaviour over time with monitoring and successful interventions for early or later signs of difficulties. Timely accurate diagnoses of ASD are important for ensuring that the child's needs in this area are appropriately understood and supported.

Key Points

✓ Children with vision impairment are vulnerable to developing social communication difficulties and ASD.

✓ From the earliest days, parents need support and guidance in their child's social communication, social relationships, and behaviour and play areas, which are all areas of risk that may continue over time.

✓ Those with profound vision impairment are most at risk of multiple developmental delays and developmental setback in the early years, which is an emerging sign of severe ASD.

✓ Children showing signs of concern should be referred to specialist paediatric services who can assess for ASD and advise on these areas of need.

✓ Development and consensus of scientifically modified assessment tools will improve diagnostic reliability, guidance to parents, and scientifically led interventions.

Acknowledgements to Dr Elaine Clark who reviewed a draft of this chapter and gave helpful suggestions.

REFERENCES

Absoud M, Parr JR, Salt A, Dale N (2011) Developing a schedule to identify social communication difficulties and autism spectrum disorder in young children with visual impairment. *Dev Med Child Neurol* 53(3): 285–288.

American Psychiatric Association (2013) Autism Spectrum Disorders. In *Diagnostic and Statistical Manual of Mental Disorders,* 5th Edition. Arlington, VA: American Psychiatric Association. https://doi.org/10.1176/appi.books.9780890425596.dsm05.

Andrews R, Wyver S (2005) Autistic tendencies: are there different pathways for blindness and Autism Spectrum Disorder? *Br J Vis Impair* **23**(2): 52–57.

Bathelt J, Dale N, de Haan M (2017) Event-related potential response to auditory social stimuli, parent-reported social communicative deficits and autism risk in school-aged children with congenital visual impairment. *Dev Cog Neurosci* **27**: 10–18.

Brambring M, Asbrock D (2010) Validity of false belief tasks in blind children. *J Autism Dev Disord* **40**(12): 1471–1484.

Butchart M, Long JJ, Brown M et al. (2017) Autism and visual impairment: a review of the literature. *Review J Autism Dev Disord* **4**: 118–131.

Butler MG, Rafi SK, Manzardo AM (2015) High-resolution chromosome ideogram representation of currently recognized genes for autism spectrum disorders. *Int J Mol Sci* **16**(3): 6464–6495. doi: 10.3390/ijms16036464.

Cass H, Sonksen PM, McConachie HR (1994) Developmental setback in severe visual impairment. *Arch of Dis Child* **70**: 192–196.

Dale N, Sonksen P (2002) Developmental outcome, including setback, in young children with severe visual impairment. *Dev Med Child Neurol* **44**(9): 613–622.

Dale NJ, Tadić V, Sonksen P (2014) Social communicative variation in 1–3-year-olds with severe visual impairment. *Child Care Health Dev* **40**(2): 158–164.

Dale NJ, Sakkalou E, O'Reilly MA et al. (2019) Home-based early intervention in infants and young children with visual impairment using the Developmental Journal: longitudinal cohort study. *Dev Med Child Neurol* **61**(6): 697–709.

de Vaan G, Vervloed MPJ, Peters-Scheffer NC, van Gent T, Knoors H, Verhoeven L (2018) Assessing autism spectrum disorder in people with sensory impairments combined with intellectual disabilities. *J Dev Phys Disabil* **30**(4): 471–487.

Do B, Lynch P, Macris EM et al. (2017) Systematic review and meta-analysis of the association of Autism Spectrum Disorder in visually or hearing impaired children. *Ophthalmic Physiol Opt* **37**(2): 212–224.

Gilbert J, Man HY (2017) Fundamental elements in autism: from neurogenesis and neurite growth to synaptic plasticity. *Front Cell Neurosci* **11**: 359.

Green S, Pring L, Swettenham J (2004) An investigation of first-order false belief understanding of children with congenital profound visual impairment. *Br J Dev Psychol* **22**(1): 1–7.

Greenaway R, Plaisted K (2005) Top-down attentional modulation in autistic spectrum disorders is stimulus-specific. *Psychol Sci* **16**(12): 987–994. doi: 10.1111/j.1467-9280.2005.01648.x.

Greenaway R, Pring L, Schepers A, Isaacs DP, Dale NJ (2017) Neuropsychological presentation and adaptive skills in high-functioning adolescents with visual impairment: a preliminary investigation. *Appl Neuropsych-Chil* **6**(2): 145–157.

Hyde KL, Samson F, Evans AC, Mottron L (2010) Neuroanatomical differences in brain areas implicated in perceptual and other core features of autism revealed by cortical thickness analysis and voxel-based morphometry. *Hum Brain Mapp* **31**(4): 556–566.

Hobson RP (2014) The coherence of autism. *Autism* **18**(1): 6–16.

Huguet G, Ey E, Bourgeron T (2013) The genetic landscapes of autism spectrum disorders. *Annu Rev Genomics Hum Genet* **14**: 191–213.

Lord C, Risi S, Lambrecht L et al. (2000) The Autism Diagnostic Observation Schedule – Generic: a standard measure of social and communication deficits associated with the spectrum of autism. *J Autism Dev Disord* **30**(3): 205–223.

Meaney M (2010) Epigenetics and the biological definition of gene x environment interactions. *Child Development* **81**(1): 41–79.

Molinaro A, Micheletti S, Rossi A et al. (2020) Autistic-like features in visually impaired children: a review of literature and directions for future research. *Brain Sci* **10**: 507. https://doi.org/10.3390/brainsci10080507.

Mukaddes NM, Kilincaslan A, Kucukyazici G, Sevketoglu T, Tuncer S (2007) Autism in visually impaired individuals. *Psychiatry Clin Neurosci* **61**(1): 39–44.

O'Reilly MA, Bathelt J, Sakkalou E et al. (2017) Frontal EEG asymmetry and later behavior vulnerability in infants with congenital visual impairment. *Clin Neurophysiol* **128**(11): 2191–2199.

Parr JR, Dale NJ, Shaffer LM, Salt AT (2010) Social communication difficulties and autism spectrum disorder in young children with optic nerve hypoplasia and/or septo-optic dysplasia. *Dev Med Child Neurol* **52**(10): 917–921.

Pijnacker J, Vervloed MP, Steenbergen B (2012) Pragmatic abilities in children with congenital visual impairment: an exploration of non-literal language and advanced theory of mind understanding. *J Autism Dev Disord* **42**: 2440–2449. doi: 10.1007/s10803-012-1500-5.

Piven J, Elison JT, Zylka MJ (2017) Toward a conceptual framework for early brain and behavior development in autism. *Mol Psychiatry* **22**(10): 1385–1394.

Pugliese L, Catani M, Ameis S et al. (2009) The anatomy of extended limbic pathways in Asperger syndrome: a preliminary diffusion tensor imaging tractography study. *Neuroimage* **47**(2): 427–434.

Salt A, Dale N (2017) *Developmental Journal for babies and young children with visual impairment (DJVI)*. Available at: <https://xip.uclb.com/i/healthcare_tools/DJVI_professional.html> [Accessed July 2021].

Tadić V, Pring L, Dale N (2009) Attentional processes in young children with congenital visual impairment. *Br J Dev Psychol* **27**: 311–330. doi: 10.1348/026151008x310210.

Tadić V, Pring L, Dale N (2010) Are language and social communication intact in children with congenital visual impairment at school age? *J Child Psychol Psyc* **51**(6): 696–705.

CHAPTER 12

Cognition

Rebecca Greenaway and Simon Ungar

INTRODUCTION

Cognition encompasses the mental processes involved in the acquisition of knowledge and understanding. It involves processing the experiences and the data received via the senses, leading to concept formation, analysis, and problem-solving. It guides meaningful and productive action in the physical and social environment. Early concept formation is concrete and based in direct experience; more abstract reasoning emerges as the child matures. Cognition includes attention, memory, and executive function processes; all of which need to be integrated for successful thinking and learning. Vision impairment impacts significantly on the learning of all infants and young children in their early years, but for some children learning challenges may persist. As vision impairment often occurs in the context of other brain differences (see Chapter 2), other factors such as intellectual disability or attention disorder may be relevant.

This chapter focuses on cognition in school-aged children and explores research and practice relevant to different areas of cognition and approaches to assessment. Early development of cognition is considered in Chapter 8.

COGNITION

Verbal and Non-Verbal Reasoning

In cognitive assessment a distinction is generally made between reasoning tasks that are 'verbal' and those that are 'non-verbal'. Verbal reasoning tasks are presented through language and generally require a spoken or written response (e.g. explaining what concepts link two words). Non-verbal reasoning tasks are language-free and typically require an individual to reason about spatial or figurative information presented through pictures or patterns; the response required is also non-verbal (e.g. drawing, pointing, and assembling objects to form a pattern). It is important to note that the distinction is based on the test materials used and the nature of the responses required. In practice, individuals often use language to help solve non-verbal problems (e.g. giving verbal labels to different parts of a pattern) and mental imagery to help solve verbal problems (e.g. creating a mental image of three named objects to help identify what they have in common).

Studies have found that children and adults with congenital vision impairment perform better on verbal perception and cognition tasks than do comparison groups with typical vision (Wakefield et al. 2004; Occelli et al. 2017). This advantage is likely to be due to a higher salience and significance of auditory verbal information when vision is not available, as well as greater verbal processing efficiency due to its enhanced neuroplastic development (see Chapter 7). In addition to studies indicating verbal strengths, there is also some evidence highlighting the greater challenge of verbal concept formation for children with vision impairment owing to reduced opportunity to directly experience certain concepts (Jaworska-Biskup 2011).

Assessment of non-verbal reasoning among individuals with typical vision usually involves reasoning with vision-based materials, such as puzzles and pictures. Other senses, such as hearing, touch, and proprioception, can also provide a rich source of information about the world. However, vision offers a number of important cues that support the processing of information in particular ways. When looking at a picture, diagram, or map, some aspects of visual information are rapidly and automatically processed simultaneously; for instance, all elements that are similar in some way (e.g. same shape) 'pop out' from all the other information. Many of these rapid perceptual processes appear not to be available when using touch alone, and it therefore becomes an additional task (and greater cognitive load) to apply deliberate strategies to substitute for this (e.g. to sequentially search a tactile diagram to find all of the features that are the same shape). Furthermore, visual experience drives us to integrate spatial information into 'cognitive maps', which provide a very flexible and economic way to process complex spatial information. Without this visual input during the early period of development, children and adults with congenital vision impairment may later show challenges with spatial reference frames (Gori et al. 2017; see Chapter 15). It is therefore not clear that non-verbal reasoning with visual stimuli is directly comparable with analogous tasks using tactile stimuli, as tactile information is often accessed in a more sequential way. This places additional demands on executive functioning skills, such as working memory (Bathelt et al. 2018).

Short-Term and Working Memory

Psychologists use the term 'short-term memory' to describe the temporary storage of information over relatively short time periods, whilst 'working memory' refers to the mental manipulation of this information in temporary storage. Working memory depends both on storage capacity and on the efficiency with which the information is processed. It involves more active processing and may place demands on executive functioning. Working memory is important for many aspects of classroom learning including following instructions, mental arithmetic, reading, comprehension, recording work, and monitoring progress through the steps of complex tasks. Research has generally found that children with vision impairment perform better on simple digit span tasks (i.e. recalling a list of numbers or digits of increasing length), which draw on short-term memory, than children with typical vision (Withagen et al. 2013). In adults, research has found this better performance to be specific to those with early-onset vision impairment and it is not found in those with later onset visual loss (Dormal et al. 2016). Some limited research is available concerning more complex working memory tasks involving manipulation of information and higher executive function demands (see below), and is of greater relevance in the classroom.

Long-Term Memory

In contrast to capacity-limited short-term memory, long-term memory is the enduring storage of knowledge and information from prior events. There is limited research in this area with children with vision impairment, though research with adults with congenital vision impairment has identified greater memory accuracy and more efficient memory retrieval on a verbal list-learning task compared to adults with typical vision (Pasqualotto et al. 2013). Children with congenital vision impairment have been found to perform similarly to children with typical vision, on memory for word pairs that are easy to visualise, and on story memory, but they performed better on memory for hard to visualise word pairs, e.g. 'near' and 'copy' (Wakefield et al. 2004). The authors suggest that this may be explained by differences in strategy use: children with typical vision were more likely to rely on visualisation, with the task becoming harder when this strategy cannot be employed.

Attention

Attention involves focussing on relevant information, whilst filtering out competing irrelevant information, and is achieved through a combination of processes. Some of these are quite automatic (in the sense that our attention is drawn to and structured by salient aspects of our environment) while others are more consciously and deliberately directed. Currently, there have been relatively few studies of attention in children with vision impairment and those studies available have focussed on auditory attention. Children with vision impairment and no additional needs have been shown on average to perform in line with or better than peers with typical vision (e.g. Wakefield et al. 2004; Greenaway et al. 2017). However, children and young people with vision impairment often report difficulty in focussing on a learning task in a noisy environment. In a large national telephone survey conducted in the USA, parents of children with non-correctable vision problems reported a higher prevalence of attention-deficit/hyperactivity disorder compared to those without vision problems, particularly among children with milder vision impairment (DeCarlo et al. 2016). The explanation for this association is not clear and the aetiology and nature of these vision problems was not reported.

Executive Function

Executive function skills are the mental processes necessary for the control of behaviour, including processes such as planning, attentional control, inhibition, working memory, and flexibility. These are increasingly recognised to be important in academic success and adaptive skill development. Other than working memory research, there is minimal research involving direct assessment in children with vision impairment, because most available assessment measures involve visual materials and are not suitable for use with this population. Studies using parent-report measures have found higher reported difficulties in everyday executive abilities among children with vision impairment compared to those without vision impairment, including planning skills, performance monitoring, and the ability to shift from one activity to another (Greenaway et al. 2017; Bathelt et al. 2018).

ASSESSMENT AND PRACTICE

The Multidisciplinary Team

For children with vision impairment of school age, parents and teachers, including specialist teachers for children with vision impairment, play a primary role in assisting and monitoring the child's learning and cognitive progress. If there are concerns about the child's progress, detailed formal assessment of cognitive functioning may be required, and this can be carried out by educational/school psychologists, clinical psychologists, or neuropsychologists. Teachers are also involved in curriculum-based assessments. Assessment should be preceded by liaison with parents and other professionals involved, in particular the child's teacher and specialist teacher for vision impairment, who can advise on learning and cognition and access needs. For example, it may be appropriate to use haptic (i.e. active touch) measures of cognition for children familiar with tactile learning materials, whilst for children with mild or moderate vision impairment, cautious use of non-verbal assessment materials can be appropriate. Multidisciplinary working is vital to consider cognition and learning alongside other abilities and needs, such as language and motor abilities, to provide a holistic assessment of the child.

Assessment

Cognitive assessment is undertaken to understand the child's strengths and needs in relation to their cognitive functioning. This can help to ensure that learning potential is not underestimated and that learning needs are appropriately supported. Deficits in areas of cognitive functioning important for classroom learning and everyday adaptive functioning, including intellectual, attention, working memory, and executive functioning limitations, can coincide with vision impairment. When a child is struggling in school, it is important to consider the possibility of co-occurring difficulties and not solely attribute all challenges to the child's vision impairment.

The cognitive assessment should be driven by the referral question and presenting concerns. These may include concerns about general progress or about specific aspects of learning and other challenges, including possible intellectual disability, limited independence skills, under-performance in the classroom, difficulties concentrating or working independently, and behavioural or emotional difficulties associated with schooling or school refusal. Alternatively, the referral may be driven by medical concerns. The child may have experienced a brain injury or illness or have a neurological condition with a known impact on cognitive development. In any of these concerns, an assessment may be indicated to gather baseline information, to evaluate cognitive functioning, to track areas of cognitive development, to support decision-making around the curriculum or habilitative interventions, to inform neurodevelopmental or medical diagnoses, and to evaluate intervention outcomes.

Assessment Methods

The psychologist conducts a detailed interview with parents, including a detailed developmental history, as well as consulting other practitioners involved in the child's care and education, in particular teachers. Older children and young people also need to be consulted regarding their learning experiences.

Psychologists may use a combination of assessment methods to provide an individualised approach, including direct observation, consultation with adults who are familiar with the child (which may be guided by checklists or questionnaires), and direct work with the child, for example asking the child to carry out curriculum-based or more abstract problem-solving or reasoning tasks. Such approaches will be informed by a detailed knowledge of models of cognition (e.g. information-processing models).

The psychologist may undertake standardised assessment measures of cognition (i.e. tools such as intelligence tests where an individual receives a score that can be compared with a normative sample drawn from the same age group) or non-standardised cognitive assessment tools (e.g. the Cognitive Abilities Profile – Deutsch and Mohammed, 2010). They may also include aspects of curriculum-based assessment, for example evaluating the child's conceptual development in relation to age-related expectations. Careful theory-driven observation and skilled questioning is essential to detect the specific strengths and needs of the child in different aspects of their cognitive functioning.

Standardised measures include those specifically developed for assessing children and young people with vision impairment (e.g. Comprehensive Vocational Evaluation System, Dial et al. 1991; and the Intelligence Test for Visually Impaired Children, Dekker 1993) and measures normed on the general population with typical vision, that are accessible for children with vision impairment by involving auditory rather than visual tasks. It is helpful to have a combination of both auditory and haptic measures to gather a fuller picture of the child's profile, including both verbal and non-verbal reasoning skills. It is also important to consider tests or subtests that draw more on 'fluid reasoning' (i.e. the ability to think flexibly and to problem-solve) as well as what the child already has learned, or acquired knowledge (see Fig. 12.1).

Owing to the rarity of vision impairment and heterogeneity in the population (see Chapter 2), normative cognitive data are challenging to develop. This has meant there are only very limited measures available for children with vision impairment and where such measures exist (e.g. Intelligence Test for Visually Impaired Children) they are limited in availability. Moreover, the norms have become outdated over time and may include a mixed population with additional needs. Therefore, many psychologists rely on auditory measures taken from standard general child population assessments. This provides information on how the child is able to perform relative to normative expectations for their peers with typical vision, and can help identify a child's strengths and needs as part of a broader assessment (Greenaway et al. 2017). Some questions may need to be omitted or reworded because they rely entirely on visual information. Caution in interpretation is required as these measures have not been normed on children with vision impairment,

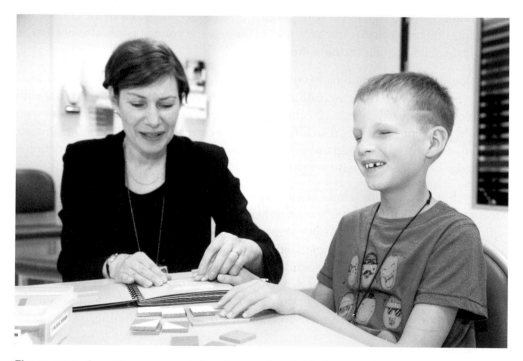

Figure 12.1 Cognitive assessment. (A colour version of this figure can be seen in the colour plate section)

which may reduce their validity. Concerns have been raised, including the risk that the assessment may not validly assess the child's true ability, as some verbal items may draw on visual knowledge or ask about concepts that the child with vision impairment experiences and learns differently as a result of their differing perceptual experience.

It is important to recognise the value and any limitations of available cognitive standardised assessments, and to consider these in a broader perspective that considers testing alongside the child's actual learning, progress, and performance in the school environment. For further guidance in undertaking cognitive and neuropsychological assessment in child vision impairment, see Goodman et al. (2009), Greenaway and Dale (2021).

Practical Support

Assessment of a child's profile of cognitive abilities helps explain a child's learning and behaviour and improves understanding of the child and their needs. On this basis the psychologist gives guidance and makes recommendations for supporting any identified areas of need as well as fostering strengths. Children who are struggling in the classroom need greater understanding of their cognitive profiles, as well as modifications for their needs, including individualised interventions or strategies tailored to their needs. Without these essential modifications, participation in education and development of independence skills throughout childhood and into adulthood may be more constrained.

The greater challenges for any child with vision impairment in the classroom has long been recognised and needs to be considered within the context of reduced opportunity for incidental learning via observation. Of high interest nowadays is an additional vision-impairment specific extra-curriculum. This is a necessary addition to the general curriculum, for the child with vision impairment, to learn skills that need direct and specific teaching and to give broader opportunities that might otherwise be missed (see Chapters 14 and 20).

Verbally conveyed information holds particular significance for the child with vision impairment and therefore teaching which includes rich descriptions of the environment and all relevant aspects of a situation in the classroom to support learning is important. Teachers and parents need to be advised to avoid language that requires the child to be able to see in order to make sense of what is said. It is also vital to consider the auditory environment in the classroom and to reduce extraneous sounds and speech, which may be distracting and interfere with the child's concentration. This is particularly relevant for children with vision impairment and auditory attention difficulties who find it difficult to concentrate if the environment is noisy, possibly because they are so dependent upon their soundscape to orientate themselves and to know what is going on.

It is often suggested that the child with vision impairment in the classroom has greater demands on their cognitive load/working memory resources as they cannot rely on visual cues and information. There is also evidence that short-term memory capacity for information acquired through touch is less than for visual information, potentially due to the more sequential nature of tactile information (Picard and Monnier 2009). Therefore, teaching strategies that reduce working memory load (see Gathercole and Alloway 2008) may benefit learning, particularly for a child with vision impairment and co-occurring weakness in working memory. This will be particularly important in preparing children to make effective use of tactile graphics (e.g. maps and technical diagrams) where the use of 'chunking' strategies has been shown to improve the capacity to organise and use information from these sources (Ungar et al. 2004), and forms part of a more general 'tactile graphicacy' approach (Aldrich et al. 2003).

In order to support concept formation including the move from concrete to more abstract concepts, it is crucial that the child has the relevant experiences, opportunities, and access to adapted materials to support this. Presenting information in multisensory formats is associated with improved learning in the general population (Shams and Seitz 2008). Recent research has explored multisensory learning approaches to support children with vision impairment to access the academic curriculum more fully, for example using adaptive materials (Rule et al. 2011), sonification (use of non-speech sounds) (Lahav et al. 2018), and low vision aid technology (see Chapters 15 and 16).

The additional demands for the child with vision impairment learning in a school designed for children with typical vision creates challenges and may at times be very tiring and elicit stress, for instance if the child's learning materials are not suitably adapted for their vision level (see Chapter 21). Difficulties with learning can lead to anxiety and the child's wellbeing and mental health in the learning environment needs consideration (see Chapter 18). Promoting a positive self-concept as an individual with vision impairment is also important for the child or young person to fully engage with meeting their goals and engaging with accessibility adaptations (see Chapter 19). Involvement of the young person in finding better strategies or adaptations that work, is important.

IMPLICATIONS FOR RESEARCH AND PRACTICE

Existing cognitive assessment tools for children with vision impairment have limited or outdated norms. The field is in urgent need of updated cognitive tests for this population. It is therefore important that the psychologist is knowledgeable about vision impairment and can access the opinion and advice of other psychologists in the field, if possible, to be confident that their assessment and interpretation of results is sound. Furthermore, given the limitations of certain tools in this population, a more holistic and broader assessment, including observations and consultation with other practitioners, is important.

Much of the research exploring cognitive processing in individuals with vision impairment has been carried out with adults. Future research with children is needed and will help elucidate whether 'sensitive' periods of development exist as well as the differing needs of children with congenital versus acquired vision impairment. Further research understanding how different cognitive processes develop (e.g. executive function, auditory and haptic attention) in children with vision impairment will be important for the design and evaluation of interventions that may target cognitive needs more successfully.

SUMMARY

Children with vision impairment may acquire strong verbal and auditory processing and reasoning skills, but they may differ in the way they mentally represent non-verbal information. Ongoing assessment of the child in the classroom by teachers is the most important way of monitoring the child's responses to educational opportunities and their ability to problem-solve and think flexibly. Parents also notice and support how their child uses cognitive strategies in their everyday environment. On occasion, individual children with vision impairment need access to cognitive assessment to establish whether they have general or specific cognitive difficulties. Multidisciplinary assessment involving cognition plays an important role in supporting children with vision impairment as they advance through education.

Of key importance is to understand the child's needs in the context of vision impairment to ensure these are appropriately met and to motivate while maintaining high expectations, so that optimal potential is reached.

Key Points

- ✓ There is a complex relationship between vision impairment and cognitive development, with the differing perceptual experience leading to differences in strategy use, strengths, and needs.
- ✓ Consultation between health, education, and parents and young people are important for shared understanding and problem-solving.
- ✓ Individualised specialised and mainstream habilitation and educational strategies are needed to support progress and help the child reach optimal potential.
- ✓ Some children will require clinical or educational assessment, taking into account the impact of vision impairment, to detect strengths and needs (including intellectual disability and specific learning difficulties).
- ✓ Research is advancing understanding of how children with vision impairment develop cognitive processes and learn, and future developments will enhance learning approaches and participation in society.

REFERENCES

Aldrich F, Sheppard L, Hindle Y (2003) First steps towards a model of tactile graphicacy. *The Cartographic Journal* **40**: 283–287.

Bathelt J, de Haan M, Salt A, Dale NJ (2018) Executive abilities in children with congenital vision impairment in mid-childhood. *Child Neuropsychology* **24**: 184–202.

DeCarlo DK, Swanson M, McGwin G, Visscher K, Owsley C (2016) ADHD and vision problems in the National Survey of Children's Health. *Optometry and Vision Science* 93: 459.

Dekker R (1993) Visually impaired children and haptic intelligence test scores: Intelligence Test for Visually Impaired Children (ITVIC). *Dev Med Child Neur* 35: 478–489.

Deutsch R, Mohammed M (2010) *The Cognitive Abilities Profile*. London: Real Group.

Dial JG, Chan F, Mezger C et al. (1991) Comprehensive vocational evaluation system for visually impaired and blind persons. *Journal of Visual Impairment and Blindness* 85: 153–157.

Dormal V, Crollen V, Baumans C, Lepore F, Collignon O (2016) Early but not late blindness leads to enhanced arithmetic and working memory abilities. *Cortex* 83: 212–221.

Gathercole SE, Alloway TP (2008) *Working Memory and Learning: A Practical Guide for Teachers*. London: Sage Publishing.

Goodman SA, Evans C, Loftin M (2009) *Intelligence Testing of Individuals Who Are Blind or Visually Impaired*. Available at: <https://sites.aph.org/accessible-tests/laws-guidelines/intelligence-testing/> [Accessed July 2021].

Gori M, Cappagli G, Baud-Bovy G, Finocchietti S (2017) Shape perception and navigation in blind adults. *Frontiers in Psychology* 8: 10.

Greenaway R, Pring L, Schepers A, Isaacs DP, Dale NJ (2017). Neuropsychological presentation and adaptive skills in high-functioning adolescents with visual impairment: a preliminary investigation. *Applied Neuropsychology: Child* 6: 145–157.

Jaworska-Biskup K. (2011). The world without sight. A comparative study of concept understanding in Polish congenitally totally blind and sighted children. *Psych of Lang and Comm* 15: 27–48.

Lahav O, Hagab N, El Kader SA, Levy ST, Talis V (2018). Listen to the models: sonified learning models for people who are blind. *Computers & Education* 127: 141–153.

Occelli V, Lacey S, Stephens C, Merabet LB, Sathian K (2017) Enhanced verbal abilities in the congenitally blind. *Exp Brain Res* 235: 1709–1718.

Pasqualotto A, Lam JS, Proulx MJ (2013) Congenital blindness improves semantic and episodic memory. *Behav Brain Res* 244: 162–165.

Picard D, Monnier C (2009) Short-term memory for spatial configurations in the tactile modality: A comparison with vision. *Memory* 17: 789–801.

Rule AC, Stefanich GP, Boody RM, Peiffer B (2011) Impact of adaptive materials on teachers and their students with vision impairments in secondary science and mathematics classes. *International Journal of Science Education* 33: 865–887.

Shams L, Seitz AR (2008) Benefits of multisensory learning. *Trends in Cog Sciences* 12: 411–417.

Ungar S, Simpson A, Blades M (2004) Strategies for organising information while learning a map by blind and sighted people. In: Heller M, Ballasteros S, editors, *Touch, Blindness and Neuroscience*. Madrid: Universidad Nacional de Educacion a Distancia, pp. 271–280.

Wakefield CE, Homewood J, Taylor AJ (2004) Cognitive compensations for blindness in children: an investigation using odour naming. *Perception* 33: 429–442.

Withagen A, Kappers AM, Vervloed MP, Knoors H, Verhoeven L (2013) Short term memory and working memory in blind versus sighted children. *Res in Dev Dis* 34: 2161–2172.

CHAPTER 13

Experience of Parenting a Child with Vision Impairment

Christopher Clark and Kate Clark

We are an average nuclear family of four, and we have a daughter, Ellie, with a severe vision impairment. Ellie has a sister who is 4 years younger, and we live with an assorted collection of animals!

When Ellie was just 4 weeks old we noticed she had significant nystagmus (involuntary to and fro movement of the eyes). Ellie could see and follow bright light, particularly in the dark, but nothing more. She was diagnosed with Leber congenital amaurosis at 7 months. At 7 years she was diagnosed as having autism spectrum needs within the context of profound visual impairment, which led to greater understanding of her current needs. Ellie is now 9 years old, doing very well, and attends our local main-stream primary school.

INFANCY AND EARLY YEARS

As an infant, Ellie was extremely sensitive to noise and disliked change, including being laid down in a new place for a nappy change. She would become upset easily, and would cry at any sudden noise, becoming anxious from any vocalisation from other infants/children. This made attending activities and going out in public very challenging. Once Ellie was upset, it was very difficult to distract her so she could calm down. In contrast, at home she was a happy and content baby, enjoying music and toys whilst lying on her back. Despite this, we tried to live as 'normally' as possible, taking her to infant groups, swimming, and other activities. It was a very difficult time for us all; we grieved Ellie's sight loss and worried about her future.

Over time, things got easier as we started to understand Ellie and her needs. We learnt she liked routine and structure, needed time to get used to new things such as going outside (particularly making sense of the wind), touching new textures, hearing new sounds, new environments, and people. Ellie loved books, music, and language and we spent a lot of time patiently answering the endless 'why?' questions. This thirst for knowledge undoubtedly helped Ellie form her early understanding of the world.

GETTING HELP AND SUPPORT

We turned to the Internet to search for answers and practical help to guide us through the very difficult early years. We were not only raising our first born with no prior experience of infants/children, but we were also learning to teach a child with a severe vision impairment. Without Internet-based support groups leading to strong friendships in many parts of the world, we definitely would not have felt able to cope with life. These friendships offer us very valuable emotional and practical support.

A very important part of both our and Ellie's early life was our wonderful health visitor. She listened and took the time to make a difference to our lives, including visiting us at home to check her weight as Ellie could not cope with the noise of the infant clinic. Following Ellie's diagnosis at 7 months, we were introduced to our local specialist teacher for the vision impaired. This was a huge relief after waiting for what seemed to be an eternity for someone to help our family. We needed to know what we should expect from Ellie, where she should be in terms of following milestones, and how to encourage her to move and explore, amongst many other things. The specialist teacher gave us practical ideas, support, and hope for the future. Ellie's mum made a commitment to learn basic braille and the specialist teacher provided a Perkins brailler to practise on.

We attended a local 'meet and greet' evening when Ellie was almost a year old. We needed to meet other local families with older children with vision impairment, and this event was invaluable for us. We are still in contact with some of these families and meet regularly for the children to enjoy the company of their peers on an equal footing.

Ellie attended our local mainstream day nursery, and Ellie was supported by a one-to-one assistant. We were upset and overwhelmed when we first visited, but the nursery was fabulous, giving us emotional and practical childcare advice. The nursery staff listened to us as we educated them about Ellie and they took advice from the specialist teacher to ensure Ellie had an inclusive and relevant experience. Ellie learnt her braille alphabet whilst still at nursery. She struggled socially to interact with other children but flourished with adults.

We attended the Developmental Vision clinic at Great Ormond Street Hospital annually when Ellie turned 1 year old until the age of 5 years. This gave us access to clinicians who were able to assess and record Ellie's abilities and track her progress. This allowed us to see her progress not only against other children but also her peers who had visual impairment, something we did not have from any other source. A report from each visit was written; we were able to share these with others working with her and continue our focus on maintaining high expectations for Ellie. We were also involved in two research projects from the hospital team, including evaluation of early intervention (OPTIMUM) and assessment of social communication needs (DAiSY), and we got reports on Ellie's performance and learned about the research.

FIRST SCHOOL YEARS

Ellie has attended two mainstream schools. Her first year in school was the most stressful year of our lives, consumed with frustration, anxiety, and guilt. Changes in teaching staff caused immense difficulties, and so we worked with another school preparing for Ellie to move. She learned routes around the new school and met the teacher and other children. This second school made an audiobook for her of her classmates' voices and appointed two teaching assistants who learned braille over the summer holidays. The transition could not have gone better. Her teaching assistants continue to be her biggest support, following her through the school and providing the most wonderfully adapted work and inclusive activities to support the teacher and Ellie's learning. Ellie is very settled, enjoys school, has friends, and is well supported.

SOME CHALLENGES AND GROWTH

Ellie lacked motivation to move and explore and did not crawl and walk until later than average. Ellie's mum left a career in mechanical engineering to retrain as a habilitation specialist when Ellie turned 3 years old to support her and other children in this area.

Ellie has always pressed her eyes. As an infant this was almost constant but is much less significant today, although she still presses in various situations. She also has various head rolling, stepping (from one foot to the other), and hand flapping tendencies that she tries to manage.

Ellie's eating has always been of concern to us, not having a strong appetite and never asking/wanting food or drink. She still rarely asks for food or drink, and struggles to know when she is full, preferring to ask if her plate is empty.

Ellie is very outgoing but finds it hard to maintain the interest of another child, often talking in riddles or make-believe that is hard to follow. She finds it difficult to listen and take on other opinions. Her peers will choose to walk away rather than discuss things like an adult would. Her relationships remain strong with adults around her. Ellie has struggled with social interactions, but she now has made a few closer relationships with school friends, which we hope will remain strong. Ellie has a strong bond with her sibling and this developing relationship has definitely helped her social interactions with others. She still struggles to anticipate outcomes of her words or actions, but can now play cooperatively rather than needing to dictate play on her terms.

We have found the processes involved in establishing the support that Ellie needs for her education and learning frustrating and challenging as processes and provision vary across the country, and we have to campaign for things to meet Ellie's needs. Access to adapted physical education in school, and provision of orientation, mobility, and independence skills outside of school are other problems we have faced. It can be a lonely road to tread; we have often felt there is no 'professional' advocate for our child and that we have only our own perseverance and intuition to guide us.

Shortly after starting school Ellie started pulling her hair out with anxiety and worries. She was unable to express herself but her anxiety showed in her mood, attitude, and behaviour. We struggled to find anyone that had experience of mental health in a child with severe vision impairment. In the end, we did manage to find the right person (a clinical psychologist with expertise in visual impairment) and this support has been invaluable to Ellie. Not only to address challenges in the here and now and to give strategies for handling them but to give Ellie that confidence of knowing there is someone there to listen and help should she need it.

JOINING IN AND PARTICIPATING

We gain vital support from events and charities, seeking out every opportunity that becomes available to our family. Sporting events such as 'have a go' days helped Ellie try new things. She reluctantly tried judo at one of these events and is now in her third year and enjoying every second. Ellie (and her sibling) have completed many activities that she/they would have not been able to experience had Ellie not had a vision impairment. Ellie has abseiled, rock climbed, canoed, skied, been to tennis festivals, met Paralympians, competed in a swimming gala for children with vision impairment, and met and handled a huge number of animals. We regularly attend family science days. These are adapted and inclusive and allow us to engage in society as a family, knowing both children are catered for.

We have gained friendships with many adults with vision impairment, including professional athletes, international mobility specialists, and cat and guinea pig enthusiasts, and they act as role models for Ellie and give her invaluable knowledge and experience.

What is important to us as parents?

✓ Informed and specialist support from as early as possible in our child's life including early intervention to help us help our child's progress and learning.

✓ Shared understanding of success, aspirations, and the highest possible expectations set for our child.

✓ A proactive partnership between medical, education, and specialist practitioners in vision impairment, including identifying and overcoming needs and challenges for our child.

✓ Appropriate and timely mental health support, as and when needed by our child.

✓ Social networks and peer support for our child and us as a family including for siblings.

✓ The support and opportunities from many visual impairment organisations, networks, and children and adults with visual impairment – parent groups, Internet networks, charities and voluntary organisations, sport camps, adult role models.

✓ Opportunities for Ellie and our family to feel 'normal' and to be able to participate in all activities available for other children and their families.

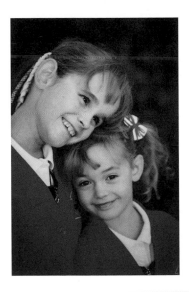
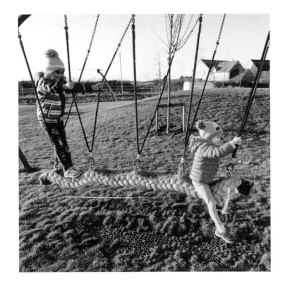

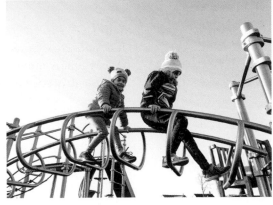

PART 3

Further Approaches to Habilitation

CHAPTER 14

Orientation, Mobility, and Independence Skills

Habilitation Approaches

Jessica Hayton and Susan Mort

INTRODUCTION

Habilitation for independence is the process of maximising independence in children with vision impairment. This includes supporting the functional performance of motor, cognitive, and psychological developmental milestones in everyday life (Hayton and Dimitriou 2019). Specialist professionals in 'habilitation' aim to bring together and promote positive outcomes in orientation and independence skills in children with visual impairment.

Mobility is the ability to physically move and navigate around any given environment (Miller et al. 2011). Orientation skills emerge from mobility skills and knowing your position in space. Independence skills complete the triad of the habilitation for independence approach as they also depend on mobility and orientation. Independent living skills associated with daily living in domestic and social contexts are expressed through adaptive behaviours (Greenaway et al. 2017; Bathelt et al. 2019). Examples of independence skills include communication, socialisation, dressing, self-feeding and personal care like toileting and tooth-brushing in home, educational, and public settings (Fairnham et al. 2002; Bardi 2014). Independence in mobility is positively associated with wellbeing in adolescents with vision impairment (Kef et al. 2000; see also Chapter 19). The acquisition of independence skills and presentation of adaptive behaviours depend on the chronological age and developmental stage of the child with vision impairment, who may lag behind typically developing peers of the same age.

HABILITATION AND VISION IMPAIRMENT

Definition of Issues

All children with vision impairment, whatever their diagnosis and variable needs, require and are entitled to habilitation for independence provision. As the population of children with vision impairment include those who have additional needs (such as intellectual disability, autism spectrum disorder, motor impairment, and mental health needs), the habilitation specialist will need to be able to cover the full range of needs whilst working in a multidisciplinary team and context.

Habilitation for independence is operationalised as the combination and teaching of mobility, orientation, and independence skills from birth, through childhood to adulthood (Miller et al. 2011). Habilitation is distinguished from rehabilitation, as it adopts a child-centred developmental approach to equip children and young people with essential and transferable skills that are fundamental for daily living (Hayton and Dimitriou 2019). Habilitation accounts for the developmental history and trajectory of each child when planning structured, systematic support to maximise the independence of the child in achieving their individual potential.

The practical strategies incorporated for habilitation depend on an understanding of typical and atypical infant and childhood development. The child who is typically sighted tends to learn and acquire independence and autonomy skills incidentally via visual observation, imitation of others, practice, and habitual learning (Wall 2019). For children with vision impairment, access to incidental learning may be absent or very compromised depending on their level of vision. This removes their immediate access to observing, learning, and practice; the achievement of all skills underpinning independence are delayed. Habilitation programmes seek to compensate for these developmental delays and barriers to learning associated with lack of vision through specialist formal systematic teaching and practical support.

Adaptive Behaviour

Adaptive behaviour skills draw on mobility, orientation, and independence skills. They may be lower than the child's chronological age or cognitive abilities (Bathelt et al. 2019), which can lead to challenges in relation to expectations in the environment. Using education as an example, children joining at first school entry are expected to have achieved basic independence skills like self-dressing (for physical education class) or independent toileting at recreation times. However, the child with severe vision impairment is not necessarily developmentally ready to undertake these tasks independently. They may lack the readiness in motor coordination, body awareness, sensory, and cognitive planning skills to begin to learn this task or to master it proficiently without assistance.

There have been very few studies reported of adaptive behaviour skill development in children with vision impairment under the age of 8 years, so the degree and extent of delays and challenges are not well known. It is anticipated that those with profound vision impairment or very severe vision impairment will be the most affected. A study (based on parental-report) examining adaptive behaviours in children with vision impairment found that children with vision impairment performed only 44% of 101 daily living skills compared to 84% performed by peers who are typically sighted (Lewis and Iselin 2002). The contrast between the two groups was most prominent in elements of personal care, such as drying hair (with towel/hairdryer) and applying a plaster to cuts, and relating to time, such as using a watch/alarm clock. These differences revealed the potential impact of vision impairment on independence and adaptive behaviour.

In middle childhood and adolescence, some small-scale studies exist. A study of 8 to 12-year-olds with congenital disorders of the peripheral visual system (of average verbal intelligence) found significantly reduced adapted behaviour on the parent-reported Adaptive Behaviour Assessment System, 2nd Edition (ABAS-II) in children with profound-severe vision impairment compared with peers who are typically sighted; effects were smaller for children with moderate vision impairment (Bathelt et al. 2019). Another study of adolescents with congenital vision impairment and average verbal intelligence performed below the average range on all subscales of the ABAS-II, with the exception of 'communication' and 'leisure' skills. The adaptive behaviour domains of 'functional academics' (literacy/numeracy skill), and 'home living' (cleaning, organisation, and food preparation) were identified as areas that required much improvement (Greenaway et al. 2017). However, adaptive behaviour was a 'mediating' factor for quality of life at school; those children with higher scores on the ABAS-II had higher quality of life even if their vision level was more severely reduced (Bathelt et al. 2019). This highlights the importance of specialist provision that can work with young people and their parents to enhance their adaptive behaviour skills.

Habilitation for Independence and Outcomes

Habilitation for independence links to the International Classification of Functioning, Disability and Health: Children and Youth (ICF-CY) model (World Health Organization 2013; see Chapter 1) as it accommodates the biopsychosocial factors of a child with vision impairment, in addition to the bidirectional interactions between the child and the persons/object within their environment. Habilitation for independence has a particular focus on the 'function' and 'participation' domains of the ICF-CY model.

To date, little empirical research has examined these outcomes and the effectiveness of habilitation approaches for independence in children with vision impairment. This may be due to the re-introduction of the concept of 'habilitation for independence', the specialist discipline being relatively new (Hogg et al. 2017), and a general confusion of the term 'habilitation' and its objectives (Miller et al. 2011). Any available published works tend to include small sample sizes, are not safe to generalise (due to the heterogeneous nature of the sample), and are rarely replicable. However, the importance of starting habilitation for independence as early as possible is now well established (Skellenger and Sapp 2010; Keil et al. 2017).

Parents/caregivers and educators have a crucial role in the development and acquisition of independence and adaptive behaviours, both in supporting and fostering this development and influencing the timing of different independence opportunities. There are cultural and societal differences in expectations of autonomy and independence at different ages, which will need to be considered (Taverna et al. 2011). A further influence is parental perception and expectations towards their child regarding how independent they can or should be at each age level. In typically developing children (mean age 10 years), parents' willingness and perception of their child's autonomy are predictors of greater independent mobility to school (Ayllón et al. 2019). In relation to children with vision impairment, qualitative focus group research has shown some differences in perspective between parent, specialist professional, and young people with vision impairment and their views and expectations on 'independence and autonomy' (Tadić et al. 2013; Rainey et al. 2016). Although the evidence is still limited, research suggests that parent and teachers make important contributions to the development and acquisition of adaptive behaviours. However, there are tensions and contradictions in the discourse and practices of risk-taking for children, young people, and adults with disabilities and education, health, and social care settings may be risk-averse with vulnerable children (Seale et al. 2013). Habilitation practice therefore requires a conceptual framework that incorporates creativity and resilience for positive risk-taking (as proposed by Seale et al. for special and inclusive education practices). This can enhance 'readiness' and commencement of independence skills and adaptive behaviours in line with expectations of autonomy.

ASSESSMENT AND PRACTICE

Globally, access to habilitation for independent living provision varies according to country and context (Wall 2019). Habilitation is proposed as the key to empowering and supporting children with vision impairment, yet some inconsistencies in practice, communication, and funds detrimentally affect accessibility and quality of provision (Hogg et al. 2017).

Habilitation needs to account for the child's holistic functioning. Realistic objectives and strategies are designed to accommodate individual need in collaboration with the child and parent/caregiver as key partners. The habilitation practitioner works closely with the multidisciplinary team, including ophthalmology, child development/neurodisability health team, educational staff including specialist teacher for the visually impaired, and family support organisations and social care staff so that the child's level of vision, and additional child and family needs, if present, are understood as part of the habilitation programme.

The Quality Standards for Habilitation (UK; Miller et al. 2011) offer a basis for the professional training and delivery of habilitation for independent living, indicating the crucial need for collaborative and multidisciplinary working to support and maximise the independence of children and young people with vision impairment (see Chapter 20). The commencement of a habilitation programme by qualified habilitation practitioners can occur as young as possible, supporting mobility, orientation, and independence skill development from infancy and early years, through childhood into adolescence and adulthood (Keil et al. 2017; see Chapter 20). This develops good practice from the outset, avoiding the possibility of developing practice or habits that may later require modification, such as cane skills for mobility (Miller et al. 2011).

Assessment

The process for receiving formal habilitation support begins with referral. After referral, a habilitation specialist will observe the child in familiar and unfamiliar settings (notably, home, education, and public contexts). The observations and assessment include mobility, orientation, and independence skills in addition to how the child accesses age appropriate, non-curriculum-based information and their social skills to inform the habilitation programme.

The importance of working with the parent as partner is recognised, as the parent/caregiver plays the primary role in the development of mobility, orientation, and independence skills. As a result, it is crucial that the child, parent/caregiver, and family are consulted and involved in the assessment and decision-making process underpinning the programme (Miller et al. 2011). One of the essential practical elements of habilitation is harnessing the child's motivation toward tasks and this requires effective verbal and non-verbal communication with the child.

To assess emerging, developing, and acquired skills or skills that need to be fostered, a variety of methods and schemes can be used. From a practitioner stance, a comprehensive detailed list of age/stage appropriate skills designed specifically for 'Habilitation for independence' (Australia; Do it Yourself) (Fairnham et al. 2002) and MISE (UK; Mobility and Independence Specialists in Education 2016) are available, as well as those covering all areas of development. The scientifically evaluated Developmental Journal for babies and young children with visual impairment (DJVI; UK; Salt and Dale 2017; Dale et al. 2019) has a domain on 'Towards Independent self-care' including milestones and goals for feeding/eating, dressing, toileting, washing, bedtime routine, and sleeping pattern, covering the early months to 3 years 7 months (see further Chapter 8). It is integrated with all other areas of development including 'Movement and mobility' and 'Social and emotional development'. The Oregon Project (USA; Anderson et al. 2007) is valuable for the older preschool range, which is not covered by the DJVI. These materials assess the developmental stages of a child with vision impairment, assist in target setting, identify strengths and weaknesses, and record skill acquisition and developmental progress. They are useful in coordinating habilitation programmes based on individual level of need, task analysis, and strategies for support.

The parent will have knowledge of the child's skills in everyday settings and their observations need to be incorporated when using developmental tracking records. The DJVI, for example, is designed to be used in partnership with the parent and the materials including guidance Activity cards are written for the parent and to focus on positive and realistic progress of the individual child in their everyday setting. The tracking checklists also highlight if a child is not making steady progress and may require referral to specialist health services for further assessment (see Chapter 8). Parents need to be supported through this process.

For assessment of habilitation skills as the child becomes older and is functioning in different environments (e.g. home, school, organisation), it is important to record the transferability of skills (e.g. to different contexts or unfamiliar environments) and identify any potential barriers that could impact the successful execution of the skill (Table 14.1). This is because the child may need to learn environment-specific strategies for particular skills to maintain independence in particular domains (e.g. eating a meal at home vs in a restaurant). Learning alternative strategies can help overcome obstacles that cannot be mitigated within the particular environment.

To reduce the potential impact of barriers, scaffolding skills support a child in moving from simplified play-based activities to complex independence tasks. For example, rolling and cutting playdough is a useful pre-requisite to spreading and cutting a sandwich. This

Table 14.1 Transferability and barriers of skill learning

Examples of transferable skills	The potential barriers impacting on the learning of the skill
Problem solving	Lack of initiative Poor choice making Low confidence
Assessing risk	Acting rashly Lack of environmental awareness Unknown consequences
Following instruction	Unpredictable behaviour Understanding of concepts/language
Sequencing	Lack of concepts/exposure

is due to concept formation and sensory-motor development associated with learning the skill initially through play. Exposure to appropriate experiences, developing, and rehearsing skills builds the knowledge to develop simple snack-making techniques, through to accessing recipes, purchasing ingredients, and cooking hot dinners. Each stage requires consistency, routine, and organisation, ensuring maintenance of skill whilst prioritising specific techniques.

Task Analysis and Programme Design

After observations and assessment of initial skills, an individualised programme is designed in conjunction with parents/caregivers, the child, and the multidisciplinary team. Strategies for support, agreed outcomes, and responsibilities (e.g. who will be undertaking what) are detailed. The habilitation specialist leads the design and implementation of the programme, supported by assistants and other key partners working closely with the specialist. The habilitation specialist supports the overall running of the programme by providing environmental audits and risk assessments for all activities. The child is also involved in the risk assessment process to encourage self-understanding in areas of risk and problem-solving to mitigate the risks posed.

The habilitation programme is designed for the individual needs of the child, accommodating aspirations and environmental contexts. The programme is monitored and reviewed periodically and adapted where necessary. Adaptations arise from changes in visual or other learning need, skill acquisition, and transitions to different settings. The habilitation programme needs to account for the cognitive, physical, psychological, and social development of the child. Consistent and structured interventions based on task analysis is essential for habilitation training in all contexts. Task analysis supports the development of habilitation for independence skills, splitting the whole activity into smaller, nuanced, yet observable stages. Regular reviews examine the ongoing impact of the habilitation programme, monitoring the transition from dependence to independence.

The habilitation approach covers many different pre-requisite and transferable skill-learning areas such as gross and fine motor skills suited to independent living (i.e. route planning, independent travel, and long cane work) or other activities such as personal care (see Table 14.2). Within a habilitation programme, mobility, orientation, and independence skills are systematically taught over developmental phases, age and stage appropriate to the individual child (Bardin 2014; Fazzi 2014; Wall 2019).

Key Salient Strategies to Support Habilitation for Independence

Adopting the principle that 'habilitation begins at home', there are salient strategies to support and identify areas for development. Underpinning these skills are

Table 14.2 Habilitation skill-learning

Examples of skills taught by a habilitation specialist
Engaging with self, others, and the environment
Planning and learning identified routes
Using a cane to travel independently
Managing own personal care
Independently dressing, shopping, and managing laundry
Eating and table skills
Food storage and preparation
Simple household tasks including organisation and labelling
Developing and maintaining relationships
Access to information to promote independence
Being able to self-advocate

communication, love and support, consistency, patience, inspiration, playfulness, and strong role modelling (see Table 14.3).

The practical utility of such strategies varies depending on context and provision. To meaningfully assess child readiness and development, communication must be appropriate and understood by the child. Before assessing (in)formally, a parent or associated professional must gauge the child's conceptual comprehension. Concept formation and the ability to understand and follow instructions are essential to habilitation and preparation for exploring the world. Strategies and habilitation programmes are child-led, increasing in complexity alongside the demands of daily living. The strategies and questions outlined do not replace professional input, rather are considerations prior to formal provisional arrangements, and will also assist those working with children in countries where highly specialist support is not available.

IMPLICATIONS FOR RESEARCH AND PRACTICE

Research and practice in habilitation for independence are evolving. Mobility and orientation and new technological aids are advancing in research and practice (see Chapter 15), yet independence is less developed. Multidisciplinary collaborative work is needed between habilitation practitioners, other service providers, and scientific researchers to develop evidence-based practice. An evidence-based approach could lead to a more integrated means of delivery, improved training for practitioners, and shared understandings for the future.

There remains a global lack of prioritisation of the need for habilitation for independence for children and young people with vision impairment. This remains a high clinical

Table 14.3 Functional strategies to support mobility, orientation, and independence

Targeted skills	Eliciting and assessing current skills Does/Can the child...?	Practical developmental strategies
Sensory skills	• Turn their head or respond positively to certain stimuli compared with others? • Actively seek sensory stimulation?	Observe and record sensory preferences to create play-based activities focussing on multisensory stimulation.
Body awareness	• Name and locate the parts of their body? • Know how the body connects, e.g. limbs? • Know the boundaries of their body? • Demonstrate good posture and balance?	Develop motor skills and body awareness through songs and play. Teach the name and location of body parts and motions on self and others.
Knowing the environment	• Understand the different functions and purposes of space(s)? • Name and recognise geographical and man-made features?	Systematic learning of rooms within the home and educational setting. Community visits to explore outdoor and public locations.
Orientating and navigating	• Identify clues and landmarks on a familiar route? • Initiate finding and identifying clues and landmarks? • Use senses to orientate themselves?	Practice using sighted guide or mobility device. Create tactile, sensory, and mental maps of short routes. Teach clues and landmarks on routes. Involve the child in route planning to achieve their goals.
Making and maintaining relationships	• Co-operate and demonstrate cultural etiquette when requested? • Show empathy for others? • Demonstrate awareness of turn-taking in conversation? • Actively listen to others and respond accordingly given context? • Respect personal space?	Practise and role model positive social behaviours. Discuss strategies for managing body language and absence/reduced eye contact. Develop peer groups to converse, turn take, and play. Role play scenarios and settings commensurate to the needs of the child. Allow the child to make mistakes and learn from them.

(Continued)

Table 14.3 Functional strategies to support (Continued)

Targeted skills	Eliciting and assessing current skills Does/Can the child...?	Practical developmental strategies
Self-advocacy	• Understand their specific need(s)? • Know what support will meet that need? • Have the skills to ask for the support they need? • Can the child explain their needs to peers?	Encourage communication. Praise when help is requested. Role model respect for self and others. Develop a sense of ownership. Discuss strengths and weaknesses.
Personal care	• Show readiness for physical independent tasks? • Understand what the task is, the rationale, and the steps taken from start to finish? • Initiate activities, i.e. remove items of clothing or begin to take ownership of sequences, taking over from adult support?	Grow food, shop, discuss nutrition, and practise cooking and table skills. Encourage self-care, hygiene, and dressing daily. As the child takes on more responsibility, introduce the concepts of time and time management and linked responsibilities such as healthy choices.
Risk management	• Understand the concept of 'stop'? • Understand associated risks with activities? • Express management of risk, e.g. knowing to wait at a roadside? • Actively explore their environment in a safe and purposive way? • Know when to ask for help and from whom?	Climb mountains, paddle in streams, and dream big. Role model how to assess and manage personal risk in controlled situations.
Problem-solving	• Explore varied approaches independently? Are alternative strategies safe and meaningful relative to the goal?	Allow plenty of time for consideration before intervening in difficult or challenging situations.
Accessing information	• Show awareness of signage in shops, streets, as well as home and educational setting? • Demonstrate awareness of printed materials? • Have preferred technology to enable access to printed materials?	Access to talking books, magazines, and radio. Provision of home and community information in preferred medium.

priority to maximise the potential and participation of all children and young people with vision impairment.

Habilitation underpins opportunities for independent living, higher education, employability, and self-realisation in adolescence and adulthood. Longitudinal research studies could monitor the effectiveness of training and provide increased evidence to underpin public spending and policy decisions in this area. The ICF-CY framework is giving impetus to child, parent, and practitioner stakeholder research and new methods of measuring 'activity' and 'participation' domains as potential meaningful outcome measures (Rainey et al. 2016).

SUMMARY

Children with vision impairment need support and habilitation for independence and autonomy. Habilitation programmes can start from birth, initially provided at home, and should continue through the school years with specialist and multidisciplinary support. The variable visual and developmental needs and environmental factors affect habilitation provision, so individualised programmes need to be collaboratively developed by habilitation specialists, the child, and their family to maximise independence. There is no single way of teaching or developing habilitation skills, but consistency and collaboration are fundamental to ensure the needs, abilities, and aspirations of the child and family are incorporated into the design.

Key Points

✓ Globally, all children with vision impairment are entitled to habilitation for independence provision.

✓ Structured interventions teach children with vision impairment essential self-care, self-organising, and problem-solving strategies.

✓ The importance of the family partnership should be built into and inform habilitation design and delivery.

✓ Empirical and longitudinal research is required to understand the impact of habilitation programmes on the development of mobility, orientation, and independence skills in children with vision impairment.

✓ Collaborative and multidisciplinary work is essential to support holistic habilitation for children with vision impairment and to close the research to practice gap.

REFERENCES

Anderson S, Boigon S, Davis K, DeWaard C, South Oregon Education Service District (2007) *The Oregon Project for Preschool Children Who Are Blind or Visually Impaired*, 6th Edition. Medford, OR: South Oregon Education Service.

Ayllón E, Moyano N, Lozano A, Cava MJ (2019) Parents' willingness and perception of children's autonomy as predictors of greater independent mobility to school. *International journal of Environmental Research and Public Health* **16**(5): 732.

Bardin JA (2014) Independent living. In: Allman CB, Lewis S, editors, *ECC Essentials: Teaching the Expanded Core Curriculum to Students with Visual Impairments*. New York: American Printing House for the Blind, pp. 283–310.

Bathelt J, de Haan M, Dale NJ (2019) Adaptive behaviour and quality of life in school-age children with congenital visual disorders and different levels of visual impairment. *Res in Dev Disabilities* **85**: 154–162.

Dale NJ, Sakkalou E, O'Reilly MA (2019) Home-based early intervention in infants and young children with visual impairment using the Developmental Journal: longitudinal cohort study. *Dev Med & Child Neurol* **61**(6): 697–709.

Fairnham M, Johnston C, Kain S, Kaine N, McCauley A, Steele E (2002) Do it yourself: Encouraging Independence in Children who are blind. In Flavel R, Lunn H, Johnston C, editors, *Vision Australia (Blindness and Low Vision Services)*. Sydney: University of Sydney.

Fazzi D (2014) Orientation and mobility. In: Allman CB, Lewis S, editors, *ECC Essentials: Teaching the Expanded Core Curriculum to Students with Visual Impairments*. New York: American Printing House for the Blind, pp. 248–272.

Greenaway R, Pring L, Schepers A, Isaacs DP, Dale NJ (2017) Neuropsychological presentation and adaptive skills in high-functioning adolescents with visual impairment: a preliminary investigation. *Applied Neuropsychology: Child* **6**(2): 145–157.

Hayton J, Dimitriou D (2019) What's in a word? Distinguishing between habilitation and re-habilitation. *Int Journal of Orientation & Mobility* **10**(1): 1–4.

Hogg K, Thetford C, Wheeler SL, York S, Moxon R, Robinson J (2017) Habilitation provision for children and young people with vision impairment in the United Kingdom: a lack of clarity leading to inconsistencies. *British Journal of Visual Impairment* **35**(1): 44–54.

Kef S, Hox JJ, Habekothe HT (2000) Social networks of visually impaired and blind adolescents. Structure and effect on well-being. *Social Networks* **22**: 73–91. doi: 10.1016/S0378-8733(00)00022-8.

Keil S, Fielder A, Sargent J (2017) Management of children and young people with vision impairment: diagnosis, developmental challenges and outcomes. *Archives of Disease in Childhood* **102**(6): 566–571.

Lewis S, Iselin SA (2002) A comparison of the independent living skills of primary students with visual impairments and their sighted peers: a pilot study. *Journal of Visual Impairment & Blindness* **96**(5): 335–344.

Miller O, Wall K, Garner M (2011) Quality standards: delivery of habilitation training (mobility and independent living skills) for children and young people with visual impairment. Mobility and Independence Specialists in Education, 2016. Available at http://www.ssc.education.ed.ac.uk/resources/vi%26multi/habilitation.pdf.

Mobility and Independence Specialists in Education (2016) *Mobility and Independence, Assessment and Evaluation Scheme: Early Years*. Available at Mob & Ind 28.2.07 final.indd (habilitationviuk.org.uk).

Rainey L, Elsman EBM, van Nispen RMA, van Leeuwen LM, van Rens GHMB (2016) Comprehending the impact of low vision on the lives of children and adolescents: a qualitative approach. *Quality of Life Research* **25**(10): 2633–2643.

Salt A, Dale N (2017) *Developmental Journal for Babies and Young Children with Visual Impairment (DJVI)*, 2nd Edition. Available at: <https://xip.uclb.com/i/healthcare_tools/DJVI_professional.html> [Accessed July 2021].

Seale J, Nind M, Simmons B (2013) Transforming positive risk-taking practices: the possibilities of creativity and resilience in learning disability contexts. *Scand Journal of Dis Res* **15**(3): 233–248.

Skellenger AC, Sapp WK (2010) Teaching orientation and mobility for the early childhood years. *Foundations of Orientation and Mob* 2: 163–207.

Tadić V, Cooper A, Cumberland P, Lewando-Hundt G, Rahi JS (2013) Development of the functional vision questionnaire for children and young people with visual impairment: the FVQ_CYP. *Ophthalmology* **120**(12): 2725–2732.

Taverna L, Bornstein MH, Putnick DL, Axia G (2011) Adaptive behaviors in young children: a unique cultural comparison in Italy. *Journal of Cross-Cultural Psychology* 42(3): 445–465.

Wall K (2019) Habilitation and rehabilitation. In: Ravenscroft J, editor, *The Routledge Handbook of Visual Impairment: Social and Cultural Research*. Abingdon and New York: Routledge, pp. 333–359.

World Health Organization (2013) *How to Use the ICF: A Practical Manual for Using the International Classification of Functioning, Disability and Health (ICF). Exposure Draft for Comment*. Geneva: WHO.

CHAPTER 15

Technological Aids for Spatial Perception and Mobility

Monica Gori and Giulia Cappagli

INTRODUCTION

Spatial perception is a person's ability to be aware of and internalise relationships between the body and the environment. Therefore, it is a prerequisite for independent navigation and mobility. Vision is the sensory modality that provides the most accurate and reliable information about the external world's spatial properties. Therefore, even a temporary lack of visual information may significantly affect spatial cognition in people with typical sight. The assessment of spatial abilities in children and young people with vision impairment gives a significant opportunity to learn about this development process in the absence of vision, and to support children and young people in their spatial understanding. This chapter discusses spatial perception in children and young people with vision impairment and technological aids that can be employed to enhance their spatial perception and mobility. It covers knowledge about developmental stages that might be potentially delayed and technological aids to support the acquisition of perceptual and motor abilities in this context. The creation of new technological devices that can be adopted early in life can improve these abilities, reduce disability, and increase the child or young person's independence, autonomy, and participation in the environment and society.

SPATIAL PERCEPTION

Children with vision impairment tend to manifest problems in the motor domain (Hallemans et al. 2011; Rogge et al. 2021), and also in several perceptual aspects, including localisation in the auditory domain (Fazzi et al. 2011; Cappagli and Gori 2016; Vercillo et al. 2016), localisation in the tactile domain (Cappagli et al. 2017a), and orientation discrimination in the tactile modality. It has been suggested that having a profound vision impairment challenges spatial perception because it prevents exploratory activities with objects and locomotor experiences and therefore constrains the acquisition of self-knowledge in the environment. Recent behavioural and neurophysiological studies suggest that there are some limits to compensation in the case of vision sensory loss (Amadeo et al. 2019). However, psychophysical evidence suggests that tactile and auditory skills can be enhanced in individuals with congenital profound visual impairment, such as localising a sound source in the horizontal plane or discriminating between different pitch sound (Doucet et al. 2005; Fortin et al. 2008). Animal (Petrus et al. 2014) and human (Thaler et al. 2011; Arnott et al. 2013; Norman and Thaler 2019; Thaler et al. 2020; Tonelli et al. 2020) studies confirm this view, suggesting that the visual cortex is activated for sound processing after visual deprivation. For instance, Norman and Thaler (2019) demonstrated that blind expert echolocators who perceive space through sound echoes using clicks show the retinotopic-like mapping of sound echoes, indicating that the functional topography of the visual cortex can encode auditory stimuli for a localisation task. For further details related to the studies assessing visual area activation following a visual loss, see Chapter 7.

Presenting Features

Visual perception acquisition through auditory means is of fundamental importance for children with vision impairment, especially those with severe and profound vision impairment because it supports the ability to navigate in the environment independently. It may also support the engagement in positive social interaction with peers. While visual feedback represents the most important incentive for intentional actions and thus for the development of mobility for children with typical sight (Vasilyeva and Lourenco 2012), children and adults with vision impairment rely strongly on auditory cues and landmarks to encode spatial information. For instance, they might rely on sound-producing objects in the room to find the exit door. Spatial perception emerges gradually in infants who are typically sighted due to the reciprocal influence between visual perception and the execution of movements (Bremner et al. 2008). In contrast, infants and young children with vision impairment lack not only the visual input necessary to establish the sensory-motor feedback that typically promotes early spatial development but also manifests a general delay in the acquisition of important locomotor and proprioceptive (i.e. sense of self-movement and position of a body in space) skills. As they get older, this may cause them to accumulate much less spatial experience compared to their peers with typical sight.

Scientific research has provided mixed results about the development of spatial cognition and spatial perceptual abilities in the child with vision impairment. Developmental delay in sound localisation abilities and motor responses to sound have been observed in studies of infants and young children with severe vision impairment. For instance, children with vision impairment show worse performance compared to children with typical sight in an auditory bisection task requiring understanding of the spatial relation of three sounds differently positioned in space (Vercillo et al. 2016), and in an audio depth task requiring them to identify which of two consecutive sounds was closer to their body (Cappagli et al. 2017a). These difficulties seem to be related to an important role of visual input during the first years of life as proposed by the 'cross-sensory calibration theory' (Gori et al. 2013). Other studies indicate that children learn to compensate for their lack of vision after initial delays by developing good manipulatory and walking skills through an interest in and exploration of sound-producing objects in the environment (Fazzi et al. 2011). Moreover, studies of proprioceptive localisation (where proprioception, also referred to as kinesthesia, is the sense of self-movement and body position of immediate and memorised stimuli) have shown that early visual deprivation does not necessarily prevent the development of spatial representations in children with profound visual impairment but that it might disrupt the ability to represent space from different perspectives other than the one from their own body. This could even impact on social development and social perspective-taking (see Chapter 11). Moreover, it has been recently demonstrated that visually impaired children show a developmental delay in the ability to update spatial coordinates, further confirming the pivotal role of vision in shaping allocentric spatial coding across development (Martolini et al. 2020). Conversely, several works have shown that blind individuals who rely on echolocation for their spatial judgments may not present such developmental delays and impairments observed in visually impaired individuals who do not echolocate (Teng et al. 2012; Vercillo et al. 2015; Kolarik et al. 2017; Tonelli et al. 2020). Such evidence indicates that perceptual competencies in visually impaired and blind individuals strongly depend on training and rehabilitation experiences across their lifespan. As recently demonstrated, an early multisensory and multidimensional rehabilitation intervention can improve overall neuropsychomotor development in children with congenital visual impairment (Morelli et al. 2020) and the early introduction of physical activities can improve postural stability and navigation performance in children who are blind and visually impaired (Rogge et al. 2021).

Short- and Long-Term Outcomes

Challenges and constraints in spatial perception and cognition may have short and long-term impacts on children and young people and their ability to participate in society. These may include difficulties developing spontaneous creative play with objects, navigating the playground to find peers to play with, and learning to go out and navigate independently and autonomously. The inability to find objects that disappear or reliance on others to localise objects or navigate to a particular place independently may cause immediate frustration for the child, and dependence on adults for assistance. This may have longer-term implications for self-autonomy, independence, peer relationships, academic and occupational success, and mental health. Therefore, the development of spatial perception and cognition must be given systematic attention and appropriate habilitation and support throughout childhood and as appropriate for the child's needs. The children who remain most at risk in this area are those with severe to profound vision impairment, who lack sufficient vision to aid spatial cognition.

Assessment of needs and technological aids and interventionist training are potentially important to support the development of spatial perceptual abilities in children with vision impairment. However, there are research issues that need resolving. Until now, the lack of standard and validated behavioural assessment tests available to measure spatial perception and spatial cognition has limited the systematic measurement of developmental progress and identification of needs that would benefit from assistance. Moreover, lack of awareness of which spatial perceptual abilities are affected in children and young people with vision impairment and which children are most 'at risk', has limited the development of evidence-led habilitative intervention strategies. Technological aids and interventionist training that may be augmentative for spatial perception and navigation are likely to be beneficial, but very few technological devices have been developed and validated so far for children with vision impairment (Gori et al. 2016).

Efforts have been put towards the development of sensory substitutions devices that aim at substituting the missing sense (i.e. vision) by conveying the information generally transmitted by the missing sense with a different sensory channel (i.e. tactile or auditory). An example of this is the vOICe (Meijer 1992), which permits 'listening' to images by converting them into a sound pattern via a special computer connected to a standard television camera. While sensory substitutions devices can provide support for specific spatial perceptual tasks in adults' object localisation and recognition (Auvray et al. 2007), they have never been tested in children principally because their use might overwhelm children's attentional resources and they require extensive training from adults (Gori et al. 2016). Therefore, their transferability to children is not known, including the age at which they could be beneficial, if at all. In the next section, we provide evidence that from an improved definition and understanding of spatial perceptual development and developmental challenges in the child with vision impairment, it is possible to create new habilitation tools to support their growth and maturation.

Intervention strategies using multisensory training and audio training have now been trialled. New multisensory technological solutions have been developed to address this important aspect, including the Audio Bracelet for Blind Interaction (the ABBI device), an audio-motor system to improve spatial, motor, and social skills of children with profound and severe vision impairment from 3 to 18 years of age (see Figs 15.1 and 15.2).

SUPPORT AND MANAGEMENT

Assessment

As children with vision impairment show delays in developing a spatial representation of the environment that can impact other areas of development and participation in society (including navigation and mobility and interacting with peers), it is valuable for the clinician or educator to assess spatial perception and cognition systematically. A standardised clinical tool to assess spatial perception in the developing child with vision impairment would provide the criterion standard to identify spatial challenges and rate of progress and focus habilitation and intervention strategies on areas requiring support. With this aim, our research group developed and demonstrated the reliability of a battery of six spatial tasks to provide the first criterion standard for assessing spatial cognition deficits in children with visual impairment (Blind Spatial Perception – BSP) (Finocchietti et al. 2019). Thirty children with visual impairment (6–17 years old) participated in two identical sessions, at a distance of 10 weeks, in which they performed six spatial tasks: auditory bisection (listening to three sounds and reporting whether the second sound was closer in space to the first or to the last one presented), auditory localisation (listening to one sound and pointing towards its spatial location), auditory distance discrimination (listening to three sounds and reporting whether the first or the second presented is closer to their body), auditory reaching (listening to one sound and reaching for it in space), proprioceptive reaching (repeating a memorised arm movement towards a specific spatial position), and general mobility (walking straight for 3 metres and coming back at their own pace). We assessed the test–retest reliability of the battery, which showed good-to-excellent reliability for all six tests, demonstrating that the BSP is a reliable tool to identify spatial impairments in children with vision impairment.

Intervention

The development of technologies to support children and adults with vision impairment is a major societal and global challenge. Despite the huge recent progress in technological designs, many of the devices developed for people with vision impairment are not accepted by final users because of their complexity and lack of adaptability to the everyday context and situations that users may encounter (Gori et al. 2016). Several participatory user studies show that technological products need to be relatively simple to be adopted by final users. For instance, aids for people with vision impairment that are based on a simple, practical principle, where training is relatively straightforward and builds on everyday normative activity, are generally accepted and adopted by users. This is the case for the white cane and the guide dog to augment natural independent mobility. Echolocation tools requiring more sustained training and development of enhanced auditory ability for echo perception and localisation have also had acceptability for navigation and orientation needs of those who can learn these skills. Starting from these observations, our research group developed a new rehabilitation device called ABBI. ABBI is a sonorous (sound-producing) bracelet based on the idea of conveying spatial information related to the body through audition. The bracelet can generate continuous or intermittent sounds at the technical level depending on the user's need, and sound settings can be modified through an Android/Apple application designed for the mobile phone. The sounds could be pure tones adjustable in volume and frequency or playback sounds stored in the bracelet memory as WAV files. Similar to the experience of children with typical sight when moving and observing limbs in space, this bracelet provides children with vision impairment the opportunity to experience audio-motor correspondences when moving limbs on which the sonorous bracelet is attached. In this way, ABBI's audio feedback can substitute the visual feedback typically used by children to develop a coherent sense of space. Thus, the most important aspect of ABBI is that it allows the creation of a new association between body movement and sound.

Unlike most existing sensory substitution devices that are introduced in late childhood or adulthood, the approach proposed in ABBI does not require learning new ways of processing sensory information. Therefore, it can be applied in and is designed for use in the first years of life. The ABBI device is manufactured for public usage and it has been now certified with the CE mark. ABBI is a medical device that is undergoing the optimisation process to commercialise the device. A kit has been developed, including the pre-evaluation, training, and post-evaluation tests to make the device usable in every day and rehabilitation settings. Using the ABBI kit and without requiring any prior knowledge of the technology or specialised training, the practitioner will be able to adopt the intervention training and the measures with the child that have been performed originally in the clinical trial.

The ABBI device has been validated as a clinical habilitation tool with a clinical trial on 44 children with vision impairment aged 6 to 17 years (Cappagli et al. 2019). In the clinical trial, two groups of children were tested: first, an experimental group performing training with the bracelet, and second, a control group performing classical habilitation training without the use of ABBI. The experimental-training group engaged in an intensive but entertaining habilitation over 12 weeks. They performed audio-spatial exercises with the ABBI bracelet; the control-training group performed classical habilitation activities (such as psychomotor activities based on motor, tactile, and/or visual stimulation) for the same period. The BSP assessment battery was administered before and after the training period; results indicated that the children using ABBI in the experimental-training group significantly improved in almost all of the spatial aspects considered whilst the control group did not show any improvement. These findings confirm that spatial perceptual development in the case of vision impairment can be fostered by providing the child with multisensory contingencies such as the audio-motor experiences provided by ABBI. Therefore, the early or childhood introduction of a tailored audio-motor training could prevent spatial developmental delays and ongoing difficulties in these children. Further research may answer whether the ABBI device could be used as a tool to encourage individuals with vision impairment to rely on environmental sounds (including their own generated sounds) to better comprehend spatial coordinates. Given its simplicity, the sonorous bracelet of ABBI can be used at earlier stages of development. We have shown that ABBI has beneficial effects for younger children with vision impairment aged 3 to 5 years old (Cappagli et al. 2017b) and for adults with congenital profound vision impairment (Finocchietti et al. 2017) (see Fig. 15.2).

Service Implications

Our results suggest that using an audio-feedback habilitation strategy associated with body movements can help improve spatial, motor, and social skills when visual information is not available. This approach may become an integrated part of clinical support in the future, although it is still at the research stage and not yet integrated into practice. It could become a useful part of the habilitation and orientation specialists' repertoire (see Chapter 14), including assessing spatial perceptual abilities and an augmentative habilitation programme involving audio-motor feedback starting from a young age. Specialist teachers of children with vision impairment, occupational therapists, and physiotherapists may also be relevant practitioners to support this area of development and participation, with children and young people and their parents as key partners.

IMPLICATIONS FOR RESEARCH AND PRACTICE

This chapter highlights the need to increase scientific knowledge of the spatial abilities that can be compromised or vulnerable in children with vision impairment in order to tailor clinical intervention strategies according to the areas of need. It emphasises the importance of developing and validating new assessment methods and technologies to support habilitation interventions for children with vision impairment and to increase their social inclusion and participation (Gori et al. 2016). Intervention training commonly adopted in relation to spatial perception has been mostly unimodal, focussing on reinforcing residual vision through intensive and repetitive visual activities without including concurrent auditory or tactile stimulation. Alternatively, the training has substituted visual input with a vicarious auditory or tactile input through sensory substitution devices that transform the visual properties into sonorous or tactile stimuli (Velázquez 2010; Maidenbaum et al. 2014; Sorgini et al. 2017). Our research has shown that multisensory audio-motor training effectively improves spatial abilities in children or adults with vision impairment. Very few studies have yet validated the new technological products with clinical trials and participatory user-centred studies and these are the important next steps before final testing with users. Early introduction of multisensory and sensorimotor training activities such as those performed with ABBI could increase learning opportunities for children with vision impairment. Further research may answer whether the ABBI device could be used as a tool to encourage individuals with vision impairment to rely on environmental sounds (including their own generated sounds) to better comprehend spatial coordinates.

SUMMARY

This chapter presents current research evidence about the spatial perception and spatial abilities of children with vision impairment, including abilities that may be enhanced and those that are delayed or constrained. The case for greater attention and focus on this area of development is given, including an assessment tool for measuring spatial abilities and a summary of modern technological products designed to support spatial development in children with vision impairment. Effort is now being put into the development of simpler technological devices that can be used by children with vision impairment from the first years of life, including the ABBI. This is a validated sonorous bracelet that provides auditory feedback of body movements and enhances the spatial and potentially social interactional abilities of children with vision impairment by helping them couple auditory and motor information conveyed by their own body. The direction forward is to assess spatial perceptual skills systematically and to support multisensory habilitation strategies that can help build spatial abilities for immediate and longer-term participation in society.

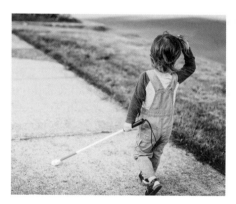

Figure 15.1 Photo ID: 1192950880. Blind or Visually Impaired Child/Kid/Toddler/Preschooler/Boy Walking Through Neighborhood with Long White Cane; Back to Camera (Copy Space) By Tracy Spohn

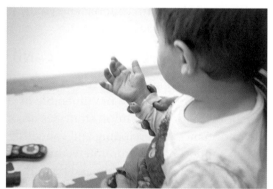

Figure 15.2 The Audio Bracelet for Blind Interaction (the ABBI device). Photo by Laura Taverna

Key Points

✓ Scientific evidence indicates that vision impairment in children can lead to spatial delays and constraints.

✓ Most of the technological products developed for people with vision impairment may not be applicable to children with vision impairment because of their complexity and inadaptability.

✓ Habilitation practice would benefit from systematic assessment of spatial perceptual and spatial cognitive abilities, leading to individual goal-focussed intervention.

✓ Technological devices should support the habilitation practices of children with vision impairment by reinforcing their multisensory and sensorimotor abilities throughout childhood.

✓ The ABBI device is a technological device that can enhance children's spatial abilities by providing auditory feedback of their body movements and could be introduced from a young age.

REFERENCES

Amadeo MB, Campus C, Gori M (2019) Impact of years of blindness on neural circuits underlying auditory spatial representation. *NeuroImage* **191**: 140–149.

Arnott SR, Thaler L, Milne JL, Kish D, Goodale MA (2013) Shape-specific activation of occipital cortex in an early blind echolocation expert. *Neuropsychologia* **51**: 938–949.

Auvray M, Hanneton S, O'Regan JK (2007) Learning to perceive with a visuo–auditory substitution system: localisation and object recognition with 'The Voice'. *Perception* **36**: 416–430.

Bremner AJ, Holmes NP, Spence C (2008) Infants lost in (peripersonal) space? *Trends in Cognitive Sciences* **12**: 298–305.

Cappagli G, Cocchi E, Gori M (2017a) Auditory and proprioceptive spatial impairments in blind children and adults. *Developmental Science* **20**(3): e12374.

Cappagli G, Finocchietti S, Baud-Bovy G, Cocchi E, Gori M (2017b) Multisensory rehabilitation training improves spatial perception in totally but not partially visually deprived children. *Frontiers in Integrative Neuroscience* **11**: 29.

Cappagli G, Finocchietti S, Cocchi E (2019) Audio motor training improves mobility and spatial cognition in visually impaired children. *Scientific Reports* **9**: 3303.

Cappagli G, Gori M (2016) Auditory spatial localization: developmental delay in children with visual impairments. *Research in Developmental Disabilities* **53**: 391–398.

Doucet ME, Guillemot JP, Lassonde M, Gagne JP, Leclerc C, Lepore F (2005) Blind subjects process auditory spectral cues more efficiently than sighted individuals. *Exp Brain Res* **160**: 194–202.

Fazzi E, Signorini SG, Bomba M, Luparia A, Lanners J, Balottin U (2011) Reach on sound: a key to object permanence in visually impaired children. *Early Human Development* **87**: 289–296.

Finocchietti S, Cappagli G, Giammari G, Cocchi E, Gori M (2019) Test–retest reliability of BSP, a battery of tests for assessing spatial cognition in visually impaired children. *PloS One* **14**: e0212006.

Finocchietti S, Cappagli G, Gori M (2017) Auditory spatial recalibration in congenital blind individuals. *Frontiers in Neuroscience* **11**: 76.

Fortin M, Voss P, Lord C et al. (2008) Wayfinding in the blind: larger hippocampal volume and supranormal spatial navigation. *Brain* **131**: 2995–3005.

Gori M, Cappagli G, Tonelli A, Baud-Bovy G, Finocchietti S (2016) Devices for visually impaired people: high technological devices with low user acceptance and no adaptability for children. *Neuroscience & Biobehavioral Reviews* **69**: 79–88.

Gori M, Sandini G, Martinoli C, Burr DC (2013) Impairment of auditory spatial localization in congenitally blind human subjects. *Brain* **137**: 288–293.

Hallemans A Ortibus, E, Truijen S, Meire F (2011) Development of independent locomotion in children with a severe visual impairment. *Research in Developmental Disabilities* **32**: 2069–2074.

Kolarik AJ, Scarfe AC, Moore BC, Pardhan S (2017) Blindness enhances auditory obstacle circumvention: assessing echolocation, sensory substitution, and visual-based navigation. *PloS One* **12**: e0175750.

Maidenbaum S, Abboud S, Amedi A (2014) Sensory substitution: closing the gap between basic research and widespread practical visual rehabilitation. *Neuroscience & Biobehavioral Reviews* **41**: 3–15.

Martolini C, Cappagli G, Luparia A, Signorini S, Gori M (2020) The impact of vision loss on allocentric spatial coding. *Frontiers in Neuroscience* **14**: 565.

Meijer PB (1992) An experimental system for auditory image representations. *IEEE Transactions on Biomedical Engineering* **39**: 112–121.

Morelli F, Aprile G, Cappagli G (2020) A multidimensional, multisensory and comprehensive rehabilitation intervention to improve spatial functioning in the visually impaired child: a community case study. *Frontiers in Neuroscience* **14**: 768.

Norman LJ, Thaler L (2019) Retinotopic-like maps of spatial sound in primary 'visual'cortex of blind human echolocators. *Proceedings of the Royal Society B* **286**(1912).

Petrus E, Isaiah A, Jones AP et al. (2014) Crossmodal induction of thalamocortical potentiation leads to enhanced information processing in the auditory cortex. *Neuron* **81**: 664–673.

Rogge A-K, Hamacher D, Cappagli G et al. (2021) Balance, gait, and navigation performance are related to physical exercise in blind and visually impaired children and adolescents. *Experimental Brain Research* **239**(4): 1111–1123.

Sorgini F, Caliò R, Carrozza MC, Oddo CM (2017) Haptic-assistive technologies for audition and vision sensory disabilities. *Disability and Rehabilitation: Assistive Technology* **13**(4): 394–421.

Teng S, Puri A, Whitney D (2012) Ultrafine spatial acuity of blind expert human echolocators. *Experimental Brain Research* **216**: 483–488.

Thaler L, Arnott SR, Goodale MA (2011) Neural correlates of natural human echolocation in early and late blind echolocation experts. *PLoS One* **6**: e20162.

Thaler L, Zhang X, Antoniou M, Kish DC, Cowie D (2020) The flexible action system: click-based echolocation may replace certain visual functionality for adaptive walking. *Journal of Experimental Psychology: Human Perception and Performance* **46**: 21.

Tonelli A, Campus C, Gori M (2020) Early visual cortex response for sound in expert blind echolocators, but not in early blind non-echolocators. *Neuropsychologia* **147**: 107617.

Vasilyeva M, Lourenco SF (2012) Development of spatial cognition. *Wiley Interdisciplinary Reviews: Cognitive Science* **3**: 349–362.

Velázquez R (2010) Wearable assistive devices for the blind. *Wearable and Autonomous Biomedical Devices and Systems for Smart Environment* **75**: 331–349.

Vercillo T, Burr D, Gori M (2016) Early visual deprivation severely compromises the auditory sense of space in congenitally blind children. *Developmental Psychology* **52**: 847.

Vercillo T, Milne JL, Gori M, Goodale MA (2015) Enhanced auditory spatial localization in blind echolocators. *Neuropsychologia* **67**: 35–40.

CHAPTER 16

Low-Vision Aids and Assistive Technologies for Reading, Learning, and Education

Michael Crossland, Annegret Dahlmann-Noor, and Ngozi Oluonye

INTRODUCTION

Vision habilitation aims to allow children to gain independent access to visual information as far as is possible within the limits of their vision impairment and other disabilities. Low-vision aid technology and the support of a multidisciplinary team can enable many children with vision impairment to access education in mainstream schools, and support the development of better reading and literacy skills (Douglas et al. 2011; Gyawali and Moodley 2018). The team can also help the child to access more visual information in their everyday life and with the support of parents in the early years, thereby potentially increasing participation in society. Children with no vision or very severe vision impairment require training in braille (see Chapter 17), but it is important to distinguish children who can access and be well supported by low-vision aid technology (Pal et al. 2006).

Low-vision aids (LVAs) are broadly defined as any device that enables a person with low vision to improve their visual performance. This chapter gives an overview of currently available optical low-vision and aids and assistive technologies to improve visual performance, including the assessment which helps the practitioner and family decide which strategies to adopt.

THE EVIDENCE BASE

LVAs include optical aids, such as high-power glasses, magnifiers, and telescopes, and, more recently, electronic assistive technologies. Non-optical methods can also be helpful, such as the enlargement of printed material, and occasionally tinted or filter lenses, for example for children with ocular albinism (Barker et al. 2015).

Until the 1980s, no low-vision services existed for preschool children in the UK. Developmental research in the 1980s established that young children learn through vision and so should be encouraged to use their vision as early as possible in order to maximise developmental outcomes (Sonksen 1983). At the same time, evidence emerged that children from a developmental age of 2 years could benefit from the introduction of simple optical aids, such as stand magnifiers, monoculars, and binoculars by a developmental age of 4 years (Ritchie et al. 1984). These findings led to the development of multidisciplinary paediatric preschool low-vision services, using a holistic approach with a paediatrician working alongside a specialist optometrist (Gould and Sonksen 1991).

LVAs are known to provide an effective means to improve visual performance, though most studies report only the change in font size that children can read with LVAs rather than more complex functional outcomes such as reading speed, accuracy, and comprehension (Barker et al. 2015). In younger children, training in performing a visual task such as following a line with the use of a magnifier is superior to visual task training only (Cox et al. 2009). Few studies report the impact of LVAs on children's quality of life, although instruments for measuring this exist, such as the validated Vision-Related Quality of Life (Tadić et al. 2016) and the Low Vision Prasad Functional Vision Questionnaire (Gothwal et al. 2012). The score on the Prasad instrument increases with training and use of telescopes, reading stands, and large-print books (Ganesh et al. 2013; Kavitha et al. 2015). Qualitative research has shown that children value the support offered by paediatric low-vision clinics (Tadić et al. 2015).

Limited motor skills and sensory-motor integration, and, in older children, peer pressure and the fear of 'standing out' can affect usage of LVAs by children and young people (Mason 1999; Monteiro et al. 2006; Cox et al. 2009).

SUPPORT AND MANAGEMENT

The Multidisciplinary Clinic

The multidisciplinary team should include skilled optometrists, ophthalmologists, paediatricians, dispensing opticians, and counsellors, alongside community services such as teachers for visual impairment, habilitation specialists, and technology advisors. In order to support children in the use of LVAs, especially at a young age, it is ideal if a paediatrician and optometrist work together with the child and family. In this context a paediatrician can provide understanding of the developmental, educational, and health issues that may impact on use of LVAs. Other key practitioners include the specialist education or habilitation practitioner (see Chapter 14), bringing education, habilitation, and health together in an integrated manner. The parent and child are also crucial partners in this process.

It is important at the start of the assessment to enquire about the child's health, sleep, tiredness, mobility, social integration, participation at home and school, and the child's access to help and support through education and habilitation specialists and practitioners. Emotional difficulties are discussed, such as challenges in 'fitting in' and stigma issues around using aids, and may require referral to appropriate services as required (see Chapter 18). Liaison with the school helps with acceptance and understanding of LVAs, and with gaining a greater understanding of the child's needs and challenges in access to materials at school and at home.

Occupational therapists can provide advice on handwriting and postural management and so their advice should be sought. Parental understanding and feedback is also vital, particularly to help support their child in usage of the aids at home or the outside environment, and parents may be signposted to other support organisations and services.

Ongoing support and encouragement may be required and sensitivity to the needs of the young person and acceptability of their aids. The developmental appropriateness of the aids and the ability of the child to use them functionally is also a key issue.

LOW-VISION ASSESSMENT

Refraction

Spectacle correction of refractive error should always be considered for children with visual impairment. Refraction alone improves visual acuity by at least two lines in more than 10% of people with low vision (Sunness and El Annan 2010). In younger children, cycloplegic retinoscopy provides the most accurate method of refraction (Royal College of Ophthalmologists 2012), whilst above the age of 8 years a combination of retinoscopy and subjective refraction is preferred. Poor or absent accommodation is well recognised in certain conditions including cerebral palsy and Down syndrome (McClelland et al. 2006; Watt et al. 2015). It can be identified by dynamic retinoscopy and treated with a bifocal or varifocal correction. Amblyopia treatment should not be overlooked (see Chapter 2).

Spectacles are generally well tolerated by children, although contact lenses may be preferred for those with high prescriptions or a dislike of spectacles. Contact lenses create a larger image than spectacles in children with high myopia, which can increase the visibility of small objects. Conversely, children with hypermetropia or aphakia may see better in spectacles than in contact lenses, due to spectacle magnification. A further advantage of contact lenses is that, as they move with the eye, there are fewer peripheral distortions than in high-power spectacle lenses.

It has long been suggested that contact lenses can control nystagmus in some children (see e.g. Allen and Davies 1983), although there are currently no randomised controlled trial data to show the benefit of this in children.

Magnification

The easiest way to increase the visibility of an object is to enlarge it. There are four ways to magnify an image. *Relative-size magnification* involves increasing the physical size of the object. This can be through asking the teacher to write in larger print of appropriate line width on the whiteboard, to use large print books, or to use optimally enlarged font sizes for worksheets. Electronic books enable easy manipulation of font size on a tablet computer or laptop. The increased use of computers in education means that text is enlarged to an appropriate size on the screen and when printed out, and large print keyboards can be of great use.

Relative distance magnification reduces the distance between the object and the eye, either by moving the child closer (asking them to sit nearer the whiteboard), moving the task closer (using a relay screen for the whiteboard), or by moving the image of the object closer to the child (using a hand or stand magnifier). Positive spectacle lenses reduce the need to accommodate for close objects, enabling the child to see comfortably at a short distance for a prolonged period. These are prescribed as single-vision reading glasses, bifocals, or varifocals.

Angular magnification uses a telescopic system to increase the visual angle of the object at the eye. Finally, *digital magnification* uses electronics to magnify the image of an object, such as on a closed circuit television (CCTV) magnifier, or the camera and zoom function on a tablet computer or smartphone or screen-sharing software with an interactive whiteboard (see below).

Table 16.1 shows examples of each type of magnification for two common classroom tasks.

Optical Low-Vision Aids

High-powered reading spectacles can be prescribed to allow the child to hold the print closer, providing relative distance magnification. These lenses typically have an addition power of between 4 and 20 dioptres. With increasing magnification, the distance between spectacles and text is reduced, from 25cm for a 4 dioptre addition to 5cm for a 20 dioptre addition. These lenses will blur distance vision, so they are prescribed either for reading only, or in a bifocal with the distance prescription incorporated in the top segment of the lens. High-powered bifocal spectacles can

Table 16.1 Examples of magnification strategies for two common classroom tasks

	Viewing interactive whiteboard	Book reading
Relative size magnification	Larger screen used	Large print book
		Reading on electronic computer, tablet, or laptop
Relative distance magnification	Relay screen	High-power reading spectacles and holding close
	Tablet or laptop with screen-sharing software	Stand magnifier (e.g. 'dome')
Angular magnification	Binoculars	Near spectacle mounted telescope (not recommended)
	Monocular telescope	
Digital magnification	Distance electronic magnifier connected to laptop	Desktop CCTV
	Tablet with zoom	Portable video magnifier

have a negative effect on mobility, by blurring the lower visual field, so are generally used only when sitting.

Handheld (Fig. 16.1) and stand magnifiers (Fig. 16.2) are the most commonly used types of near-vision LVAs used by children with vision impairment (Özen Tunay et al. 2016). From a young age, children can be taught how to use simple magnifiers, such as dome magnifiers (Fig. 16.2), which they can rest on a page of pictures or text and then slide across the page (Haddad et al. 2006). Even before the age of reading print,

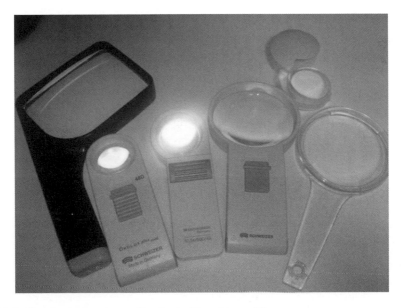

Figure 16.1 Illuminated and non-illuminated hand magnifiers

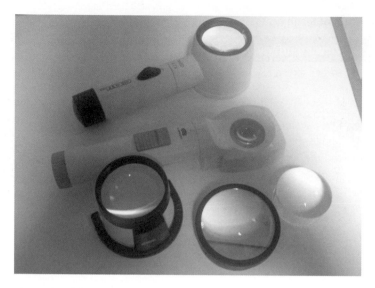

Figure 16.2 Illuminated and non-illuminated stand magnifiers. (A colour version of this figure can be seen in the colour plate section)

handheld aids can be used to look at small objects that are not easily magnified (such as veins on a leaf, patterns on stones and shells), which their peers who are typically sighted see and understand effortlessly.

Most children and young people will be introduced to a telescopic lens system such as binoculars or a handheld monocular telescope to magnify objects viewed at a distance (Fig. 16.3; Kavitha et al. 2015; Özen Tunay et al. 2016). For older children this

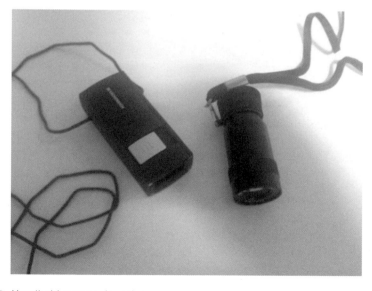

Figure 16.3 Handheld monocular telescopes

will increase independence by enabling signs to be read and helping navigation. For younger children, they can be used for days out such as trips to the zoo and distinguishing between a cow and a sheep in a field, for instance.

In all children, and particularly in younger children, motor skills must be taken into account when prescribing LVAs. In older children and teenagers, concerns will change and the fear of 'standing out' may lead to LVAs being abandoned (Mason 1999). Qualitative research using drama enactment research methodology has demonstrated that young people at 10 to14 years with vision impairment may minimise their own difficulties, be uncomfortable using LVAs in public, and often suffer from a lack of participation in decisions about their own health (Monteiro et al. 2006). This highlights the importance of children and young people as participatory partners in health decision-making regarding their use of LVAs.

Electronic Low-Vision Aids

Electronic LVAs have several advantages over optical magnifiers. They have the facility to produce high amounts of magnification without the distortion and optical aberration created by high-powered optical lenses. Image brightness can be manipulated and the text contrast can be reversed, so that text is presented as white on a black background, for example. These manipulations are particularly helpful for children who suffer from glare, such as those with retinal disease, aniridia, or opacities in the ocular media.

However, electronic magnifiers are generally heavier, more cumbersome, and far more expensive than optical devices. They are increasingly being superseded by consumer devices such as tablet computers (see below).

Desktop Electronic Magnifiers

Desktop electronic magnifiers, popularly known as CCTVs, enable very high levels of magnification over a relatively large area. They are intuitive to use, even for young children. Their large size makes them more suitable for primary school students who are based in one classroom. The large screen enables a parent, carer, or teacher to read alongside the child. Some models include a distance camera too.

Handheld Video Magnifiers

Handheld video magnifiers are smaller devices, with a screen of around 10cm to 30cm. In common with desktop magnifiers, they can alter the contrast and brightness of the image, in addition to providing high levels of magnification.

Consumer Electronic Devices

Smartphones are now almost ubiquitous, particularly with high school students, in many parts of the world. All smartphones allow the font size, font colour, and screen brightness to be adjusted, enabling the user to read text messages and to access the Internet and social media. Text-to-speech is usually incorporated in the operating system (e.g. Voiceover), allowing messages to be read through the device speaker or headphones. Although designed for users who are profoundly or very severely visually impaired, about half of adults with low vision also use text-to-speech systems (Crossland et al. 2014).

People who have vision impairment use a large variety of smartphone apps. Transport apps announce what the next bus will be at a specific bus stop or which platform to go to for a certain train. GPS maps give step-by-step walking directions, reducing the need to identify street signs. Navigation apps such as Soundscape give audio commentary about nearby places. Barcode scanner apps identify food packets and give details on the ingredients and cooking instructions. Children and young people can be introduced to these systems from an early age, to help find the correct platform for a train, or to help a parent with shopping. This can be integrated with the input of their habilitation specialist (see Chapter 14).

Smartphone apps can use the phone camera to read printed or handwritten text, to identify colours and to recognise banknotes. These apps use either human or artificial intelligence to decode the images. In 2021 the most comprehensive low-vision app is Seeing AI, which includes text-to-speech reading, face recognition, colour, and brightness identification (see Resources).

People with low vision also use basic smartphone features. Teenagers are usually more willing to use the camera and zoom facility than to use a telescope to read a menu over the counter of a fast food restaurant. The built-in camera flash can also be used as a torch to illuminate dim print.

Tablet computers are widely used in the classroom in many countries, starting from 6 years upwards for children with vision impairment. Children will also be introduced to laptops in the later primary or elementary school years. They can be used to present written information and also to relay information from the interactive whiteboard at the front of the classroom. A particular strength of these systems is that the content on the whiteboard from the teacher's computer is transmitted directly to the pupil's laptop or tablet via the Internet or Wi-Fi, using screen-sharing software like TeamViewer or join.me or paid for use programmes and apps. This gives the pupil a remote monitor that they can use to zoom in and out permitting them to adjust the screen angle contrast, colour, and magnification settings on their own device. Pupils report that the lower visual demand helps reduce visual fatigue. The viewing distance, screen brightness, and text size can be manipulated by the child. If every child in the classroom uses a tablet computer then this removes the sense of 'otherness' that some young people with vision impairment experience.

Children should also be encouraged to learn to touch-type (often facilitated by big buttons and enlarged keys on the keyboard), and be allowed to type answers in exams and tests. As well as being an important life skill, this ensures that their school performance is not limited by lower ability to read their own handwriting.

For children and young people who sing or play instruments, a particular challenge is viewing music on a piano or music stand, typically at 60cm to 100cm. Large print music is cumbersome, and intermediate distance telescopes are difficult to use. Nowadays, digital music displays and electronic tablet apps (e.g. AirTurn – see resources) can be used to display large print music, using a foot pedal to advance to the next section of the musical score.

Wearable Electronic Low-Vision Aids

Head-mounted electronic LVAs have been available for more than two decades, but only recently have they become light and versatile enough to be more widely used. OrCam MyReader (see Resources) is a spectacle-mounted camera that reads text aloud through an earpiece. It can also recognise faces, identify products from barcodes, and tell the time.

There are various augmented reality-based head-mounted magnifiers available in 2021, including eSight, SightPlus, OXSIGHT, and IrisVision (see Resources). These perform digital magnification and contrast enhancement in real time. They significantly improve visual acuity and contrast sensitivity (Wittich et al. 2018) but remain very expensive and cannot be worn when walking as they interfere with balance and mobility. Future development of these devices will include making them smaller, lighter, and more cosmetically acceptable.

Visual Field Expansion

Reduced visual fields significantly affect reading, finding objects in a room, and safe orientation and mobility. Mobility training and eye movement training are the major habilitation and rehabilitation approaches for children and young people with reduced visual fields. Where children have good central vision, reversed telescopes or handheld minifiers can be used to compress information into the remaining part of the visual field. In contrast to a magnifier, a minifier makes the scene smaller and expands the field of view.

Prisms can be used to relocate images for people with hemianopia. Some people can use high power Fresnel prisms in the peripheral part of a spectacle lens to detect obstacles and to navigate more safely (Peli 2000). In specialist low-vision clinics at Moorfields Eye Hospital in London (UK), we have had some success with this technique in children with hemianopia following stroke or epilepsy surgery. Eye movement training can also help these children (Ivanov et al. 2018).

IMPLICATIONS FOR RESEARCH AND PRACTICE

Long-term outcomes of low-vision habilitation and rehabilitation in children are difficult to quantify due to the ethical problems of withholding intervention from a control group. Randomised trials can be used over the short-term to quantify the effect of an additional intervention: for example, assessing the benefit of routine supply of a consumer electronic tablet (iPad) for education (Gothwal et al. 2018). Outstanding questions requiring further research include the best types of devices to be used by children with vision impairment, the impact of new technology on their education, and when children with low vision should be encouraged to read print as their primary means of education, and when audio support or braille should be introduced (see Chapter 17). With the more extensive use of electronic technology, this research becomes more urgently required so that future habilitation and use of new assistive technology is evidence-based.

A recommended theoretical framework consists of three interacting relations between LVA, child, and task. This may facilitate future research into LVA use by children, by defining the implementation problem children face when using an LVA in terms of discovering and controlling the relations between themselves, the LVA, and the task (Schurink et al. 2011). This might include the synchronised motor skills required to move a magnifier along a page (Cox et al. 2009). Further research is needed into the social and emotional factors that may influence LVA use. Systematic interventions to encourage the use of assistive technology by young people with low vision should be introduced and evaluated, such as routine psychosocial training and counselling (see Chapter 18).

SUMMARY

All children with vision impairment need to receive the input of a multidisciplinary low-vision rehabilitation team. Even children with no vision should be provided with advice and training in text-to-speech systems and assistive technology. The child and young person and parents are key partners in the process. There is evidence that the support of low-vision clinics improves visual function and some domains of quality of life. Further research is needed to identify additional strategies to best habilitate and rehabilitate children with vision impairment.

Key Points

- ✓ A multidisciplinary integrated health-education approach is needed for effective use of LVAs and assistive technology.
- ✓ Children and young people and parents are key partners in decision-making for effective use of assistive technology.
- ✓ Simple optical magnifiers such as hand and stand magnifiers can be introduced from preschool age.
- ✓ LVA acceptance is limited by many factors, including the fear of appearing different and 'standing out'.
- ✓ Developments in consumer electronic technology, apps, and wearable LVAs will provide important opportunities for children and young people to achieve their aspirations and participate fully in society.

REFERENCES

Allen ED, Davies PD (1983) Role of contact lenses in the management of congenital nystagmus. *Br J Ophthalmol* **67**: 834–836.

Barker L, Thomas R, Rubin G, Dahlmann-Noor A (2015) Optical reading aids for children and young people with low vision. *Cochrane Database Syst Rev* **3**: CD010987.

Cox RF, Reimer AM, Verezen CA, Smitsman AW, Vervloed MP, Boonstra NF (2009) Young children's use of a visual aid: an experimental study of the effectiveness of training. *Dev Med Child Neurol* **51**: 460–467.

Crossland MD, Silva RS, Macedo AF (2014) Smartphone, tablet computer and e-reader use by people with vision impairment. *Ophthal Physl Opt* **34**: 552–557.

Douglas G, McLinden M, Farrell AM, Ware J, McCall S, Pavey S (2011). Access to print literacy for children and young people with visual impairment: implications for policy and practice. *Eur J Spec Needs Edu* **26**: 39–46.

Ganesh S, Sethi S, Srivastav S, Chaudhury A, Arora P (2013) Impact of low vision rehabilitation on functional vision performance of children with visual impairment. *Oman J Ophthalmol* **6**: 170–174.

Gothwal VK, Sumalini R, Bharani S, Reddy SP, Bagga DK (2012) The second version of the LV Prasad-functional vision questionnaire. *Optom Vis Sci* **89**: 1601–1610.

Gothwal VK, Thomas R, Crossland M et al. (2018) Randomized trial of tablet computers for education and learning in children and young people with low vision. *Optom Vis Sci* **95**: 873–882.

Gould E, Sonksen PM (1991) A low vision aid clinic for preschool children. *Br J Vis Impair* **9**: 44–46.

Gyawali R, Moodley VR (2018) Need for optical intervention in children attending a school for the blind in Eritrea. *Clin Exp Optom* **101**: 565–570.

Haddad MA, Lobato FJ, Sampaio MW, Kara-Jose N (2006) Pediatric and adolescent population with visual impairment: study of 385 cases. *Clinics (Sao Paulo)* **61**: 239–246.

Ivanov IV, Kuester S, MacKeben M et al. (2018) Effects of visual search training in children with hemianopia. *PLoS One* **18**: e0197285.

Kavitha V, Manumali MS, Praveen K, Heralgi MM (2015) Low vision aid – a ray of hope for irreversible visual loss in the pediatric age group. *Taiwan J Ophthalmol*, **5**: 63–67.

Mason H (1999) Blurred vision: a study of the use of low vision aids by visually impaired secondary school pupils. *Br J Vis Impair* **17**: 94–97.

McClelland JF, Parkes J, Hill N, Jackson AJ, Saunders KJ (2006) Accommodative dysfunction in children with cerebral palsy: a population-based study. *Invest Ophthalmol Vis Sci* **47**: 1824–1830.

Monteiro GB, Temporini ER, de Carvalho KM (2006) Use of optical aids by visually impaired students: social and cultural factors. *Arq Bras Oftalmol*, **69**: 503–507.

Özen Tunay Z, Çalışkan D, İdil A, Öztuna D (2016) Clinical characteristics and low vision rehabilitation methods for partially sighted school-age children. *Turk J Ophthalmol* **46**: 68–72.

Pal N, Titiyal JS, Tandon R, Vajpayee RB, Gupta S, Murthy GV (2006) Need for optical and low vision services for children in schools for the blind in North India. *Indian J Ophthalmol* **54**: 189–193.

Peli E (2000) Field expansion for homonymous hemianopia by optically induced peripheral exotropia. *Optom Vis Sci* **77**: 453–464.

Ritchie JP, Sonksen PM, Gould E (1984) Low vision aids for preschool children. *Dev Med Child Neurol* **31**: 509–519.

Royal College of Ophthalmologists (2012) *Guidelines for the Management of Strabismus in Childhood.* London: Royal College of Ophthalmologists.

Schurink J, Cox RF, Cillessen AH, van Rens GH, Boonstra FN (2011) Low vision aids for visually impaired children: a perception-action perspective. *Res Dev Disabil* 32: 871–882.

Sonksen PM (1983). The assessment of 'vision for development' in severely visually handicapped babies. *Acta Ophthalmologica* 157 *(Suppl.)*: 82–90.

Sunness JS, El Annan J (2010) Improvement of visual acuity by refraction in a low-vision population. *Ophthalmology* 117: 1442–1446.

Tadić V, Hundt GL, Keeley S, Rahi JS, Vision-related Quality of Life (VQoL) group (2015) Seeing it my way: living with childhood onset visual disability. *Child Care Health Dev* 41: 239–248.

Tadić V, Coope, A, Cumberland P, Lewando-Hundt G, Rahi JS (2016) Measuring the quality of life of visually impaired children: first stage psychometric evaluation of the novel VQoLCYP instrument. *PLoS One* 11: e0146225.

Watt T, Robertson K, Jacobs RJ (2015) Refractive error, binocular vision and accommodation of children with Down syndrome. *Clin Exp Optom* 98(1): 3–11.

Wittich W, Lorenzini M-C, Markowitz SN et al. (2018) The effect of a head-mounted low vision device on visual function. *Optom Vis Sci* 95: 774–784.

RESOURCES

Seeing AI (Microsoft Corporation, Redmond, WA, USA).

Soundscape (Microsoft Corporation, Redmond, WA, USA).

AirTurn (AirTurn Inc, Boulder, CO, USA).

OrCam MyReader (OrCam, Jerusalem, Israel).

eSight (eSight Corp, Toronto, Canada).

SightPlus (GiveVision, Birmingham, UK).

OXSIGHT (OXSIGHT Ltd, Oxford, UK).

IrisVision (IrisVision Global, Inc., Pleasanton, CA, USA).

CHAPTER 17

Reading Approaches for Braille Readers

M Cay Holbrook and Kim T Zebehazy

INTRODUCTION

Reading and writing are essential academic attainments for all children, including those with vision impairment. Despite a current misconception that technological access to text (e.g. listening to digital text-to-speech output) may replace the need to learn braille, braille remains the best option for literacy for some children with significant vision impairments, including those who have insufficient vision to access enlarged print for fluent reading. Braille is an essential medium for 'active' reading and writing, providing the means for accessing the educational curriculum and participating in learning and society. This chapter explores the evidence for and practice methods for instruction in braille, and future directions for braille understanding and developments.

BRAILLE READING AND INSTRUCTION

Braille is a system of reading and writing that uses a six-dot cell and was developed initially by Louis Braille (1809–1852), who was a student at the first specialised school for students who were blind in Paris. Each cell or set of cells represents a letter, combination of letters, or a word

The current braille system used by English-speaking countries is called 'Unified English Braille' (UEB). UEB symbols and rules are governed by the International Council

Braille Alphabet

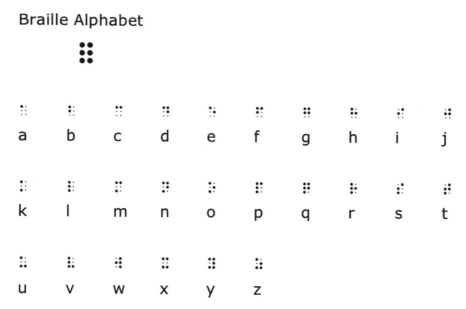

Figure 17.1 Braille alphabet graphic

on English Braille, an international board of braille readers, transcribers, and other professionals. The current code is unified across English-speaking countries and across subject matter text (literary and mathematics/science), permitting materials written in UEB and electronic braille files to be shared between different countries. The USA also uses the Nemeth code for mathematics as an additional option for technical materials.

Closely linked to braille reading and overall literacy is the ability to acquire and interpret information represented through tactile graphics. A comprehensive programme for developing braille reading should include instruction around graphics. Guidelines exist for the creation of quality tactile graphics (International Council on English Braille 2014) but a precise system with definitive rules does not exist (compared to the braille code). As with braille reading, similar considerations are needed to help children and young people develop their graphic literacy including symbol discrimination, quality of hand movements and exploration, and comprehension of graphic types. In addition, quality systematic direct instruction and early and frequent exposure to graphics is fundamental to their ability to understand graphics in the tactile format (Zebehazy and Wilton 2014).

Braille reading and writing has been studied from educational, psychological, neurological, and physical perspectives. While research to date has not been extensive enough to meet evidence-based practice standards (e.g. replication), each aspect of research brings greater understanding to the process of braille reading and writing.

Learning Braille

At the early literacy level of education, learning the letter configurations and rules of braille cannot be separated from learning to read and write. Children and young people with vision impairment go through a developmental process that parallels the process followed by children who are typically sighted as they learn to read print. This includes acquisition of phonemic awareness, phonics, vocabulary, fluency, and comprehension (National Reading Panel 2000). However, for braille readers, there are additional considerations and skills that must be learned and developed, including tactile discrimination, tactile identification, systematic introduction of the symbols that make up the braille writing system, and concept development of the world to support reading comprehension (Holbrook et al. 2017). An understanding of the intersection between the development of the reading process, individual child characteristics, and mechanics of braille reading is critical for teachers to select effective instructional approaches.

Whether a person has early- or late-onset blindness will be a factor in the type of instruction selected and may also affect braille mechanics and other factors requiring special attention (Oshima et al. 2014). Braille mechanics include instruction in the procedures used for writing braille on a manual Perkins braille writer (e.g. paper insertion, setting margins, use of backspace, and line advance keys) and smooth, efficient finger and hand movements. Throughout early instruction in braille reading, students are taught proper hand movements, using two hands in a scissor approach in which the two hands move together approximately halfway along the line of braille and then the right (lead) hand continues to the end of the line while the left hand retraces the line and moves to the next line where it starts moving and is met by the right hand to continue to the end of the line (Wright et al. 2009).

Children who are congenitally blind learn braille differently from children who have experienced visual loss during later childhood. For example, concept development in children who are congenitally blind needs to be directly experiential to compensate for what is not learned incidentally through visual observation and to take into account the range of cognitive abilities in children with vision impairments and additional disabilities (see Chapter 10 and Chapter 12).

Within first grade school entry through to school-leaving grade (or K-12, USA), children who need braille from the outset learn to read and write along with their peers who are typically sighted; however, they need to master braille as their native writing system. This system is internalised with no direct connection to print since their experience with the written word is entirely or almost entirely tactual. On the other hand, children or young people requiring braille instruction after they have learned to read and write through print, mainly due to trauma or later eye or brain disorder or progressive vision loss, will need to map their developing braille reading and writing onto their previous knowledge and skill as a print reader. Their previous level of proficiency with print reading is important to consider in determining the best instructional approach.

In addition, some children will learn to read both braille and print, mastering them simultaneously from the beginning. These children have sufficient visual function to access some print in the environment and in texts, through magnification or enlargement, but they also benefit from the use of touch for access to other text (such as lengthy passages needing a faster rate of reading). When and where they will use braille or print will be context dependent and may change, depending on expectation and environment (Lusk and Corn 2006).

The 'system' of parents and families, schools, and communities, who initially may have limited knowledge and experience with blindness and vision impairment, needs to be an integral part of literacy development for the child who will become a braille reader. Parents can be assisted to become confident and clear of their role in their child's learning, such as learning braille alongside the child and working with the teacher of students with vision impairments to find ways to encourage meaningful literacy, home activities such as bedtime reading, and writing letters to family members. The school must also embrace and support the 'normalcy' of braille reading. Communities become valuable partners when they understand how to promote full participation by children and individuals with access needs that include braille and other alternative methods.

Developmental Factors

The limited neuropsychology research available using brain magnetic resonance imaging indicates that braille readers who are congenitally blind use similar parts of their brain (the occipital lobes) while reading compared to readers who are typically sighted. However, specialisation is less distinct in braille readers with the original visual word formation area and the ventral occipito-temporal cortex of the brain responding to both tactile and auditory inputs (Kim et al. 2017; Lane et al. 2017; Rączy et al. 2019). For further information on brain plasticity, see Chapter 7.

The learning of braille will also be affected by individual child characteristics. Many children with vision impairments have additional disabilities including cognitive and motor disorders that will impact on the possibility and rate of learning braille. Some children have difficulties with tactile discrimination and struggle with differentiating the individual cells. As in children who are typically sighted, a minority have an additional reading disorder of a dyslexic nature, which needs identifying and managing. An earlier study by Greaney and Reason (1999) compared braille readers aged 7 to 12 years who were progressing well with those who were struggling to read, and found that the latter had greater difficulty with phonological skills and their approaches to learning, analogous to developmental dyslexia in sighted children.

SUPPORT AND MANAGEMENT

The Role of the Multidisciplinary Team

Blindness and vision impairment is considered a 'low incidence' disability for children in high-income countries, which affects the distribution and availability of skill expertise for teaching braille. Planning and implementing instruction will need to ensure the appropriate resources and expertise to support the child developing and using braille. The key members of the team are the specialist teacher in vision impairment, who works closely with other educational practitioners including the classroom or curriculum subject teacher, special needs coordinator, and teaching assistants. Other key partners are the child or young person, and their parent and the habilitation specialist (see Chapter 14). If concerns regarding reading or literacy progress or general learning arise, then referral to assessment by the educational or clinical neuropsychologist and the paediatric neurodisability/neurodevelopmental team may be required.

Assessment

Learning Media Assessment (LMA) is a data-driven process by which decisions are made. Annual review concerning the appropriateness of using braille, print, or a combination of both is carried out for a child with vision impairment in the USA and other English-speaking and non-English speaking countries (Koenig and Holbrook 1995). LMA gathers data from the child's educational team and a variety of sources, including clinical and functional vision assessments. It contains two phases: Phase I (Initial Selection) uses observations of a child's use of sensory information and targeted sensory tasks to support decision-making prior to the beginning of formal reading and writing instruction; it provides information about which media a young child should use to begin reading and writing. Phase II (Continuing Assessment) is conducted with students for whom a learning and literacy media has been selected and supports data-gathering on the student's current level of reading acquisition (e.g. fluency and comprehension) to provide information about whether changes in media and literacy tools are needed. Ongoing progress monitoring of acquisition of literacy skills is important for creating an effective educational plan that meets the unique needs of each student.

Planning Instruction for Braille Literacy

Planning an instructional programme for a beginning reader should include a systematic comprehensive balanced literacy programme that focuses on reading and writing and addresses all areas identified as important by the National Reading Panel (2000). Use of braille contractions for early readers should be infused into instruction in each of these areas along with the unique skills identified for efficient braille reading, including reading speed, mechanical skills, tactile perception and discrimination, and concept development (Holbrook et al. 2017). Early braille literacy programmes must include all of these components and be supported by qualified teachers who know how to teach reading and writing and the implications of reading by touch.

READING SPEED

Tactile readers read more slowly than print readers on average (Radojichikj 2015), although there are students who read at equivalent speeds to peers who are typically sighted. While the vision sensory system can take in information simultaneously (e.g. a whole word or several words at one time), the tactile sense works sequentially building up elements into a whole (i.e. stringing together braille cells to read each word). Some research suggests that the sequential nature of braille limits lexical (whole word) engagement (Veispak et al. 2012), whereas other research suggests that at least adult readers of braille can engage at the sub-lexical (parts of a word) level of reading words (Fischer-Baum and Englebretson 2016). Despite the inherent differences in sensory input that could affect reading speed, systematic instruction to develop tactile discrimination and mechanical skills such as effective hand movements can help students optimally develop their speeds. For example, North American, Greek, and Chinese studies have found that certain hand movement patterns support faster reading speeds (Wright et al. 2009; Papadimitriou and Argyropoulos 2017; Chen et al. 2019).

MECHANICAL AND DISCRIMINATION SKILLS

Mechanical skills and tactile discrimination includes the ability to consistently and accurately recognise braille cells, and to follow lines of braille efficiently. Common issues with mechanical or tactile skills include 'scrubbing' and reversals. Scrubbing refers to rapid up-and-down finger movement on a braille cell instead of light touch passing from left to right. Reversals occur when a reader perceives a braille cell from a different spatial rotation than is actually present, possibly causing the reader to identify the cell as a different letter. For example, the letters d, h, j, and f all have three dots in the upper part of the cell but are rotated differently. Targeted instruction helps readers overcome reversal issues to improve decoding, comprehension, and reading speeds. In addition, the code itself requires targeted instruction.

UEB contains 187 symbols that represent more than one letter, a word or part of a word. These are called braille contractions and are categorised into nine rule-based areas. Some contractions have unique meaning (e.g. if all dots of the 6-dot cell are raised, this represents the word or part-word 'for'), while other contractions hold different meanings depending on their position in a word (e.g. the contraction for the stand-alone word 'child' represents 'ch' when located within a word). Limited longitudinal research suggests that learning contractions (versus reading only uncontracted braille, that is all words spelled out letter by letter) might facilitate better literacy overall (Wall Emerson et al. 2009).

CONCEPT DEVELOPMENT

All readers need background knowledge in order to comprehend and understand when reading text (Cervetti and Hiebert 2015). For braille readers, direct hands-on experiences contribute and enhance knowledge, otherwise gained visually, so that related themes encountered in text have been given a basis for greater understanding (Koenig and Farrenkopf 1997). Similarly, vocabulary development should be directly targeted in instruction. One longitudinal study in North America found that braille readers' vocabulary knowledge development at grade four (approximately 8–9 years old) was reduced and behind that of their peers who were typically sighted (Wall Emerson et al. 2009). These issues are considered further in relation to conceptual development (Chapter 12) and language development (Chapter 10).

INSTRUCTIONAL TIME

With the additional considerations for braille reading development, duration and frequency of instructional time is an area of consideration. A Delphi study of 40 experienced teachers and recognised experts indicated that the level of direct instruction from a qualified teacher of students with vision impairments for braille-reading students is at least equal (2 hours per day, 5 days per week) to that needed by children who are typically sighted and learning to read and write using print (Koenig and Holbrook 2000).

INSTRUCTIONAL STRATEGIES AND MATERIALS

One effective strategy for ensuring all components of a balanced literacy programme are met, is to use a curriculum specifically written for braille readers. There are few programmes that meet the high standards of incorporating the comprehensive curriculum needed to optimise early literacy skills of braille readers. One such programme, *Building on Patterns*, is available from The American Printing House for the Blind for children just entering formal schooling (about 4 years) through the first few years of school (about 8 years). *Building on Patterns* was written by teachers of students with vision impairments who have had experience of teaching braille reading and writing. In this programme, the introduction of braille contractions is carefully controlled and based on logical sequence of instruction. Different countries use a variety of curricula, some commercially produced and more widely available. Some literacy instruction relies on an approach and philosophy rather than a set curriculum with predefined lessons.

Another effective strategy for teaching initial reading and writing through braille is to create a partnership between the general education classroom teacher and teacher of students with vision impairments to use literacy materials being used in the general classroom and to introduce braille contractions as they naturally occur in text written for readers who are typically sighted. In this situation contractions should be taught prior to exposure in storybooks or textbooks since printed texts will contain contractions in random sequence. This also means that the teacher of students with vision impairments needs to be closely involved in ensuring that the unique skills needed by the braille reader are fully addressed.

Teaching strategies for proficient print readers who are required to later learn braille will be more code-based. Students will be learning braille as a code that represents print and will, for a transitional period of learning, need to translate the braille symbols into their print equivalents. With time and practice, however, the braille contractions should be easily readable without this mental transcription. These students will also need considerable support from qualified teachers to work with them on the unique mechanical and tactile discrimination skills described above.

Assistive Technology and Independence

Braille can be written and read using a variety of technology options including computer and smart devices paired with a refreshable braille display. Children and adults who are blind can study throughout school levels and into higher education level and employment using digital braille, alongside other new technologies such as screen readers with text-to-speech output. Braille is a fast and efficient way to take notes in lessons and meetings, and is also useful for reading and reviewing various texts. Increased participation in society and independence is enabled by environmental labelling in braille, such as food and medicine labels and signage. The habilitation specialist (see Chapter 14) can assist in increasing independence in the environment using braille assistive technology. Continued advocacy for braille readers to have access to resources and tools in this electronic age is crucial.

Most children begin braille reading and writing instruction using either a Perkins Brailler or a Mountbatten Brailler because both of these options provide the opportunity for them to have immediate hard-copy access to what they have written. The child's educational team, through the process of LMA, routinely examines the need for additional literacy tools including use of appropriate technology with the ultimate goal of preparing students to move seamlessly across available devices to accomplish literacy tasks.

IMPLICATIONS FOR RESEARCH AND PRACTICE

Further research is needed to increase our understanding of effective braille reading and instructional approaches (Marcet et al. 2016), including greater understanding of the cognitive processes associated with braille reading. Current limitations of studies include often looking at words in isolation, or braille reading on an electronic display, which allows only for one hand to be used (Marcet et al. 2016). Whilst these issues are important, future research should also look at cognitive processes in more applied contexts such as reading sentences and paragraphs with both hands, and when quality and type of materials differ (e.g. Lei et al. 2019).

Future research that combines investigation of brain plasticity with different instructional interventions could support improved educational approaches for braille readers (Glyn et al. 2015; see Chapter 7). Gaining a better understanding of how braille readers engage with words will also be important for improving instruction. Some research indicates that tactile readers are predominantly sequential in their processing, but additional investigation into lexical potential is still needed as well as replication studies.

Intervention studies are mainly limited to educational research focussing on braille reading. More systematic studies are needed to investigate how evidence-based practices within the general reading instruction literature, such as repeated reading (Stanfa and Johnson 2017) and vocabulary instruction (Savaiano et al. 2016), can apply to braille readers. Investigations into medium-specific interventions for improved braille mechanics, speed, and efficiency are also needed.

It is very difficult to determine the number of braille readers in many specific countries around the world (Graves 2018), for example the USA lacks a national registry. However, investment is required to ensure that all children who need to learn braille have access to expert specialist instruction and also the assistive technology and electronic aids that are crucial for participation in learning and society. Although people who are blind face many barriers in getting a job, research shows that trained braille users who also maintain daily usage of their skill are more likely to be in employment and earning a higher income (Bell and Mino 2015).

SUMMARY

Children and young people who read and write through braille comprise a diverse group with a range of learning characteristics. These students, their parents, and teachers, along with other members of the education support system, participate in deliberate instructional efforts that are designed to result in highly developed and proficient literacy skills, founded upon in-depth understanding. Braille reading and writing abilities develop in a related parallel process to abilities of print readers but also require direct targeted instruction in skills unique to tactile reading. The importance of comprehensive and balanced instruction is emphasised.

Key Points

- ✓ Braille reading and writing are the means of literacy for individuals with significant vision impairments.
- ✓ Approaches to teaching braille reading must consider characteristics of the student including age of onset of vision impairment, and whether the student is learning both print and braille.
- ✓ Braille reading and writing includes unique mechanical and tactile discrimination skills that must be addressed for efficient reading and optimal reading speeds.
- ✓ More research is needed to better understand the braille reading and writing process, and to continue to identify evidence-based effective practices.
- ✓ Increased participation and independence in society is enabled by braille assistive technology and environmental labelling.

REFERENCES

Bell EC, Mino NM (2015) Employment outcomes for blind and visually impaired adults. *Journal of Blindness Innovation and Res* **5**(2).

Cervetti GN, Hiebert EH (2015) The sixth pillar of reading instruction: knowledge development. *The Reading Teacher* **68**(7): 548–551. doi: 10.1002/trtr.1343.

Chen X, Liang L, Lu M, Potmesil M, Zhong J (2019) The effects of reading mode and braille reading patterns on braille reading speed and comprehension: a study of students with visual impairments in China. *Res in Dev Dis* **91**: 103424. doi: 10.1016/j.ridd.2019.05.003.

Fischer-Baum S, Englebretson R (2016) Orthographic units in the absence of visual processing: evidence from sublexical structure in braille. *Cognition* **153**: 161–174. doi: 10.1016/j.cognition.2016.03.021.

Glyn V, Lim VK, Hamm JP, Mathur A, Hughes B (2015) Behavioural and electrophysiological effects related to semantic violations during braille reading. *Neuropsychologia* **77**: 298–312. doi: 10.1016/j.neuropsychologia.2015.09.008.

Graves A (2018) Braille literacy statistics research study: history and politics of the 'braille reader statistic': a summary of AFB Leadership Conference session on education. *Journal of Visual Impairment and Blindness* **112**(3): 328–331. doi: 10.1177/0145482X1811200314.

Greaney J, Reason R (1999) Phonological processing in braille. *Dyslexia* **5**(4): 215–226.

Holbrook MC, D'Andrea FM, Wormsley DW (2017) Literacy skills. In: Holbrook MC, McCarthy T, Kamei-Hannan C, editors, *Foundations of Education for Students with Visual Impairments, Volume II: Instructional Strategies*. American Foundation for the Blind.

International Council on English Braille (2014) *Unified English Braille: Guidelines for Technical Materials*. Available at: <http://www.iceb.org/guidelines_for_technical_material_2014.pdf> [Accessed 22 August 2021].

Kim JS, Kanjlia S, Merabet LB, Bedny M (2017) Development of the visual word form area requires visual experience: evidence from blind braille readers. *Journal of Neuroscience* **37**(47): 11495–11504. doi: 10.1523/JNEUROSCI.0997-17.2017.

Koenig AJ, Holbrook MC (1995) *Learning Media Assessment: Guidelines for Teachers*, 2nd Edition. Austin, TX: The Texas School for the Visually Impaired.

Koenig AJ, Farrenkopf C (1997) Essential experiences to undergird the early development of literacy. *Journal of Visual Impairment and Blindness* **91**(1): 14–24.

Koenig AJ, Holbrook MC (2000) Ensuring high-quality instruction for students in braille literacy programs. *Journal of Visual Impairment and Blindness* **94**(1): 677–694.

Lane C, Kanjlia S, Richardson H, Fulton A (2017) Reduced left lateralization of language in congenitally blind individuals. *Journal of Cognitive Neuroscience* **29**(1): 65–78. doi: 10.1162/jocn_a_01045.

Lei D, Stepien-Bernabe NN, Morash VS, MacKeben M (2019) Effect of modulating braille dot height on reading regressions. *PLoS One* **14**(4): 1–17. doi: 10.1371/journal.pone.0214799.

Lusk KE, Corn AL (2006) Learning and using print and braille: a study of dual media learners, Part 2. *Journal of Visual Impairment and Blindness* **100**(11): 653–665.

Marcet A, Jiménez M, Perea M (2016) Why braille reading is important and how to study it /Por qué es importante la lectura en braille y cómo estudiarla. *Cultura y Educación* **28**(4): 811–825. doi: 10.1080/11356405.2016.1230295.

National Reading Panel (2000) *Teaching Children to Read: An Evidence-Based Assessment of the Scientific Research Literature on Reading and Its Implications for Reading Instruction.* Washington, DC: National Institute of Child Health and Human Development. Available at: <https://www.nichd.nih.gov/sites/default/files/publications/pubs/nrp/Documents/report.pdf> [Accessed 22 August 2021].

Oshima K, Arai T, Ichihara S, Nakano Y (2014) Tactile sensitivity and braille reading in people with early blindness and late blindness. *Journal of Visual Impairment and Blindness* **108**(2): 122–131. doi: 10.1177/0145482X1410800204.

Papadimitriou V, Argyropoulos V (2017) The effect of hand movements on braille reading accuracy. *Int Journal of Educational Res* **85**: 43–50. https://doi-org.ezproxy.library.ubc.ca/10.1016/j.ijer.2017.07.004.

Rączy K, Urbanczyk A, Korczyk JM, Sumera E, Szwed M (2019) Orthographic priming in braille reading as evidence for task-specific reorganization in the ventral visual cortex of the congenitally blind. *Journal of Cognitive Neuroscience* **31**(7): 1065–1078. doi: 10.1162/jocn_a_01407.

Radojichikj DD (2015) Students with visual impairments: braille reading rate. *Int Journal of Cog Res in Science, Eng & Ed (IJCRSEE)* **3**(1): 1–5.

Savaiano ME, Compton DL, Hatton DD, Lloyd BP (2016) Vocabulary word instruction for students who read braille. *Exceptional Children* **82**(3): 337–353. doi: 10.1177/0014402915598774.

Stanfa K, Johnson N (2017) Improving reading fluency in braille readers using repeated readings. *Journal of Blindness Innovation and Res* **7**(1): 1.

Veispak A, Boets B, Ghesquière P (2012) Parallel versus sequential processing in print and braille reading. *Research in Developmental Disabilities* **33**(6): 2153–2163. doi: 10.1016/j.ridd.2012.06.012.

Wall Emerson R, Holbrook MC, D'Andrea FM (2009) Acquisition of literacy skills in young blind children: results from the ABC braille study. *Journal of Visual Impairment and Blindness* **103**(10): 610–624.

Wright T, Wormsley DP, Kamei-Hannan C (2009) Hand movements and braille reading efficiency: data from the ABC Braille Project. *Journal of Visual Impairment & Blindness* **103**(10): 649–661.

Zebehazy KT, Wilton AP (2014) Charting success: the experience of teachers of students with visual impairments in promoting graphic use by students. *Journal of Visual Impairment and Blindness* **108**(4): 263–274.

PART 4

Social Relationships and Participation

CHAPTER 18

Psychological Wellbeing, Mental Health, and Behaviour

Clare Jackson

INTRODUCTION

Children and young people with chronic conditions that can affect their health are at increased risk of developing emotional and behavioural difficulties; these difficulties need to be addressed alongside medical, social, and educational care. Vision impairment has a significant impact on the life of a young person and their family. This chapter will consider some of the psychological challenges it presents and the evidence base for and practical methods of assessing and intervening in ways that promote psychological wellbeing and support mental health.

PSYCHOLOGICAL WELLBEING AND MENTAL HEALTH

Living with a vision impairment impacts on all areas of a child's life, for example education, family and peer relationships, and independence. Grasping the immediate and long-term implications of a diagnosis is complex for both the family and the child. The task that the family faces in incorporating the vision impairment into their world to successfully make the necessary physical and emotional adaptations, should not be underestimated.

Research has demonstrated that children with a chronic physical health condition are at increased risk of developing psychological difficulties (e.g. Meltzer et al. 2000). Although some features of conditions (such as pain, cognitive difficulties, visibility, and appearance-related factors) increase the risk of psychological difficulties, there remains considerable individual variation. Although the majority do not manifest a psychological disorder, a significant minority experience difficulties with adjustment, or symptoms of psychological distress. It is estimated that 8% of children and young people aged 5 to 19 years in England have clinically diagnosed anxiety or depression (Sadler et al. 2018); however, rates among those with chronic physical health conditions are known to be higher (Meltzer et al. 2000).

Various factors related to having a vision impairment, such as mobility challenges (including accidents or near misses), barriers to learning, greater dependence on help from others, and potential lack of confidence in social situations due to the vision impairment precluding picking up facial expression and body language, may lead to young people being at greater risk of emotional disorders. When considering psychological wellbeing and mental health, most research investigates symptoms such as anxiety and depression. However, it is also important to think more broadly about young people's self-concept, adaptation to their condition, and their resilience. In terms of predictors of psychological distress in children and young people with physical health conditions, research has often shown that the level of self-esteem, social support, and ability to cope are more important predictors of psychosocial outcome than medical factors. A high level of psychological distress is associated with poorer quality of life and can result in an increased use of medical resources, such as frequent appointments or presentations to hospital.

The research base for the prevalence of psychological wellbeing and mental health in children and young people with vision impairment is relatively limited, but studies have suggested elevated levels of emotional distress in some individuals, for example, high levels of anxiety (Bolat et al. 2011). There is also some evidence that those with a severe vision impairment report greater anxiety and fears than those with a moderate impairment (Visagie et al. 2013). As in all children, fears are adaptive and potentially protective from real or perceived fear, but the nature of the fears may be intensified or specific to vision impairment. In two related studies in Jordan, 5- to 7-year-olds with profound vision impairment were described by their parents as being fearful of loud unpredictable noises that they could not see the source of, and having people-related fears (arguments, criticism, or teasing) (Al-Zboon 2017). The child's fear of the unknown, environment, transportation, people-related fear, and fear of animals were reported by teachers who also had vision impairment (Al-Zboon et al. 2017).

In a systematic review of mental health among children and young adults with vision impairments, two-thirds of the studies identified report an increased incidence of emotional problems in children with a vision impairment, with females experiencing depression more frequently than males (Augestad 2017). There is good evidence that resilience and strength are significant factors contributing to there being little apparent negative effect on emotional wellbeing among young people with vision impairment. For example, Pinquart and Pfeiffer (2014) found elevated levels of emotional problems in adolescents with vision impairment compared to matched controls, but the group with vision impairment reported the greatest improvement in symptoms during their follow-up 2 years later. This raises the important questions of who to target for intervention, and how to assess and encourage the factors that promote resiliency.

Very little research has compared the mental health needs of children with congenital versus acquired vision impairment. Furthermore, some studies in this population have not provided information on age of vision loss of children within their sample. In the longitudinal study by Pinquart and Pfeiffer (2014), those children with earlier, as compared to later, onset of vision loss showed less improvement in emotional difficulties over the length of the study, indicating that children with congenital vision impairment may have more enduring difficulties. Acquired vision loss is more common during later adulthood and there is more research on the mental health needs of this population. A systematic review identified high levels of depression in adults with irreversible vision loss and that the effects of vision loss on mental health tended to remain over time (Senra et al. 2015). Better adjustment to vision loss in this population was associated with various factors, including acceptance of vision loss, instrumental coping, and social support.

Individual variation in resilience reflects the influence of relative risk and protective factors; however, very little is known about these. In a systematic review of the literature on risk and protective factors for mental health disorders in children with vision impairment, the only risk factor established was co-occurring intellectual disability; there is very limited research on protective factors (MacKechnie et al. 2018). A study of parent-reported mental health disorder in 34 children aged 8 to 11 years old, with congenital disorders of the peripheral visual system and no known neurological disorders, found that significant minority proportions were at high risk of 'internalising' disorder (e.g. anxiety, depression) or 'externalising' disorder (e.g. aggression, defiant, or oppositional behaviour), including risk of separation anxiety. These rates were substantially higher than that of the typically developing population. A number of risk factors for mental health disorder were identified including severity of vision impairment and degree of social communication and associated behavioural difficulties (MacKechnie et al. 2018).

As suggested by Augestad (2017), early detection of potential mental health disorders and appropriate intervention will promote emotional wellbeing. The general literature on mental health difficulties in children and young people shows that experiencing these symptoms in childhood is a risk factor for the development of adult mental health difficulties, with evidence showing that adults with vision impairment are at increased risk of emotional disorders (e.g. Nyman et al. 2010; Moschos et al. 2015).

Complex Behaviour Issues

Greater emotional reactivity (such as sudden distress outbursts) are often reported by parents particularly in the home environment; these appear to be associated with greater frustration and may be triggered by having a sibling remove one's favourite object or getting stuck when making a model (see Chapter 8). Some medical conditions associated with vision impairment, for example, septo-optic dysplasia or hypothalamic tumours, have a higher likelihood of complex behaviour difficulties such as sleep disturbances, self-directed behaviour, anger outbursts, and oppositional defiance. Septo-optic dysplasia, which has hypothalamic, pituitary, and adrenal disorders and neuroendocrine deficiencies, as well as optic nerve hypoplasia, has also been associated with more repetitive and restricted behaviours (Parr et al. 2010). An increased likelihood of behaviour problems is associated with greater brain reduction in the ventral cingulum network in children with isolated optic nerve hypoplasia and mild to moderate or no vision impairment (Webb et al. 2013).

A significant proportion of children with vision impairment have additional needs or intellectual disability. A number of studies have shown that the risk of behaviour difficulties is highest in those with vision impairment and additional special educational needs or intellectual disability (Alimovic 2013; Harris and Lord 2016). This also corresponds with the greater risk for mental health disorders in children with increased social communication/autism spectrum disorder (ASD) problems but no other known neurological impairment or intellectual disability (MacKechnie et al. 2018).

ASSESSMENT AND MANAGEMENT

Role of the Multidisciplinary Team

Quality standards of care for children with chronic health conditions have been introduced in some countries; these highlight the importance of services addressing the psychological wellbeing and mental health of children and their family as a part of providing high-quality patient-centred services. One of the ongoing challenges for paediatric services is how best to deliver these.

Psychological support of children is provided by their family members, community, and team around them as part of their everyday care. For children with vision impairment, this may include support by parents, nursery, and school staff including teaching assistants, special needs teaching coordinators, the classroom teacher, educational psychologists, specialist teachers for visual impairment, and habilitation specialists. The child and parents may also be receiving support and guidance from the community or hospital paediatrician including early years' health worker and staff from the ophthalmological department including assistive vision aids service and the paediatric family liaison service.

Preventative Support and Early Identification

From the earliest days after diagnosis, parents and infants with vision impairment need appropriate care and support. Acknowledgement of the emotional impact for a child or young person, and their family receiving a diagnosis of vision impairment, and living with this, is essential. Home-based early intervention, with effective developmental materials delivered in partnership with parents, has been shown to improve parental wellbeing by reducing parenting stress and increasing satisfaction with practitioner involvement (Dale et al. 2019; see Chapter 8). Parents seek knowledge to support them in how to enhance their child's progress, handle any behaviour challenges, and promote psychological adaptation.

Many families of children with vision impairment show significant resilience, especially those showing a positive attitude towards the disability. Practitioners can contribute significantly by encouraging adaptive coping styles, and recognising the need for and helping to implement social support, other services, and leisure activities. Open communication and collaboration between family members is beneficial, as is the active use of available resources. The acceptance of help, as well as the sense of accomplishment that can accrue, have also been found to enhance resilience (de Klerk and Greeff 2011).

For the majority of children, psychological support within their usual environments is appropriate most of the time; however, at certain times, more detailed clinical assessment and, potentially, further intervention is required. The need to seek a referral to a mental health specialist or service usually indicates that a problem has reached a point where a young person or family feels that it is interfering in their quality of life. As the research has indicated, there are indicators that intervening early is likely to help in terms of preventing more chronic emotional difficulties. This makes it important to thoroughly assess and screen for emotional difficulties and any early signs of concern, and offer appropriate intervention at the earliest opportunity. Staff who are involved may include trained community health workers, behaviour support workers, clinical psychologists, neuropsychologists, and child psychiatrists.

Assessment

Any specialist assessment of wellbeing and mental health needs to take into account the context of the family, health system, school, peers, and community, as well as the potential impact of the vision impairment on the child and family.

A developmental perspective should be considered when formulating the origin of any difficulties (e.g. the normative and expected challenges of increased independence in adolescence). Assessment aims to gather relevant information to make sense of the presenting problem, and to formulate the difficulties, so that an intervention plan can be made. When formulating emotional difficulties there is a need for identification of pre-existing risk and resilience factors (e.g. social situation, cultural background, degree of vision impairment, additional or potential diagnoses such as ASD, developmental stage, and cognitive and language level) and psychological factors (such as beliefs and previous experiences) underpinning the emotional symptoms (Edwards and Titman

2010). The aim is to reach a shared understanding with the young person and family and to be collaborative in developing a plan of intervention.

During assessment of any anxiety symptoms, a developmental perspective is needed, as children tend to feel anxious about different things at different ages and many of these worries are a normal part of growing up. For example, young children often display behaviour suggesting separation anxiety; however, this tends to ease off as they get older. Anxiety at certain times, such as transition to school or exams, can be expected, but careful assessment is needed to identify those young people who are experiencing enduring unpleasant anxiety symptoms, potentially impacting on their everyday lives, harming self-esteem and emotional wellbeing. A child or young person with vision impairment may be prone to experiencing greater anxiety about separation from parents or teaching support staff, as they are more dependent on assistance in the physical environment. They may be more anxious about transitions, as they will have many additional challenges during a transition period to a new setting, for example, mapping routes around a school and classrooms, ensuring any necessary equipment is in place and getting to know new peers.

A further assessment by the paediatric neurodisability/neurodevelopmental team may be needed to consider factors that may be playing an additional role, such as undiagnosed social communication/ASD and mismatch between school expectations and child's potential abilities raising anxiety (see Chapter 11).

Similar assessment is required for children and young people presenting with symptoms of low mood and depression. Feeling sad is a normal reaction to stressful or upsetting experiences; however, those with enduring feelings of sadness that take over their usual self, and interfere with everyday life, may be experiencing depression. Depression can affect how a young person feels (e.g. sadness, irritability, lack of energy, or motivation) and behaves (e.g. missing school, self-harm, or withdrawing from social contact).

Support Across Settings

Means of supporting the young person and their emotional symptoms across different settings must be considered, for example liaison with the education setting or the medical team; there is a need for integration across these services. For example, when a child is presenting with medical procedural distress, some direct psychological work around exposure to the setting, planning ways of coping with the child and parent, and liaison with key medical professionals involved may greatly reduce a child's (and parental) anxiety. A further example illustrating the importance of inter-agency working is anxiety relating to a transition to secondary school. Providing the young person themselves with strategies for managing their anxiety symptoms is beneficial but careful liaison with the education setting is also vital, so the transition can occur in a graded, thoughtful way that addresses the anxieties of the young person and provides them with clear lines of support within the school setting. For building resilience and overcoming environment-related fears, support for families as well as orientation and mobility training, independence training, and environmental adaptation by habilitation specialists will be important (Al-Zboon 2017; see Chapter 14).

Interventions

There is very little research into preventative and clinical interventions for young people with vision impairment and emotional difficulties. In South Africa, Visagie et al. (2017) used a focus group to develop an adapted cognitive behavioural therapy-based anxiety intervention for 9- to 13-year-olds with vision impairment. Augestad (2017) highlights the importance of multi-agency working and the role that leisure activities and peer support can play in promoting wellbeing and reducing the risk of emotional disorders. Experiences of group membership and shared emotional connection to others with vision impairments have been found in a supportive sport context (Goodwin et al. 2011). The wider paediatric psychology literature on supporting children and young people with chronic medical conditions and mental health needs is also applicable to this group, providing adaptations are made where necessary.

For some young people an opportunity to discuss their adjustment to their diagnosis and vision loss provides a safe setting to consider their feelings and the emotional impact of their eye condition. For example, some talk about their sense of loss, their worries about the future, and their feelings about how their sight loss impacts on their social life and education. The experience of growing up with a vision impairment from the young person's perspective is explored by Tadić et al. (2015).

When a child or young person with vision impairment presents with clinically significant mental health symptoms, interventions may include psychoeducation about the physical response (e.g. physical symptoms of anxiety, the 'fight or flight' response) and also about some of the cognitive behavioural links between thoughts, feelings, and behaviours associated with the emotional symptoms. When working with children with vision impairments, care needs to be taken to ensure that resources are adapted appropriately so they are fully accessible. Systemic factors are also relevant and need considering in any intervention, for example parental ability to support and reassure, the education system making changes to increase accessibility, or the medical team making adjustments to their clinic setting to reduce anxiety. The normative developmental task of increasing independence in adolescence can be a difficult transition that can cause significant anxiety and frustrations on both sides and needs to be managed gradually, with attention to systemic factors such as parental anxiety about safety, versus the young person's desire for independence and increasing reliance on self and peers rather than parents (see Chapter 14).

When working with children and young people and their families, it is usually helpful to plan and rehearse different strategies to help manage emotional wellbeing, for example ways of monitoring emotional wellbeing, and coping strategies that help when a young person is feeling anxious or low (e.g. mindfulness, relaxation, and cognitive strategies such as 'thought challenging'). It is also important to think about who, if anyone, needs to help. For many children and young people with vision impairment, it will be necessary to be creative about applying some of the more widely used interventions, with a focus on tactile and auditory cues (e.g. a 'calm stone' in a pocket at school, a watch beep as a prompt for a breathing exercise, or the use of worry boxes or teddy 'guards' for night-time worries).

IMPLICATIONS FOR RESEARCH AND PRACTICE

There is a need for more longitudinal studies investigating mental health symptoms in children and young people with vision impairments and also studies identifying the risk and protective factors associated with increased distress or positive mental wellbeing. Furthermore, the mental health needs of children with congenital or very early onset vision impairment versus those who have vision in early development but later lose vision are likely to differ, but there is little research in this area. Information on risk and protective factors inform medical, psychological, and educational professionals of predictors of distress, and enable more proactive screening. Interventions that are offered more widely across paediatric clinical psychology can be appropriately used with those with vision impairments, providing care is taken to ensure resources are adapted appropriately and the clinician remains sensitive to the specific challenges presented by living with a vision impairment. Evaluation of the effectiveness of such approaches with children and young people with vision impairment needs pursuing.

SUMMARY

Children and young people with vision impairment frequently demonstrate impressive adjustment to their condition. Many families manage to successfully integrate the vision impairment into their lives and make the necessary adaptations. Some children and young people with a vision impairment experience reduced emotional wellbeing and mental health difficulties, either for a brief time or over an extended period. They need to be identified early and provided with appropriate assessment and support. Services need to work together to ensure that these young people can access psychological help. They also need to provide any environmental changes required to enable the child and young person to feel supported by those around them. Further research into this topic is required, particularly longitudinal studies through childhood and adolescence and also studies examining the effectiveness of psychological interventions for mental health difficulties.

Key Points

✓ Children and young people with vision impairment and their families make significant adjustments across many aspects of everyday life.

✓ Research has shown an increased risk of emotional symptoms such as anxiety, depression, and behaviour difficulties, the latter particularly in those with additional intellectual disability, ASD, or specific medical conditions.

✓ Assessment of wellbeing and distress needs to take a developmental and holistic perspective. Most support is provided by family, community, and education settings; however, for some young people, referral on to clinicians specialising in mental health is necessary.

✓ Interventions to support young people with mental health and behavioural needs must be evidence-based and more research is required, including predictors of positive mental health.

✓ Practitioners supporting young people with mental health needs must work closely with families and other practitioners across different agencies to ensure best support is in place.

REFERENCES

Al-Zboon E (2017) Childhood fears among children who are blind: the perspective of teachers who are blind. *Early Years* **37**: 158–172.

Al-Zboon E, Al-Dababneh KA, Baibres H (2017) Fear in children with visual impairments from the perspective of their parents. *Early Child Development and Care* **187**: 1948–1959.

Alimovic S (2013) Emotional and behavioural problems in children with visual impairment, intellectual and multiple disabilities. *Journal of Intellectual Disability Research* **57**: 153–160.

Augestad L (2017) Mental health among children and young adults with visual impairments: a systemic review. *Journal of Visual Impairment and Blindness* **111**: 411–425.

Bolat N, Dogangun B, Yavuz M, Demir T, Kayaalp L (2011) Depression and anxiety levels and self concept characteristics of adolescents with congenital complete visual impairment. *Turkish Journal of Psychiatry* **22**: 77–82.

Dale NJ, Sakkalou E, O'Reilly MA et al. (2019) Home-based early intervention in infants and young children with visual impairment using the Developmental Journal: longitudinal cohort study. *Developmental Medicine Child Neurology* **61**(6): 697–709.

de Klerk H, Greeff AP (2011) Resilience in parents of young adults with visual impairments. *Journal of Visual Impairment & Blindness* **105**: 414–424.

Edwards M, Titman P (2010) *Promoting Psychological Wellbeing in Children with Acute and Chronic Illness.* London: Jessica Kingsley.

Goodwin DL, Lieberman LJ, Johnston K, Leo J (2011) Connecting through summer camp: youth with visual impairments find a sense of community. *Adapted Physical Activity Quarterly* **28**: 40–55.

Harris J, Lord C (2016) Mental health of children with vision impairment at 11 years of age. *Developmental Medicine & Child Neurology* **58**: 774–779.

MacKechnie R, Pote H and Dale N (2018) Psychopathology profiles in children with congenital visual impairment. Unpublished doctoral dissertation. Royal Holloway University of London, London UK. Available at: <https://pure.royalholloway.ac.uk/portal/en/persons/rebecca-mackechnie(773244ad-b076-4bda-a9c2-acc902df76da)/publications.html> [Accessed 2021].

Meltzer H, Gatward R, Goodman R, Ford T (2000) *The Mental Health of Children and Adolescents in Great Britain.* London: The Stationary Office.

Moschos M, Chatzirallis A, Chatziralla, I (2015) Psychological aspects and depression in patients with retinitis pigmentosa. *European Journal of Ophthalmology* 25: 459–462.

Nyman S, Gosney M, Victor C (2010) Psychological impact of visual impairment in working age adults. *British Journal of Ophthalmology* 94: 1427–1431.

Parr JR, Dale NJ, Shaffer LM, Salt AT (2010) Social communication difficulties and autism spectrum disorder in young children with optic nerve hypoplasia and/or septo-optic dysplasia. *Developmental Medicine & Child Neurology* 52: 917–921.

Pinquart M, Pfeiffer J (2014) Change in psychological problems of adolescents with and without visual impairment. *European Journal of Child and Adolescent Psychiatry* 23: 571–578.

Sadler K, Vizard T, Ford T (2018) *Mental Health of Children and Young People in England, 2017.* NHS Digital, Government Statistical Service.

Senra H, Barbosa F, Ferreira P et al. (2015) Psychologic adjustment to irreversible vision loss in adults: a systematic review. *Ophthalmology* 122(4): 851–861.

Tadić V, Hundt GL, Keeley S, Rahi JS, Vision-related Quality of Life group (2015) Seeing it my way: living with childhood onset visual disability. *Child: Care, Health and Development* 41: 239–248.

Visagie L, Loxton H, Ollendick T, Steel H (2013) Comparing fears in South African children with and without visual impairments. *Journal of Visual Impairment and Blindness* 107: 193–205.

Visagie L, Loxton H, Stallard P, Silverman WK (2017) Insights into the feelings, thoughts and behaviors of children with visual impairments: a focus group study prior to adapting a cognitive behaviour therapy-based anxiety intervention. *Journal of Visual Impairment and Blindness* 111: 231–246.

Webb EA, O'Reilly MA, Clayden JD et al. (2013) Reduced ventral cingulum integrity and increased behavioral problems in children with isolated optic nerve hypoplasia and mild to moderate or no visual impairment. *PloS One* 8: e59048.

CHAPTER 19

Self-Concept and Social Relationships for Quality of Life and Participation

Mathijs Vervloed and Sabina Kef

INTRODUCTION

Quality of life and social participation are important concepts and outcomes for rehabilitation, education, or child-rearing for children with vision impairment, whatever their levels of ability. The main goals of quality of life intervention are independence, social participation, and wellbeing (Schalock et al. 2008). 'Participation' is the desired goal of rehabilitation and child rearing according to the International Classification of Functioning, Disability and Health: Children and Youth (ICF-CY) model, with participation based on attendance (referring to physical inclusion) and involvement (referring to social inclusion) (Imms et al. 2017). Self-concept and self-esteem (the evaluative and 'feeling' part of self-concept) are factors in both quality of life and participation, which are overlapping concepts.

A child or young person's self-concept and self-esteem help to determine how one adapts to the social and physical demands of the environment. This process is influenced by the way significant others (parents, siblings, friends, and teachers, etc.) perceive and define the child. This 'reflected-self' in turn affects how the child formulates and values their personal characteristics. Self-concept and self-esteem are affected by the social relations and experiences of the child and thus are inherently interpersonal. In ICF-CY terms, indicative behaviours of self-concept can be classified as activities within the domain of interpersonal relations. As vision impairment challenges competence in life areas, the self-concept of children with vision impairment is potentially at risk when they compare themselves to others. This is exacerbated further by being perceived by others to be different, which may contribute to developing a more negative self-concept.

This chapter describes the research evidence regarding the self-concept, self-esteem, and social relations of children with vision impairment. Practical methods to support their positive development within a developmental framework and to achieve improved quality of life and participation are provided.

SELF-CONCEPT AND SOCIAL RELATIONSHIPS

Definition and Classification

Self-concept is the answer to the question, 'Who am I as an individual?' As the collection of beliefs and opinions about oneself, self-concept is the cognitive or descriptive component of one's self. Self-concept is multidimensional and refers to the totality of the child's perception about their physical, social, and academic competence, including perceptions and beliefs of their characteristics, qualities, deficiencies, capacities, limits, values, and relationships, and what self is. Self-knowledge and body awareness are part of self-concept. The evaluative part of self-concept is self-esteem, a personal judgement of worthiness expressed in the attitudes the person holds towards themself across different life areas (Harter 2012). Feeling competent in one area or domain, such as academic or sporting or social, does not always generalise to other domains or to global self-esteem; global self-esteem may stay more stable compared to individual domains. At an individual level, only those self-esteem domains that are perceived to be important to the child or adolescent may affect global self-esteem, either positively or negatively.

Self-concept appears to be a valid predictor of many aspects of behaviour and is associated with mental health in children who are typically sighted, with higher self-esteem positively associated with later improved mental health outcomes (Henriksen et al. 2017). Both self-concept and self-esteem affect the way a person deals with life's demands. Success and failure in acquiring skills and dealing with requirements of the environment in relation to one's aspirations may help shape self-esteem. This may be particularly relevant to children with vision impairment as positive self-concept can create the drive and motivation for behaviour and greater competence may underpin higher self-esteem (Datta 2014).

A sense of belonging, arising from social relations with other persons, is one of the three basic psychological needs highlighted in the self-determination theory (Ryan and Deci 2000). When children are feeling satisfied and not frustrated in this regard, their intrinsic motivation for development and their wellbeing, quality of life, and level of participation are likely to be high (Ryan and Deci 2000; Heppe et al. 2019). Several studies show increased risks for problems in social relationships due to direct consequences of vision impairment (causing difficulties with non-verbal communication or mobility) and indirect consequences (e.g. stigmatisation by others, and exclusion) (Kef et al. 2000; Heppe et al. 2019).

Presenting Features

A systematic review of the scientific knowledge (1998–2016) relating to self-concept and self-esteem in children and young adolescents with vision impairment identified 26 publications in 15 countries, meeting the inclusion criteria (Augestad 2017). This and another review paper (Datta 2014) showed that self-concept and self-esteem are often used interchangeably, despite clear conceptual differences. The research on self-concept showed mixed results; some studies found lower self-concept whilst others found no differences with children who are typically sighted (e.g. Pinquart and Pfeiffer 2011). Some studies found that the child's age and degree of vision impairment influenced perceived self-esteem (Augestad 2017). Self-esteem may potentially be lower due to limited development of social skills. Children with vision impairment may experience social exclusion and bullying, may feel isolated, and have limited contact with their peers who are typically sighted (Kef et al 2000; Pfeiffer and Pinquart 2011). All of these factors might lead to a more negative self-concept and lower self-esteem.

Some studies found a sex difference, with females having lower self-esteem than males, particularly in the domain of physical appearance (Tołczyk and Pisula 2019). However, Were et al. (2010) found females showed higher academic self-esteem. Cultural expectations, aspirations, and sex stereotypes for males and females and greater challenges for participation and acceptance may be relevant factors here.

It is of interest to consider whether having a congenital or acquired vision impairment affects self-concept and wellbeing. The evidence points towards adolescents with blindness or vision impairment not differing overall from sighted peers in identity development. However, some differences are found once the group is divided into those with congenital or acquired vision impairment. Adolescents with congenital vision impairment and a longer period of having a visual impairment have lower levels of identity exploration than those with acquired vision impairment (Pinquart and Pfeiffer 2013). Those with lower levels of identity exploration also tended to show less problem behaviours. This might mean that adolescents with congenital vision impairment have a more stable identity status, which is associated with lower levels of problem behaviour, and are therefore 'better off' or more protected than those who have a more recently acquired vision impairment. Alternatively, these children may have been more dependent on their parents and other adults and less prone to engaging in riskier behaviours involved in identity exploration and moving further away from parents and their values.

Further research such as that of Papadopoulos (2014) suggests that congenital versus acquired vision impairment also impacts on locus of control and self-esteem. Independent mobility and low vision (and not blindness) correlated positively with locus of control. However, blindness (and not low vision), congenital vision impairment, and a longer time since onset of the vision impairment correlated positively with self-esteem. The apparent protective effect of congenital onset and greater vision reduction or blindness is somewhat surprising bearing in mind that persons with congenital disabilities are more at risk of being stigmatised than those with acquired disabilities (Bogart et al. 2019). However, this may be counteracted by the grieving over loss of functioning of the person with acquired disability compared to those with congenital disability who have not experienced loss of function (Bogart 2014). Further evidence by this research team shows that congenital onset of disability and self-esteem are significant predictors of satisfaction with life, with disability identity and disability self-efficacy (i.e. perceptions of identity and one's ability to do things for one's self and be successful associated with one's disability) mediating or influencing the way that the factors affect the outcomes. Disability pride protected self-esteem by rejecting a stigmatising culture and deciding to identify with other people with disabilities (Bogart et al. 2018). This research was undertaken with people with mobility disabilities, so it is not known whether it applies in the same way to persons with blindness and low vision. It would suggest that there is a particular value for young people with blindness in meeting with others and social-ising with those who have a similar disability, at least in those who have congenital onset vision impairment.

A causal relation between self-concept and mental health and wellbeing could not be deduced from the cross-sectional studies with children with vision impairment. However, associations between low self-esteem and loneliness, anxiety, and depression were established (Augestad 2017). Kef et al. (2000) showed that network size and satis-faction with social support related positively to wellbeing. In follow-up analyses with the same sample, Kef and Deković (2004) found practical and emotional support by peers to be positively related to wellbeing, whereas parental support was not.

Independence in mobility was also positively associated with wellbeing in adolescents with vision impairments (Kef et al. 2000). It may increase the child's locus of control and make them less dependent on peers, making visiting others and maintaining contact easier. This enhancing of autonomy and fostering self-esteem as a result of increased competence was also suggested by Papadopoulos et al. (2011) and Tołczyk and Pisula (2019).

However, the current research evidence is limited to a small number of empirical studies with cross-sectional designs, and suffers from conceptual and methodological incon-sistencies that hinder comparisons across studies (Datta 2014; Augestad 2017). Studies of global self-esteem are hard to compare with others that examine specific self-esteem domains. Sampling factors like child's age, age of onset, and level of vision impairment (blindness, low vision) vary (Augested 2017). Lastly, studies differ according to the age of the sample and their developmental age of self-description, as an expression of self-concept, and what instrument can be used to capture this.

Short- and Long-Term Outcomes

In general, the social networks of children and adolescents with vision impairment seem to be smaller, with a more prominent role for parents and adults than the networks of peers who are typically sighted (Kef et al. 2000). Successful habilitation processes and access to specialised therapeutic and educational services may also be influential, as suggested by Tołczyk and Pisula (2019). They found no difference in self-esteem between young people with vision impairment and peers who were typically sighted, but the majority of the group attended special schools where they received psychological support and participated in activities designed to develop orientation and mobility skills and give independence in everyday life. These findings align with those of Papadopoulos et al. (2011), where a sense of greater independence in self-care tasks, and higher levels of orientation and mobility skills are associated with higher self-esteem. However, the higher levels of self-esteem could also be a consequence of being educated in a specialist setting (Augestad 2017); comparison of self with other people and with the reflected self of significant others may be more supportive of positive self-concept and self-esteem in specialised settings than in mainstream education.

A further consideration is that an individual's global and domain-specific self-worth may be protected from negative effects of low self-perceptions of competence, by downplaying the perceived value or importance that one places on each domain. In 43 children with vision impairments, the children discounted the importance of physical appearance, athletic competence, and social acceptance, and had moderately high ratings of global, or overall, self-worth (Shapiro et al. 2008). This could be a self-protecting coping mechanism for self-worth and wellbeing, but on the negative side it may risk the child retreating from potentially healthy or rewarding opportunities or experiences such as sporting activities. Research investigating the physical self-concept of children with vision impairment in relation to physical activity and sports is limited. An exploratory qualitative interview study with six children (10–12 years) revealed four themes: adaptations, friends, bullying, and eyes and glasses in relation to physical activity and sports. Despite the occurrence of bullying or lack of adaptations in sports or physical activity, the children were satisfied with their physical self and global self-esteem (De Schipper et al. 2017).

SUPPORT AND MANAGEMENT

The Role of the Multidisciplinary Team

The child and young person's parents and family, school staff including teaching assistants, classroom teacher, and specialist teacher (vision impairment), health practitioners and members of the community including peers, social groups, and clubs play a role in enhancing the young person's self-esteem and self-concept, in partnership with the young person. The habilitation specialist plays an important role (see Chapter 14). All should focus on creating positive environments including social interactions and relationships to support the growth of positive self-concept and self-esteem. This may include different kinds of inclusive settings, and participation with other children and young people who are typically sighted or who also have a vision impairment. Support of a positive self-concept starts from infancy, working on social interactions and relationships with the child within their family (see Chapter 8), and continues throughout childhood and through the transition to adulthood and beyond (see Chapter 20).

Assessment

Within the clinical or educational context, it may be useful to consider and systematically assess the child or young person's self-concept or self-esteem or quality of life, though this must be done sensitively with due respect to confidentiality and safeguarding.

A variety of instruments are used to measure self-concept and self-esteem in children and young people with vision impairment (Augestad 2017) in research but less frequently in clinical practice. The Harter Self-Perception Profile (for an overview see Harter 2012) and Rosenberg Self-Esteem Scale (Rosenberg 1965) are commonly used but lack normative groups and cut-off scores, which limit their use for clinical practice. As far as is known, no instruments exist specifically to assess the self-concept and self-esteem of children with vision impairment.

For considering the child's overall quality of life, social relationships, and participation in society, the self-reporting Vision-related Quality of Life can be used. This captures the child's perspectives and the dimensions that matter to them and can be used to measure service interventions and changes in outcomes (Tadić et al. 2016). This 35-item scale has shown good construct validity, correlating strongly with health-related quality of life. As part of a joint assessment, the Functional Vision Questionnaire for Children and Young People comprises 36 items to capture self-reported level of difficulty in the performance of vision dependent activities for children and adolescents and has good psychometric properties (Tadić et al. 2013). Both measures have been developed in the UK and a cross-cultural validation of the Functional Vision Questionnaire for Children and Young People in the Netherlands has shown that instrument performance was different in each country and an adapted Dutch version was developed for measurement precision (Elsman et al. 2019a).

Other measures of social relations can be utilised but have so far been mainly used in a research context and their clinical applicability is unknown. Age-specific versions of the Participation and Activity Inventory for Children and Youth across the childhood age span have been developed in the Netherlands (Elsman et al. 2019b). Participation and autonomy were affected adversely, with moderate-large effects compared to age norms, in 18- to 25-year-old adolescents and young adults with vision impairment; worse physical functioning and vision-related quality of life was associated with increased severity of vision impairment (Elsman et al. 2019c). This is relevant to adolescent and young adulthood services (see Chapter 20).

Intervention and Practical Support

In a systematic review, Augestad (2017) concludes that friendship, independence in mobility, social support, and parenting style may enhance the self-concept and self-esteem of children with vision impairment. This constitutes a practical challenge for intervention and support, as the domains, other than mobility, involve the wider circle around the child too (such as peers, teachers, and parents). Difficulty in engaging them may stem from practical, financial, or motivational reasons.

A systematic review on group interventions to improve functioning, participation, and quality of life in children with vision impairment (Elsman et al. 2019d) included 66 studies that met the inclusion criteria (including 28 randomised controlled trials). The most effective interventions appeared to be sport camps, prescription, and training in the use of low vision devices, and oral hygiene programmes. However, the results should be interpreted with caution because of moderate to high risk of bias and suboptimal reporting.

Heppe et al. (2019) applied a randomised controlled trial design to study the effectiveness of a mentoring intervention on social participation and psychosocial functioning in 76 adolescents (aged 15–22 years) with vision impairment. The intervention consisted of 12 planned face-to-face meetings near the mentees' homes. Based on shared interests, several activities were carried out to stimulate social participation in the domains of education, work, leisure activities, and social relationships. Fifty trained mentors participated in this project. Approximately half of them had a vision impairment themselves. No intervention effects were found for improving the frequency of social participation compared to adolescents who received care as usual. However, improved psychosocial functioning (higher feelings of autonomy and higher feelings of competence) were found (Heppe et al. 2020), suggesting the potential benefit of adding a mentoring programme to habilitation services (see Chapter 14).

Supporting Participation

In the curriculum of special education and guidance of children with vision impairment in inclusive settings, increasing attention is paid to self-concept, self-esteem, and social relations (Wagner 2004). Interventions are mostly based on instruction, role play, and skill training in small groups, but as yet there has been no systematic evaluation of the effectiveness of training in personal skills and competences. A broader holistic approach is also needed to prepare the child for participating and functioning in the wider social environment. This may include challenges and barriers to participation, such as people with stigmatizing beliefs, lack of opportunities for people with disabilities, and cultural, economic, and legal hindrances.

Within the family of participation-related constructs of Imms et al. (2017), participation is not only a means but also an end in habilitation. The research evidence in this chapter suggests this end can be accomplished by helping the child and young person with vision impairment in building friendships by training social competencies but also the requisite mobility skills to allow them to maintain their friendships without being dependent on parents to get in contact with friends on their behalf. Being valued as a friend is one way to feel involved during social participation. Helping and allowing children and young people with vision impairment to make their own choices fosters their autonomy, and subsequently their self-esteem.

From a clinical and educational stance, it must be recognised that the individual child or adolescent's capacity, competence, and motivation to initiate and reciprocate communication with friends is also pivotal. Children and young people with vision impairment differ considerably in this respect, as is discussed further in Chapter 11. Assessment, intervention, and habilitation will need to cater to the individual child's capability and needs.

Within the framework of participation-related constructs, a developmental perspective is needed too as children's self-concepts and self-knowledge change over time and have normative elements related to their age, cognitive and socio-emotional status, and developmentally related tasks (e.g. greater independence and autonomy expectations in adolescence). Such development evolves through a dynamic interaction between self, context, and experiences.

IMPLICATIONS FOR RESEARCH AND PRACTICE

Cross-sectional studies cannot determine causal relationships and therefore more longitudinal and randomised controlled intervention studies are required (Augestad 2017). Multiple outcome measures in existing research prevent comparisons between studies and greater consensus in this area would be useful (Augestad 2017; Elsman et al. 2019d). Future studies should focus on promising interventions for which effectiveness is still unclear (e.g. mobility and social skills), with adequately designed methodologies. Intervention studies should include multi-dimensional perspectives on self-concept as effect sizes have been higher in studies with a multi-dimensional perspective that discounted less valued domains compared to those with global perspectives (O'Mara et al. 2006). Another issue is the need to study self-concept within the role that comparative processes play in their development and maintenance. As discussed theoretically (Van Zanden et al. 2015), children may share similar objective characteristics and accomplishments but have different self-concepts due to differing frames of reference or comparison standards. Sex stereotypes and school placement may also contribute to variations in self-concept. More research is needed into the role between disability identity, self-efficacy, quality of life, and participation for persons with vision impairment.

In relation to practice, assessment and promotion of psychosocial skills should be part of service delivery offered to children with vision impairment. This includes focussing on determinants that may influence self-concept, self-esteem, and social relationships (Zebehazy and Smith 2011; Heppe et al. 2019), including significant others in the child's family and wider environment. A practical approach is to focus on increasing positive aspects such as social inclusion, and protective and resilience factors, including compensating mechanisms and enriching the social environment. This needs to start as early in the child's life as possible, including early intervention focussing on child and family (see Chapter 8), and continue through childhood and adolescence to the transition to young adulthood (see Chapter 20). A focus on promoting self-esteem should not be at the exclusion of encouraging participation in beneficial health-promoting activities like sports activities and overcoming voluntary self-exclusion.

SUMMARY

Children with vision impairment are a heterogeneous group, and self-concept and self-esteem seem to be moderately positive for a substantial proportion but a meaningful minority appear to have problems. Knowledge about their needs and factors associated with self-concept and self-esteem is still limited as the research results are mixed and contradictory making them hard to generalise from. Better-designed studies are beginning to lead to important insights with implications for practice and further research, though evidence-based practice itself is still scarce. Psychosocial skills should be a central and structural part of assessment and interventions in the services for children with vision impairment, including focus on significant others in the child's life and the wider environment to enhance participation and quality of life.

Key Points

✓ Self-concept and self-esteem are important concepts and outcomes for child wellbeing, quality of life, and participation in society.

✓ Multidimensional aspects should be considered in assessment and interventions including participation in activities that may be initially discounted or devalued by the child.

✓ Social relationships, including a sense of belonging, are essential in the development of self-concept and participation.

✓ More research is needed with better methodological designs to help identify determinants of self-concept and self-esteem and evaluate interventions for participation.

✓ More scientifically developed tools are available for use in research, clinical practice, educational settings, or habilitation contexts.

ACKNOWLEDGEMENTS

We thank Sena Öz (Erasmus summer-school student) for assisting us in the study of the literature.

REFERENCES

Augestad LB (2017) Self-concept and self-esteem among children and young adults with visual impairment: a systematic review. *Cogent Psychology* 4: 1319652. doi: https://doi.org/10.1080/23311908.2017.1319652.

Bogart KR (2014) The role of disability self-concept in adaptation to congenital or acquired disability. *Rehabilitation Psychology* 59(1): 107–115. doi: https://doi.org/10.1037/a0035800.

Bogart KR, Lund EM, Rottenstein A (2018) Disability pride protects self-esteem through the rejection-identification model. *Rehabilitation Psychology* 63(1): 155–159. doi: https://doi.org/10.1037/rep0000166.

Bogart KR, Rosa NM, Slepian ML (2019) Born that way or became that way: Stigma toward congenital versus acquired disability. *Group Processes & Intergroup Relations* 22(4): 594–612. doi: https://doi.org/10.1177/1368430218757897.

Datta P (2014) Self-concept and vision impairment: a review. *British Journal of Visual Impairment* 32(3): 200–210. https://doi.org/10.1177/0264619614542661.

De Schipper T, Lieberman LJ, Moody B (2017) 'Kids like me, we go lightly on the head': experiences of children with a visual impairment on the physical self-concept. *British Journal of Visual Impairment* 35(1): 55–68. doi: https://doi.org/10.1177/0264619616678651.

Elsman EBM, Tadić V, Peeters CF, van Rens GHMB, Rahi JS, van Nispen RMA (2019a) Cross-cultural validation of the Functional Vision Questionnaire for Children and Young People (FVQ CYP) with visual impairment in the Dutch population: challenges and opportunities. *BMC Medical Research Methodology* 19: 221. https://doi.org/10.1186/s12874-019-0875-9.

Elsman EBM, Van Nispen RMA, Van Rens GHMB (2019b) Psychometric evaluation of a new proxy-instrument to assess participation in children aged 3–6 years with visual impairment: PAI-CY 3-6. *Ophthalmic and Physiological Optics* 39: 378–391. doi: https://doi.org/10.1111/opo.12642.

Elsman EBM, van Rens GHMB, van Nispen RMA (2019c) Quality of life and participation of young adults with a visual impairment aged 18-25 years: comparison with population norms. *Acta Ophthalmologica* 97(2): 165–172. https://doi.org/10.1111/aos.13903.

Elsman E, Al Baaj M, van Rens G et al. (2019d) Interventions to improve functioning, participation and quality of life in children with visual impairment: a systematic review. *Survey of Ophthalmology* 64: 512–557. doi: https://doi.org/10.1016/j.survophthal.2019.01.010.

Harter S (2012) *The Construction of the Self: Developmental and Sociocultural Foundations,* 2nd Edition. New York: Guilford Press.

Henriksen IO, Ranøyen I, Indredavik MS, Stenseng F (2017) The role of self-esteem in the development of psychiatric problems: a three-year prospective study in a clinical sample of adolescents. *Child Adolescent Psychiatry and Mental Health* 11: 68. doi: https://doi.org/10.1186/s13034-017-0207-y.

Heppe ECM, Willemen AM, Kef S, Schuengel C (2019) Improving social participation of adolescents with a visual impairment with community-based mentoring: results from a randomized controlled trial, *Disability and Rehabilitation,* Advance online publication. doi: https://doi.org/10.1080/09638288.2019.1589587.

Heppe ECM, Willemen AM, Kef S, Schuengel C (2020) Evaluation of a community-based mentoring program on psychosocial functioning of adolescents with a visual impairment: a randomized controlled trial. *British Journal of visual Impairment,* first published 9 July 2020. doi: https://doi.org/10.1177/0264619620935944.

Imms C, Granlund M, Wilson PH, Steenbergen B, Rosenbaum PL, Gordon AM (2017) Participation, both a means and an end: a conceptual analysis of processes and outcomes in childhood disability. *Developmental Medicine & Child Neurology* 59: 16–25. doi: https://doi.org/10.1111/dmcn.13237.

Kef S, Hox JJ, Habekothe HT (2000) Social networks of visually impaired and blind adolescents. Structure and effect on well-being. *Social Networks* 22: 73–91. doi: https://doi.org/10.1016/S0378-8733(00)00022-8.

Kef S, Deković M (2004) The role of parental and peer support in adolescents well-being: a comparison of adolescents with and without a visual impairment. *Journal of Adolescence* 27: 453–466. doi: https://doi.org/10.1016/j.adolescence.2003.12.005.

O'Mara AJ, Marsh HW, Craven RG, Debus RL (2006) Do self-concept interventions make a difference? A synergistic blend of construct validation and meta-analysis. *Educational Psychologist* 41(3): 181–206. doi: https://doi.org/10.1207/s15326985ep4103_4.

Papadopoulos K, Metsiou K, Agaliotis I (2011) Adaptive behavior of children and adolescents with visual impairment. *Research in Developmental Disabilities* 32: 1086–1096. doi: https://doi.org/ 10.1016/j.ridd.2011.01.021.

Papadopoulos K (2014) The impact of individual characteristics in self-esteem and locus of control of young adults with visual impairments. *Research in Developmental Disabilities* 35: 671–675. doi: https://doi.org/10.1016/j.ridd.2013.12.009.

Pfeiffer JP, Pinquart M (2011) Attainment of developmental tasks by adolescents with visual impairments and sighted adolescents. *Journal of Visual Impairment & Blindness* 105(1): 33–44. https://doi.org/10.1177/0145482X1110500104.

Pinquart M, Pfeiffer JP (2011) Yes, I can. Self-efficacy beliefs in students with and without visual impairment. *Journal of Blindness Innovation and Research* 1: 3. doi: https://doi.org/10.5241/2F1-20.

Pinquart M, Pfeiffer JP (2013) Identity development in German adolescents with and without visual impairments. *Journal of Visual Impairment & Blindness* 107: 338–349. doi: https://doi.org/10.1177/0145482X1310700503.

Rosenberg M (1965) *Society and the Adolescent Self-Image*. Princeton: Princeton University Press.

Ryan RM, Deci EL (2000) Self-determination theory and the facilitation of intrinsic motivation, social development, and well-being. *American Psychologist* 55: 68–78. doi: https://doi.org/10.1037/0003-066X.55.1.68.

Schalock RL, Bonham GS, Verdugo MA (2008) The conceptualization and measurement of quality of life: Implications for program planning and evaluation in the field of intellectual disabilities. *Evaluation and Program Planning* 31: 181–190. doi: https://doi.org/10.1016/j.evalprogplan.2008.02.001.

Shapiro DR, Moffett A, Lieberman L, Dummer GM (2008) Domain-specific ratings of importance and global self-worth of children with visual impairments. *Journal of Visual Impairment & Blindness* 102(4): 232–244. doi: https://doi.org/10.1177/0145482X0810200408.

Tadić V, Cooper A, Cumberland P, Lewando-Hundt G, Rahi JS (2016) Measuring the quality of life of visually impaired children: first stage psychometric evaluation of the novel VQoL_CYP instrument. *PLoS One* 11(2): e0146225.

Tadić V, Cooper A, Cumberland P, Lewando-Hundt G, Rahi JS (2013) Vision-related quality of life G. development of the functional vision questionnaire for children and young people with visual impairment: the FVQ_CYP. *Ophthalmology* 120(12): 2725–2732. https://doi.org/10.1016/j.ophtha.2013.07.055.

Tołczyk S, Pisula E (2019) Self-esteem and coping styles in Polish youths with and without visual impairments. *Journal of Visual Impairment & Blindness* **113**(3): 283–294. doi: https://doi.org/10.1177/0145482X19854903.

Van Zanden B, Marsh HW, Seaton M, Parker P (2015) Self-concept: from unidimensional to multidimensional and beyond. In: Wright JD, editor, *International Encyclopedia of the Social & Behavioral Sciences,* 2nd Edition. Amsterdam: Elsevier. doi: https://doi.org/10.1016/B978-0-08-097086-8.25089-7, pp. 460–468.

Wagner E (2004) Practice report development and implementation of a curriculum to develop social competence for students with visual impairments in Germany. *Journal of Visual Impairment and Blindness* **98**(11): 1–18.

Were CM, Indoshi FC, Yalo JA (2010) Gender differences in self-concept and academic achievement among visually impaired pupils in Kenya. *Educational Research* **1**(8): 246–252.

Zebehazy KT, Smith TJ (2011) An examination of characteristics related to the social skills of youths with visual impairments. *Journal of Visual Impairment & Blindness* **105**(2): 84–95. doi: https://doi-org.ru.idm.oclc.org/10.1177/0145482X1110500206.

CHAPTER 20

Towards Autonomy and Independence in Adolescence

Graeme Douglas, Mike McLinden, and Rachel Hewett

INTRODUCTION

Adolescence is the phase of a young person's life in which they are moving from childhood to adulthood. It can therefore be a profound transition in a young person's life, particularly as they progress towards higher education, employment, adult autonomy, and independence. Independence skills as well as academic success are predictors of positive long-term outcomes for young people with vision impairment. Sustained educational intervention targeting environmental, social, and personal factors is needed to ensure that autonomy and independence develop well. They must seek to balance two inter-related approaches: 'access to learning' and 'learning to access'. Finding a balance between these approaches requires careful person-centred planning in the adolescent years. This chapter explores interventions and educational strategies that may be useful for supporting the development of independence and autonomy whilst finding a balance between access to learning and learning to access during adolescence.

AUTONOMY AND INDEPENDENCE IN ADOLESCENCE

Adolescence is defined by the World Health Organization as the phase between 10 and 19 years old, although precise definitions are debated (Sawyer et al. 2018). Within the education sector, 'transition' is the term commonly used to describe the life changes that children and young people experience as they move through educational systems and from one setting to another. In adolescence this is typified by transition periods between very different systems (compulsory secondary/high school education, higher education, early employment, and independent living), with contrasting expectations and support available for young people with vision impairment at each stage (Douglas et al. 2019a).

Vision Impairment Education

Douglas et al. (2019b) undertook a review of the effectiveness of educational interventions to support children and young people with vision impairment. They reported that 'vision impairment education' has a long tradition of focussing upon two broad areas of targeted educational outcomes and associated interventions: (1) ensuring young people have fair and optimised access to the school curriculum and (2) ensuring young people have opportunities to develop their independence and social inclusion.

The first area is concerned with equal access and participation in education. The second area is linked with maximising a young person's ability to develop as an independent learner within education systems and also part of a broader agenda of empowering learners for adult life through promoting personal agency. The two broad areas of intervention map onto the International Classification of Functioning, Disability and Health: Children and Youth framework because they are concerned with targeting both environmental and personal factors that affect young people's development and participation. The interventions target:

- *Access to learning*: inclusive or universal practice and differentiation ensuring that the child's environment is structured and modified to promote inclusion, learning and access to the core (academic) curriculum, the culture of the educational setting, and broader social inclusion.
- *Learning to access*: teaching provision that supports the child to learn independence skills and develop agency, in order to afford more independent learning and social inclusion. This recognises that there is a need to teach a broader curriculum to promote learner independence, which includes mobility and habilitation, low vision training, and social skills.

Within the USA, these distinctive 'learning to access' areas are commonly described as an 'expanded core curriculum' and refer to the knowledge, concepts, and skills generally learned incidentally by typically sighted students but which must be systematically taught to students with vision impairment (Sapp and Hatlen 2010; Allman and Lewis 2014). They are described as a body of skills needed by learners with vision impairment to fully participate in education, work, and daily life (see Fig. 20.1).

Evidence of the importance of these two educational approaches exists when considering longer-term educational outcomes, in particular employment outcomes for young people with vision impairment. One of the most significant positive predictors of their employment is the level of educational attainment (Clements et al. 2011).

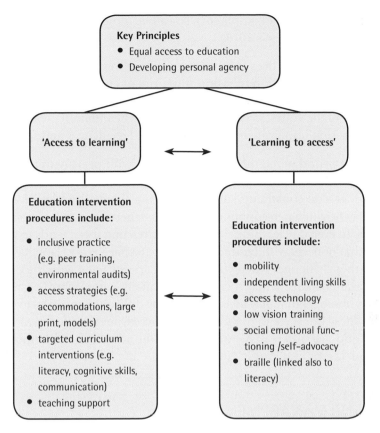

Figure 20.1 Relationship between 'learning to access' and 'access to learning' in the field of vision impairment education with examples of education intervention procedures (adapted from Douglas et al. 2019b). Contains public sector information licensed under the Open Government Licence v3.0

The presence of skills promoting greater independence, including career preparation, mobility and orientation skills, social skills, technology skills, and braille skills, are also associated with positive employment outcomes (Capella McDonnall 2011; Wolffe and Kelly 2011).

Adolescence and Vision Impairment Education

Adolescence is commonly characterised by strong peer influences, 'living in the present', and lower levels of future orientation (Patton et al. 2016). In contrast, vision impairment education is focussed on preparation for adulthood and recognition that some aspects of independence must be actively taught (e.g. mobility, independent living skills, independent study skills, and the use of access technology). Such interventions tend to be future-orientated and can highlight differences from one's peers (special lessons, additional support, specialist equipment), so can be more difficult to implement with adolescents (Allman and Lewis 2014).

Other factors will also affect the young person's experiences, reactions, and needs during this period, including variation in vision impairment and possible other learning or motor difficulties. A further challenge is the rarity of individual childhood vision disorders; those around the young person will commonly be unfamiliar with the nature of their particular vision impairment and the associated challenges and solutions.

Adolescence is a period when increased differences with peers with typical sight can become more evident and may be particularly difficult to acknowledge or accept, particularly if they lead to constraints such as not being able to learn to drive a car. These constraints may heighten perceptions of reduced independence and more limited career opportunities. In everyday learning situations, the reading speed tends to fall considerably behind that of peers with typical sight by the teenage years (Douglas et al. 2011), providing further challenges when young people are engaging with the curriculum or approaching examinations. Whilst there are augmentative approaches (e.g. magnification and speech technology) that may assist overcoming difficulties in access to learning (see Chapter 16), these can serve to highlight differences from their peers. Mobility canes, monoculars, and magnifiers may not be used if the adolescent 'attempts to pass as a sighted person' (Lewis and Wolffe 2006, p. 153).

SUPPORT AND MANAGEMENT

Navigating the complex range of interventions and services requires multidisciplinary and collaborative working with the young person and their families. The professional make-up of the teams will vary between countries, but the education team commonly includes the young person's teachers, special needs teachers including those who specialise in vision impairment, teaching support assistants, and habilitation/mobility specialists (see Chapter 14). The health teams may include the vision services (including low-vision aids), child development team, child and adolescent mental health team, or learning difficulties team. During the transition to adulthood, the independence habilitation specialist and an occupational therapist may support aspects of functional living and arrangements around housing. The availability of services and specialist professionals is inevitably context-specific, with young people in many countries having little or no access to either. Even so, some of the principles presented can be applied in any context and this is revisited at the end of the chapter.

Education interventions will be introduced to support the growth and transition through adolescence, but there is little systematic evidence concerning which interventions are the most effective (Douglas et al. 2019b). This may be because longstanding experience within existing educational practice already shows the value of teaching the use of technology, low-vision devices, and long canes. Furthermore, there is well-established knowledge that without such targeted teaching many independence skills will not develop and access to the core curriculum will be compromised (see further Chapter 14). However, the lack of research evidence means that intervention implementation lacks precision, i.e. when, with whom, and exactly how these interventions should be used (Douglas et al. 2019b). The implications of this for support services for adolescents with vision impairment are that only broad recommendations for interventions can be made and that stakeholders (teachers, parents, and young people) must actively gather evidence of what is working in the specific circumstances. McLinden et al. (2017) argue that specialist teachers have an important role to play in this process as practitioner-researchers who are 'agents of change'.

The UK-based Longitudinal Transitions Study provides a rich source of adolescent experiences and views (Hewett et al. 2016). The project has worked with a cohort of young people with profound to moderate vision impairment for 10 years. It has employed a longitudinal qualitative research design with 80 participants recruited at the age of 14 and 16 years; at that time all were supported by specialist vision impairment education services. Each participant was interviewed approximately twice a year, with many being involved in more detailed case study work. Drawing upon this study and the wider literature, several important transition strategies are recommended (see the following sections).

Transition Reviewing and Planning

Appropriate planning allows young people and services to prepare for the next phase (e.g. college or apprenticeship, independent or supported living). A formal process for young people with disabilities exists in many countries, such as the preparation of a 'Transition Plan' in England and Wales, which involves an annual meeting at school to talk about the young person's future. Such formal processes reflect a general future-orientated outlook, as exemplified by guidance of the Royal National Institute for the Blind (RNIB) UK (RNIB 2019). Such planning prepares for a specific transition to be made by giving the young person opportunity to access the information needed, make informed pathway choices, and act as independently as possible once the choice has been made (Hewett et al. 2017). For example, young adults in higher education reported benefitting from having information about their legal rights and the services available to facilitate them to study independently (Hewett et al. 2017).

Independence: Self-Esteem and Social Skills

Evidence has found a positive link between degree of independence and 'ideal' self-concept amongst adolescents with vison impairment, and concluded that increased independence is a route to improved self-esteem (Lewis and Wolffe 2006). Douglas and Hewett (2014) found that when discussing definitions of employment-based independence, adolescents with vision impairment had difficulties balancing what was their own responsibility, with what was the responsibility of others (including their legal entitlement), and when they should ask for help from others. This study highlighted the importance of teaching young people relevant skills whilst at school, which include a balance between personal independence skills and clear understanding of the accommodations and support to which they are entitled for maximum personal agency.

Nevertheless, young people's views of what they consider to be possible and 'ideal' is strongly influenced and facilitated by others (and for adolescents, their peers are particularly important; see Chapter 19). As Bailey has written in guidance for the RNIB (Bailey 2009), 'two-way interventions' supporting both the young person with vision impairment and also enabling their peers through peer group work, and general awareness training can provide further environmental support to facilitate growth of independence. In addition, meeting peers and adults who successfully live with vision impairment is identified as a potentially empowering strategy for adolescents because it can challenge stereotypes and provide role models (as proposed by Lewis and Wolffe 2006). Young people with vision impairment may often be the only person with vision impairment in their school or community and may rarely get opportunities to meet others similarly affected. The Longitudinal Transitions Study has many positive examples of young people taking part in leisure activities, including self-organised user groups. Technology also provides alternative ways of making social connection, as indicated by the finding that adolescents commonly engage in social media in similar ways to peers with typical sight (Hewett et al. 2012).

Self-Advocacy and Advocacy

During middle childhood and older, teachers and parents will commonly advocate for children by ensuring that they have the resources and opportunities that they need, making adjustments on their behalf and teaching them directly ('access to learning'). Nevertheless, they should also encourage and facilitate young people to manage their own learning and articulate their own needs ('learning to access'), and this may be particularly important during adolescence. The Longitudinal Transitions Study has identified several ways in which it is important for young people to self-advocate, such as explaining their vision impairment to others, and requesting and explaining required adjustments (Hewett et al. 2016). They found that adolescents commonly did not fully understand their vision impairment and often understood little about their entitlements. Young people describe benefitting from previous experiences of self-advocating in a safe setting in which they can develop these skills, with support from their specialist teachers and family members, and developing a thorough understanding of what they are advocating for (Hewett et al. 2017). This may include understanding more about their own vision impairment and impairment of sight, as well as understanding what typical sight is, as it is difficult to appreciate a function that one has never had experience of. Guidance is available for parents and carers to hold these 'tough talks' with their child (RNIB 2017).

Depending on their capacity to make informed decisions and take responsibility, the young person will be assisted to decide on options and organise and plan for their leisure, school, and post-school endeavours. The young person has a right for assisted 'advocacy on their behalf' if they are unable to self-advocate fully, due to learning disability or other capacity issues. This may come through parents, educators, or an independent advocate. The principles of 'self-advocacy' remain the same, whether assisted or not.

Work Experience and Employment Opportunities

Several studies have identified previous work placement opportunities (Capella McDonnall 2011) and wider work preparation training (Wolffe and Kelly 2011) as important factors for helping young people with vision impairment successfully achieve paid employment. Participants in the Longitudinal Transitions Study have highlighted prior work experience opportunities as being extremely significant when they sought employment. It gave them experience of the workplace and also opportunities to travel independently, self-advocate, and to learn about the different adjustments that they could make in a workplace setting (Hewett et al. 2017). Several employment schemes and assessment approaches have been developed for people with vision impairment (Saunders et al. 2013; Wolffe 2019).

Accessing Information

Being able to access information is a key barrier faced by people of all ages with vision impairment. Educational interventions in schools should follow the dual access approach, including first, 'access to learning' where written material is prepared and available in an accessible format (braille, electronic format, or large print as required by the young person). Second, 'learning to access' involves providing appropriate equipment and teaching to encourage efficient and independent access to information (such as teaching in the use of access technology). Skilful and efficient access to information is recognised as an important educational outcome for young people with vision impairment, and this should form a key area of assessment and decision-making; see, for example, Learning Media Assessment of students with vision impairment (Koenig and Holbrook 1995; see Chapter 17). Approaches may include the use of speech and magnification software, low vision aids, braille (hardcopy and electronic), and mobile technology. Converging technology means that many functions are increasingly provided by a single mainstream device, e.g. mobile phones, laptops, and tablets (see Hewett and Douglas 2015). Positive accounts from young people in the Longitudinal Transitions Study have come from those who have developed a range of strategies for accessing information, which has enabled them to choose the most appropriate strategy for a specific task (Hewett et al. 2017). For example, a young adult with severe vision impairment in higher education might use a braille-note device to be able to follow notes in a lecture, use a laptop to access online journal articles and write essays, and use an e-reader to read or listen to books (see also Chapter 16).

Getting Around Independently

Being able to efficiently and confidently move around the environment is recognised as an important educational outcome for young people with vision impairment. Independent travel is vital for young adults to be able to live and work independently and explains why throughout the school years, habilitation, mobility, and orientation training are so important (see further Chapter 14). While the young adults in the Longitudinal Transitions Study generally felt able to get around independently in areas that were familiar to them, a large proportion felt unprepared and unable to navigate new areas or to travel on public transport (Hewett et al. 2017). This may reflect that the mobility support that they had received in school largely focussed on enabling them to learn specific routes, rather than on more generic skills that they could apply to new situations. The most positive accounts came from young people who had knowledge of services available to support them, such as rail and airport assistance, and who were able to skilfully use mobility technology (commonly accessed via their mobile phones). The access to such services and information gave them confidence to travel independently to unfamiliar places (see also Chapter 14).

IMPLICATIONS FOR RESEARCH AND PRACTICE

Central to vision impairment education is 'starting with the end in mind' (Allman and Lewis 2014, pp. 14–15). This means having a sustained focus upon developing independence skills from an early age and setting high expectations of what is possible. Even so, the approach must be sensitive to individual differences and particular circumstances, for example later onset vision impairment or sudden changes to functional vision or additional learning, motor, or social communication needs.

The key challenge for practice is balancing the 'here and now' needs of young people with the longer-term desired outcomes, particularly whilst adolescents with vision impairment experience pressures to conform with peers and need specialist interventions which differentiate them from peers. They are motivated to explore new social and physical environments, but may be finding these difficult to navigate. Specialist vision impairment services present in many countries should be designed to overcome these dilemmas and to target these broader educational goals (Sapp and Hatlen 2010; Keil 2016). Indeed, an important role is to coordinate and recruit all involved in the young person's care and development (and the importance of developing independence and autonomy from an early age is discussed in Chapter 14). This recognition that *all* in the education process have an important role to play in the education of young people with vision impairment is true for all settings but also offers a useful link to the national contexts where specialist services do not exist. Whether through direct educational input or in an advisory capacity, specialist expertise is very important because many general educators and parents will be unfamiliar with vision impairment because it is relatively rare, and some approaches require additional training and equipment (e.g. braille, mobility, and technology). Even so, general educators can make significant positive differences by adopting overarching approaches which enable adolescents with vision impairment to be included in general classroom learning (access to learning), and by teaching them skills so they can function independently. Many of these approaches benefit all learners, not just young people with vision impairment. Examples of these are described above and captured in published guidelines (VICTAR 2019; Douglas et al. 2019c), and include:

- *Access to learning:* ensuring learning materials are in accessible visual, tactile, and auditory formats (and that this is part of everyday classroom practice); ensuring classroom exchanges are inclusive and accessible (e.g. verbal descriptions of visual presentations, the use of students' names to ensure joint-attention is established); environmental audits to ensure schools and homes are safe and accessible; recruit peers and all in the community to take responsibility for maintaining inclusive social and physical environments, and use of supportive techniques (e.g. sighted guiding); teaching about diversity and difference in the school community and wider society, and the encouragement of inclusive friendship groups.

- *Learning to access:* teach and encourage the use of specialist techniques and equipment to access learning (e.g. touch typing, low-vision devices, computer equipment); celebrate student success in the development and mastery of these skills; encourage and scaffold safe independent travel drawing upon appropriate sources of information; develop self-advocacy skills amongst young people including the articulation of access needs and understanding of one's own disability; facilitate meeting other young people and adults with vision impairment.

Irrespective of the context in which learning takes place, recognition that the young person is a key partner and that person-centred planning involves the young person is crucial. This provides opportunities for dilemmas and tensions to surface, such as conflict of perspective with parents and educators, as well as opportunities for disagreements to be resolved.

SUMMARY

The chapter reviews the evidence available in relation to developing autonomy and independence in adolescents with vision impairment. It identifies that educators must balance competing educational interventions that attend to the shorter-term 'here and now' access issues and interventions that attend to longer-term independence goals. The conceptual framework offered provides stakeholders with a means to find this balance and recognise how educational priorities must change over time. The educational approaches must be personalised to the individual needs and circumstances of the young person because of the variability in the population as well as the lack of research evidence in relation to some areas of practice. For this reason, educators must take a practitioner-researcher approach.

Key Points

✓ Young people and adolescents with vision impairment vary in their capabilities and independence and transition support must take into account their individual needs.

✓ Encouraging independence skills from an early age will lead to longer-term active agency and less risk of dependency on adult carers.

✓ A balance is required of focussing on the shorter-term 'here and now' access issues ('access to learning') and on longer-term independence goals ('learning to access'). These work closely together and require an integrated approach.

✓ The curriculum must take into account these additional areas through an expanded core curriculum, which includes active teaching for mobility, independent living skills, independent study skills, and the use of access technology.

✓ Individually focussed educational planning should be reviewed and adjusted according to current needs and forward-looking goals and objectives.

REFERENCES

Allman CB, Lewis S (2014) *ECC Essentials: Teaching the Expanded Core Curriculum to Students with Visual Impairments.* New York: AFB Press.

Bailey G (2009) *What Can You See? Supporting the Social Development of Young People Who Are Blind or Partially Sighted.* Cardiff: Royal National Institute of Blind People.

Capella McDonnall M (2011) Predictors of employment for youths with visual impairments: findings from the second national longitudinal transitions study. *Journal of Visual Impairment and Blindness* **105**(8): 453–466.

Clements B, Douglas G, Pavey S (2011) Which factors affect the chances of paid employment for individuals with visual impairment in Britain? *WORK: A Journal of Prevention, Assessment, and Rehabilitation* **39**(1): 21–30.

Douglas G, Hewett R (2014) Views of independence and readiness for employment amongst young people with visual impairments in the UK. *The Australian Journal of Rehabilitation Counselling* **20**(2): 81–99.

Douglas G, Hewett R, McLinden M (2019a) Transition from school to higher education: research evidence and best practice. In: Ravenscroft J, editor, *The Routledge Handbook of Visual Impairment.* London: Routledge, pp. 143–158.

Douglas G, McLinden M, Ellis E et al. (2019b) *A Rapid Evidence Assessment of the Effectiveness of Educational Interventions to Support Children and Young People with Vision Impairment.* Welsh Government. [online] Available at: <https://gov.wales/sites/default/files/statistics-and-research/2019-09/effectiveness-educational-interventions-support-children-young-people-vision-impairment.pdf> [Accessed 22 August 2021].

Douglas G, McLinden M, Ellis E et al. (2019c) *Support for Children and Young People with Vision Impairment in Educational Settings.* Welsh Government. [online] Available at: <https://gov.wales/

sites/default/files/publications/2019-12/191209-support-for-children-and-young-people-with-vision-impairment-in-educational-settings.pdf> [Accessed 22 August 2021].

Douglas G, McLinden M, McCall S, Pavey S, Ware J, Farrell A (2011) Access to print literacy for children and young people with visual impairment: findings from a review of literature. *European Journal of Special Needs Education* **26**(1): 25–38.

Hewett R, Douglas G (2015) Inclusive design: its impact on young people with vision impairment. *Journal on Technology & Persons with Disabilities* **3**: 277–290.

Hewett R, Douglas G, Keil S (2016) *Transition to Adulthood: The Views and Experiences of Blind and Partially Sighted Young People Transitioning into Adulthood in the UK.* University of Birmingham [online]. Available at: <https://www.birmingham.ac.uk/research/victar/research/longitudinal-transitions-study/phase-two.aspx> [Accessed 22 August 2021].

Hewett R, Douglas G, Keil S (2017) *Reflections of Transition Experiences by Young People with Visual Impairments aged 19–22.* University of Birmingham [online]. Available at:<https://www.birmingham.ac.uk/research/victar/research/longitudinal-transitions-study/phase-three.aspx> [Accessed 22 August 2021].

Hewett R, Douglas G, Ramli A, Keil S (2012) *Post-14 Transitions – A Survey of the Social Activity and Social Networking of Blind and Partially Sighted Young People: Technical Report.* University of Birmingham [online]. Available at: <https://www.birmingham.ac.uk/research/victar/research/longitudinal-transitions-study/phase-one.aspx> [Accessed 22 August 2021].

Keil S (2016) *Learner Outcomes Framework for VI Children and Young People: A Framework for Support for Young People with Vision Impairment Provided by a VI Education Service.* National Sensory Impairment Partnership (NatSIP) [online]. Available at: <https://www.natsip.org.uk/> [Accessed 22 August 2021].

Koenig AJ, Holbrook MC (1995) *Learning Media Assessment of Students with Visual Impairments: A Resource Guide for Teachers,* 2nd Edition. Austin: Texas School for the Blind and Visually Impaired.

Lewis S, Wolffe KE (2006) Promoting learning and self-esteem. In: Sacks SZ, Wolffe KE, editors, *Teaching Social Skills to Students with Visual Impairments: From Theory to Practice.* New York: AFB Press, pp. 122–162.

McLinden M, Douglas G, Cobb R, Hewett R, Ravenscroft J (2016) 'Access to learning' and 'learning to access': analysing the distinctive role of specialist teachers of children and young people with vision impairments in facilitating curriculum access through an ecological systems theory. *British Journal of Visual Impairment* **34**(2): 177–195.

McLinden M, Ravenscroft J, Douglas G, Hewett R, Cobb R (2017) The significance of specialist teachers of learners with visual impairments as agents of change: examining personnel preparation in the United Kingdom through a bioecological systems theory. *Journal of Visual Impairment and Blindness* **111**(6): 569–584.

Patton GC, Sawyer SM, Santelli JS et al. (2016) Our future: a *Lancet* commission on adolescent health and wellbeing. *The Lancet* **387**: 2423–2478.

RNIB (2017) *Tough Talks: Talking to Children About Sight Loss.* RNIB [online]. Available at: https://www.rnib.org.uk/practical-help-family-friends-and-carers-resources-parents-blind-or-partially-sighted-children> [Accessed 22 August 2021].

RNIB (2019) *Your Future, Your Choice: Bridging the Gap.* RNIB [online]. Available at: <https://www.rnib.org.uk/young-people-school-life-and-planning-ahead-making-transition-school/transition-guide-bridging-gap> [Accessed 22 August 2021].

Sapp W, Hatlen P (2010) The expanded core curriculum: where we have been, where we are going, and how we can get there. *Journal of Visual Impairment & Blindness* **104**(6): 338–348.

Saunders A, Douglas G, Lynch P (2013) *Tackling Unemployment for Blind and Partially Sighted People. Summary Findings from a Three-Year Research Project.* RNIB [online]. Available at: <http://www.rnib.org.uk/services-we-offer-advice-professionals-employment-professionals/employment-assessment-toolkit> [Accessed 22 August 2021].

Sawyer SM, Azzopardi PS, Wickremarathne D, Patton GC (2018) The age of adolescence. *The Lancet Child & Adolescent Health* **2**(3): 223–228.

VICTAR (2019) *Best Practice in Supporting Students with Vision Impairment.* Vision Impairment Centre for Teaching and Research, University of Birmingham [online]. Available at: <https://www.birmingham.ac.uk/documents/college-social-sciences/education/victar/best-practice-in-supporting-students-with-vision-impairment.pdf> [Accessed 22 August 2021].

Wolffe KE, Kelly S (2011) Instruction in areas of the Expanded Core Curriculum linked to transition outcomes for students with visual impairments. *Journal of Visual Impairment & Blindness* **105**(6): 340–349.

Wolffe KE (2006) Theoretical perspectives on the development of social skills in adolescence. In: Sacks SZ, Wolffe KE, editors, *Teaching Social Skills to Students with Visual Impairments: From Theory to Practice.* New York: AFB Press, pp. 81–121.

Wolffe KE (2019) Career education for students with visual impairments. In: Ravenscroft J, editor, *The Routledge Handbook of Visual Impairment.* London: Routledge, pp. 159–173.

CHAPTER 21

Personal Experiences from a Young Person

Holly Tuke

BACKGROUND

I was born preterm at 24 weeks, weighing 624 grams, so I was rather tiny! I developed a condition called retinopathy of prematurity, as I needed oxygen to survive, which made my retinas grow too fast and not attach properly. I have stage 5 retinopathy of prematurity as I have a detached retina in my left eye, and only light perception in my right eye, therefore I have no useful vision. With that in mind, I am a braille reader. I can read braille in English, French, and German, as well as braille music. I also use a range of assistive technology.

My mum and dad have never treated me any differently because of my vision impairment, neither have my family and friends, and I think that is very important. With the encouragement of my parents, I have always done the things my sighted friends do, even from a young age.

EDUCATION

I attended mainstream school throughout my education journey. It was definitely a rollercoaster, but I got through it and got the grades that I worked hard for. I had fantastic teaching assistants who put work into an accessible format and supported me in lessons. However, there were many occasions when teachers did not give my teaching assistants the work in time for them to make it accessible, but we tried the best we could and often had to adapt. I think being a confident and proficient user of braille and assistive technology really helped with this. I started learning braille around the age of 4 or 5 years whilst everyone in my class was learning to read and write print. I think that was a great way of doing things, I was still learning like them, just in a different way. I started using assistive technology when I was around 6 or 7 years old, so I have grown up with it. In school I used a mix of braille and digital formats, which I found very useful, I would often use a combination of both. My mum and dad would also try to learn bits of braille and use the screen-reading software alongside me, so that we were all learning together in a way and, looking back, I found that really beneficial.

As I progressed through secondary school, my independence grew, and I would often not have my teaching assistants in lessons with me. We had a system that I was able to get in contact with them if I did need some support. That worked really well; it increased my confidence and independence, but it also made my teachers more aware and hopefully widened their knowledge and experience of working with a student with a vision impairment. There were teachers who did panic at times because they were under the assumption that I had to have someone with me all the time, but when they realised that I could work absolutely fine on my own, their attitudes changed. I know that many students may need support in all lessons and throughout the school day, but it is not the case for everyone so it is very important to promote independence where possible.

School was not plain sailing all the time. I had various issues, and my mum, dad, and I often had after-school meetings with staff to try and resolve issues. If more thought had been put into making lessons more accessible, planning lesson adaptations in advance and understanding what I did and did not need as a learner with a vision impairment then I think that would have made things a lot better all-round. I think it is key to be surrounded by supportive people as this makes such a difference. The teachers who really wanted to understand my disability and took the time to do so really stood out from the rest.

I would have also benefited from more specialist equipment and software during school, including a braille display and braille notetaker, especially during my exams at high school (GCSEs, A levels – UK).

Independence is a huge part of growing up but even more so for blind and visually impaired young people, as we learn independent living skills and mobility. Getting to grips with using the long cane was something I struggled with. I felt like I stood out from everyone else and that it made my disability more visible, but that was not the case at all. The thought of using the cane filled me with dread and anxiety, and I did everything I could not to use it. However, I gradually began to see the benefits and these outweighed the negatives. Finding an extremely supportive mobility officer really changed everything for me; she understood my worries and helped me to turn them around. I think people often do not realise how daunting it can be to use a cane or learn such skills, so it is important to understand this and encourage blind and vision-impaired young people, rather than discourage or force them to do things.

To be honest – I disliked my two final years at school (sixth form – UK). I most definitely felt like an outsider and that my disability was rather prominent so that people did not see me for the person I am, instead they saw my disability. Despite this, I got good final exam results (A levels) and went on to get a place at my first-choice university.

I studied the Children, Young People and Families course at York St John University. I absolutely loved my time there, enjoying my course and making a great set of friends. I was given materials in advance (most of the time) and had support available to me. At university, I definitely got better at advocating for myself as my needs were met, and I became better understood.

EMPLOYMENT

Whilst in my third year of university, I worked for a visual impairment charity for a few hours a week helping set up projects, updating social media, and doing all sorts of tasks. When I graduated, I do not think I was fully prepared for how hard it was going to be to find a graduate job, especially as a young person with a disability. It can be very disheartening when you are job hunting and you come across many jobs that are simply inaccessible However, I did get a job within 6 months of leaving university and worked as an assistive technology advisor at the university I graduated from for nearly 4 years. I now work within the charity sector as a Social Media Officer for a sight loss charity, this is something that I have had my sights set on for the last few years. It is amazing to be able to support my community.

I have received support from the government 'Access to Work' scheme, which funded a screen-reader that I simply could not have done my job without, a braille display, and orientation and mobility training. I love my job; my colleagues understand my vision impairment and see me for the person I am, and not just my disability.

HOBBIES AND INTERESTS

Other than my vision impairment, I am pretty much your average woman in her 20s. I love music, and going to concerts. I enjoy spending time with my friends and family, and I have an interest in beauty and fashion.

When I was at primary school, I started playing the flute and that continued for many years, I was even in a band. I have many fond memories of playing at my local theatre and other venues. I did not let my vision impairment stop me from learning an instrument, and, as a result, I learnt braille music and also to play by ear.

In 2015, I started my blog 'lifeofablindgirl.com' in the hope of sharing my experiences of living with a vision impairment, tackle the common misconceptions and stigmas surrounding vision impairment and disability, and also to help other disabled people in any way I can. When I was growing up, there were not really any disabled role models that I could relate to, so I wanted to be that role model in a way. There is no denying that growing up with a disability can be difficult at times, and we all need to know that we are not alone. We all sometimes need someone to relate to or to get some advice from others in the same or similar situations.

My blog has grown a lot over the years and it has gone places I never even thought of. From being named as one of the most influential disabled people in the UK, to being on radio stations, featuring in newspapers and magazines, having the opportunity to write guest posts and articles for various organisations and websites, and becoming an ambassador for a local charity. I have had some incredible opportunities through blogging that I am so grateful for. I cannot quite put into words how it feels to have readers from all over the world!

Every person with a vision impairment is different, we all have our hobbies and interests, strengths, and weaknesses. We all have our likes and dislikes, but most importantly we are not the same. This is just a bit of a snapshot into my life as a blind woman.

What is important to me as a young person with a vision impairment

- ✓ Being encouraged to strive for success and to have aspirations; having a disability is not an obstacle for success.
- ✓ Recognising that every child or young person with vision impairment is different, just like their peers. What works for one person may not work for another.
- ✓ Being listened to and understood.
- ✓ Remembering that vision impairment is a spectrum and it is important for others to understand what a young person can or cannot see.
- ✓ Focussing on the positives of having a vision impairment such as being part of the vision impairment community and proactively acting on these positives.

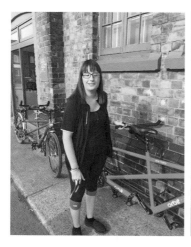
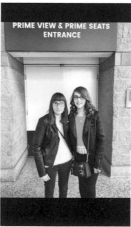
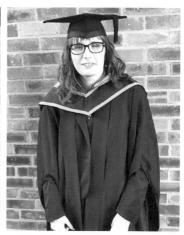

Index